Eat Smart
for a
Healthy Heart
Cookbook

BY
DENTON A. COOLEY, M.D.
Surgeon-in-Chief
Texas Heart Institute

AND
CAROLYN E. MOORE, Ph.D., R.D.
Nutrition Consultant
Texas Heart Institute

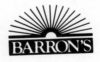
BARRON'S

New York • London • Toronto • Sydney

Credits
Color Photographs
Photography: Matthew Klein. Food styling: Andrea Swenson. Photo styling: Linda Cheverton. Props: Porcelain plates from Cerelene at Baccarat, silver flatware from Christofle at Baccarat, handthrown porcelain plates by Lynn Evans for Gordon Foster, New York City

Black and White Photographs:
Photographs on pages viii–xiv from *Essays of Denton A. Cooley, M.D.,* published 1984 by Eakin Press, Austin, Texas
Figures
Art by Bill Andrews
Book and Cover Design:
Milton Glaser, Inc.

To Matthew Smith Khourie, who inspired this guide to healthful eating.

All inquiries should be addressed to:
Barron's Educational Series, Inc.
250 Wireless Boulevard
Hauppauge, N.Y. 11788
International Standard Book No. 0-8120-5745-7
Library of Congress Catalog Card No. 86-26510

Library of Congress Cataloging-in-Publication Data

Cooley, Denton A., 1920–
  Eat smart for a healthy heart cookbook.

  Includes index.
    1. Heart—Diseases—Diet therapy—Recipes. 2. Heart—
Diseases—Prevention.   3. Low-fat diet—Recipes.
4. Low-calorie diet—Recipes.   5. Salt-free diet—
Recipes. I. Moore, Carolyn E. II. Title. [DNLM;
1. Cholesterol, Dietary—popular works. 2. Cookery.
3. Diet—popular works. 4. Heart Diseases—prevention
& control—popular works. 5. Hypertension—prevention
& control—popular works. WB 405 C774e]
RC684.D5C66 1987   616.1'205   86–26510
ISBN 0–8120–5745–7

PRINTED IN THE UNITED STATES OF AMERICA
  9 0 9683 9 8 7 6 5

CONTENTS

INTRODUCTION

If you think the *Eat Smart for a Healthy Heart Cookbook* was written only for the individual with heart disease or high blood pressure, you're wrong. Guidelines used to develop these 380-plus recipes from some of Houston's (and the nation's) finest restaurants are based on current medical recommendations for the general population.

We have incorporated lifestyle changes designed to improve your general health and increase your lifespan. Scientific evidence has shown that proper diet and weight control may prevent the most common diseases of our affluent society, namely heart disease, hypertension, and certain types of cancer. In addition to the recipes, introductory chapters discuss how our lifestyle influences the development of heart diseases, which affect more than 5 million Americans, and high blood pressure, which affects one in five adults. And while there is no single approach to increasing wellness, the *Eat Smart for a Healthy Heart Cookbook* can serve as your guide to a new, more healthful way of life, whether you dine at home or in a restaurant.

Houston has a long-standing commitment to the promotion of wellness. The city's Texas Medical Center is one of the largest and most comprehensive medical complexes in the world. With eleven hospitals and two medical schools, the Texas Medical Center enjoys an international reputation for innovation and excellence in the areas of patient care, research, and teaching. The creation of the Texas Heart Institute in 1962 clearly reflects Houston's commitment to the study, treatment, and prevention of heart disease and to the promotion of wellness.

How we live and what lifestyle we choose both influence our health and longevity. The most effective way to reduce health-care costs is to adopt a lifestyle compatible with health. Thus, a wellness approach can reduce the rising cost of medical care, and diet is certainly an important component of any wellness program.

Diet has been linked to the development of heart disease, hypertension (high blood pressure), obesity, diabetes, and certain forms of cancer. Experts now recognize that most elevations of blood cholesterol, which are associated with an increased risk of heart disease, respond favorably to reduction in saturated (animal) fat and dietary cholesterol, with a corresponding increase in the intake of polyunsaturated (vegetable) fat. In 1985, the National Institute of Health Consensus Development Conference on Lowering Blood Cholesterol to Prevent Heart Disease was convened. After hearing a series of expert presentations and reviewing the available data, the panel recommended that all Americans should reduce their intake of dietary fat from 40 percent to 30 percent of total calories. In addition, calories should be reduced overall to correct obesity and maintain ideal body weight.

We counsel patients about low-fat, low-cholesterol, and low-salt diets, as well as about weight control. But many patients making a concerted effort to lose weight or lower their blood fat levels complain that food prepared at home is tasteless and bland. A second common problem they encounter is making appropriate menu selections when eating in restaurants.

So, in response to what we perceived as a need for our patients, we decided to write a cookbook. Sixteen of Houston's finest restaurants agreed to contribute recipes. The chefs applied their creativity and developed 96 luncheon and dinner menus that are consistent with dietary guidelines to improve health and that consider color, texture, and flavor.

The recipes come from various international cuisines as well as from Southwestern cooking. Each recipe has been computer analyzed for nutrient content. For your information, the content of calories, carbohydrate, protein, fat, cholesterol, saturated fat, several minerals, and fiber are indicated for entire menus as well as for individual recipes. In addition, exchanges are provided for each recipe. The Exchange System can be used for restriction of total fat, for weight management, and for control of diabetes; it is described in Chapter 3 and on pages 357–367.

Our chefs attempted to restrict the fat content of meals to 30 percent of the total calories, and to reduce sodium. In many recipes, sugar is reduced without the use of artificial sweeteners. Luncheon and dinner menus are limited to approximately 800 and 1,000 calories, respectively. All menus are designed to provide healthful, sophisticated meals that are consistent with current medical recommendations regarding the intake of fat and sodium.

All of the Houston restaurants contributing to this cookbook are famous for their fine cuisine and excellent service. Without their contributions, this cookbook would not have been possible. During the book's development, the chefs' interest in low-fat, low-cholesterol, and low-sodium cookery increased; now, several of the restaurants include items from the *Eat Smart for a Healthy Heart Cookbook* on their regular menus.

In addition to our recipe section, the *Eat Smart for a Healthy Heart Cookbook* includes several chapters on nutrition and diet that we believe will be of interest to all people concerned about good health. The first chapter discusses the underlying causes of heart disease and provides a Coronary Risk Profile, which can be used to estimate whether your risk of heart disease is low, medium, or high. The second chapter summarizes our dietary recommendations and discusses how diet may reduce the risk of heart disease.

Today, weight control is a major health concern for many. People will go to desperate extremes to lose weight, as evidenced by the numerous fad diets we read about daily. Unfortunately, most diets are monotonous, restrictive, unbalanced, and only temporary. In the absence of permanently changed eating habits, lost pounds become weight gains. We use behavior modification techniques to control weight and to prevent its all-too-frequent regain. Chapter 3 summarizes these techniques and provides an explanation of how to calculate an appropriate calorie intake to achieve a safe rate of weight loss. Meal patterns ranging from 1,000 to 3,000 calories are also given in the Appendix.

Chapter 4 describes how to use this cookbook and gives a guide to restaurant dining. It especially considers the problems of dining in ethnic restaurants, where food selections are less familiar.

The *Eat Smart for a Healthy Heart Cookbook* is intended for people with an interest in health as well as for patients and families with heart disease. We think you will find this healthful way of eating to be one of life's enjoyable experiences. The menus can be re-created for pleasant meals at home, and the cookbook can serve as your guide to menu selection when dining in restaurants. Food has always been one of the great pleasures of life. It can and should remain so—without jeopardizing health.

ACKNOWLEDGMENTS

We are grateful to the following restaurants and individuals who developed luncheon and dinner menus that are consistent with guidelines for good health. Without the participation of these restaurants, this cookbook would not have been possible: Alex Martin of *Brennan's*, menus on pages 98, 169, 188, 219, 282, 350; Robert del Grande of *Café Annie*, menus on pages 53, 86, 108, 296, 337, 346; Ruth Meric of *Charley T's*, menus on pages 71, 95, 222, 262, 314, 354; William Edge of *Confederate House*, menus on pages 74, 146, 149, 206, 242, 279; Tony Rao of *D'Amico's*, menus on pages 80, 111, 175, 209, 258, 334; San Hwang of *Dong Ting*, menus on pages 102, 114, 184, 203, 226, 248; Gwen Barclay and Madalene Hill of *Hilltop Herb Farm*, menus on pages 156, 178, 199, 232, 271, 275; Ninfa Lorenzo and Froilan Hernandez of *Ninfa's*, menus on pages 89, 153, 166, 268, 286, 289; Max Yarbrough of *Rainbow Lodge*, menus on pages 59, 129, 160, 191, 254, 331; Ulrich Krauer of *The Remington Hotel*, menus on pages 119, 140, 172, 236, 317, 324; Edward Zielinski of *The Rivoli*, menus on pages 77, 116, 132, 212, 239, 305; Joseph Mannke of *Rotisserie for Beef and Bird*, menus on pages 56, 105, 126, 308, 340, 343; Joseph L. Lucia, Sr., of *Rudi's*, menus on pages 122, 143, 293, 311, 328; Henry Lutjens of *The Warwick*, menus on pages 68, 136, 181, 245, 302, 320; Charles Tucker of *Willie G's*, menus on pages 62, 65, 92, 195, 216, 251; and Bernard Wagner of the Wyndham Hotel, *Travis Centre*, menus on pages 50, 83, 163, 229, 266, 299.

We also would like to thank Mary Ellen Wahlheim, M.P.H., R.D., for her many hours of computer analysis and recipe modification. Ms. Wahlheim relied on her excellent culinary talents and knowledge of nutrition to make appropriate recipe modifications. We are also grateful to Marianne Kneipp and Christine Lanzisera for their editorial review of the manuscript, and appreciated the assistance of Angela Evans, Elizabeth Harris, and Nell Wells in typing the cookbook. Finally, we would like to thank Bill Andrews for his excellent illustrations.

DR. DENTON COOLEY— SURGEON-IN-CHIEF, TEXAS HEART INSTITUTE

Denton Arthur Cooley, M.D., surgeon-in-chief of the Texas Heart Institute, has been described as the world's most active cardiac surgeon as well as one of the most skilled technicians in his field. Even more important, he is an innovator in the field of cardiovascular surgery, constantly revising and improving existing procedures in addition to developing new surgical techniques to correct previously inoperable conditions. In 1969, he became the first surgeon to implant an artificial heart in man.

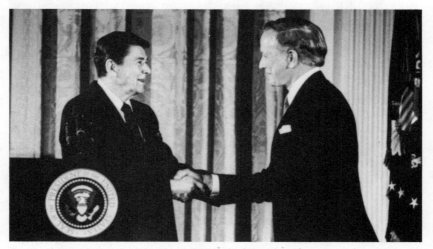

Dr. Cooley receiving the Presidential Medal of Freedom from President Reagan on March 26, 1984.

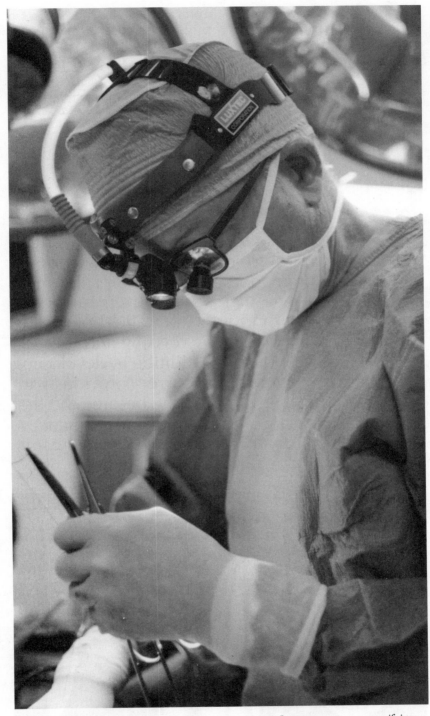

In the operating room at the Texas Heart Institute. Surgeons wear magnifying loupes and individual fiber-optic head lamps to facilitate delicate suture techniques.

Following perfection of the heart-lung machine in 1955, Dr. Cooley specialized in open-heart surgery, including surgery on infants with congenital heart defects. Cooley and his team have performed more than 63,000 open-heart operations, 19,000 vascular (blood vessel) operations, and 6,000 noncardiac operations—more than any other surgeon in the world. Cooley is a leading practitioner of the coronary bypass operation, a remedy for angina pectoris, which is the major symptom of coronary artery disease. He has contributed to the development of techniques for repair and replacement of diseased heart valves and is widely known for operations to correct congenital heart anomalies in infants and children and to repair aneurysms (sacs formed by a weakening in the wall of an artery) of the aorta. Christiaan Barnard wrote in his book, *One Life,* about Dr. Cooley's surgical skill: "It was the most beautiful surgery I had ever seen. . . . Every movement had a purpose and achieved its aim. Where most surgeons would take three hours, he could do the same operation in one hour . . . never obvious in haste, yet never going back. . . . No one I knew could equal it."

One of Dr. Cooley's most significant contributions to the field of cardiac surgery and cardiology was founding the Texas Heart Institute in Houston's Texas Medical Center. Within twenty-five years since its founding in 1962, the Institute has become a world-renowned leader in research, education, and patient care in the field of cardiovascular diseases. Arthur Hailey, celebrated author and surgical patient at the Texas Heart Institute, recently summarized Dr. Cooley's unique contribution: "What happens in the Texas Heart Institute reflects not only the exceptional skills of Denton Cooley, which are world famous and acknowledged, but also his warm humanity and the rarest of human qualities—inspired leadership which leaves its hallmark everywhere."

A native of Houston, Denton Arthur Cooley was born on August 22, 1920. His grandfather, Daniel Denton Cooley, was a founder in 1890 of the Houston Heights, a major suburb of the city. His father, Ralph Clarkson Cooley, was a prominent dentist in Houston. Dr. Cooley majored in zoology at the University of Texas and graduated in 1941 with highest honors. He was a member of Kappa Sigma fraternity (social) and Phi Beta Kappa (scholarship). While at the University, he lettered in varsity basketball three years. Athletic pursuits have continued to interest him, because Dr. Cooley believes strongly in the benefits of exercise; he is an avid golfer, tennis player, and water skier. Dr. Cooley is an expert horseman, and rides often on his working ranch near Houston.

After two years of medical studies at the University of Texas Medical Branch in Galveston, Texas, he entered Johns Hopkins University School of Medicine and graduated in 1944 at the head of his class. As a medical student, Dr. Cooley practiced his manual skill by tying surgical knots inside a matchbox. As an intern and resident under Dr. Alfred Blalock, he participated in the early de-

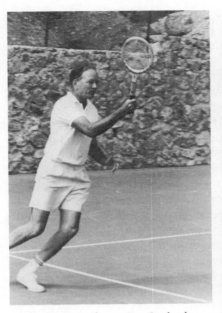

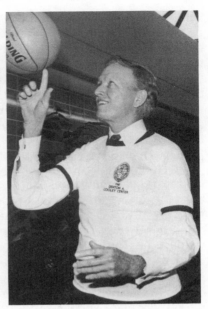

An avid tennis player, Dr. Cooley believes exercise is vital for good health.

At the sports facility of the Denton A. Cooley Center at Johns Hopkins Hospital and Medical School.

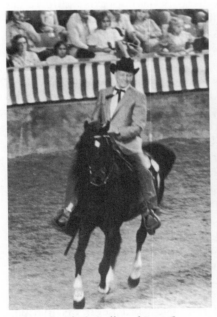

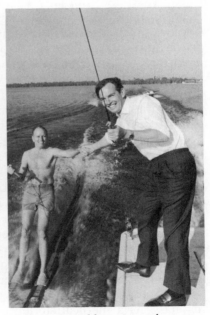

Riding the Black Stallion *horse Cass Ole, at the Pin Oak Charity Horse Show in The Astroarena.*

With renowned heart transplant surgeon Dr. Christiaan Barnard, at Cypress Gardens, Florida.

velopment of the famous Blalock "Blue Baby" operation for correction of tetralogy of Fallot, a complicated surgical procedure to correct a congenital heart defect in an infant that prevented him from obtaining enough oxygen. Dr. Cooley revealed later that it was that revolutionary operation, as well as Dr. Blalock's inspiration, that led him to make heart surgery his specialty. His military service between 1946 and 1948 was as captain in the Medical Corps and chief of surgery in Linz, Austria. After surgical training at Johns Hopkins in 1950, he spent a year with Lord Russell Brock in London, participating in the first intracardiac operations in England.

Dr. Cooley joined the full-time faculty of Baylor University's College of Medicine in 1951 and was Professor of Surgery from 1962 to 1969. He is now Surgeon-in-Chief of the Texas Heart Institute, Director of Cardiovascular Surgery at St. Luke's Episcopal Hospital, Consultant at Texas Children's Hospital, and Clinical Professor of Surgery at the University of Texas Medical School, Houston.

Cooley is a member or honorary member of more than fifty professional societies around the world and a dozen fraternities and clubs. He is the author or coauthor of more than nine hundred scientific articles and several texts. Among his forty-five honors and awards are the Rene Leriche Prize, the highest honor of the International Surgical Society; the Vishnevsky Medal from Vishnevsky Institute in Russia; the "Grande Medaille" from the University of Ghent, Belgium; the John H. Gibbon Award for outstanding contribution to perfusion technology; the Presidential Citation from the American College of Chest Physicians; and Ten Outstanding Young Men in the United States Junior Chamber of Commerce. He has been decorated by the governments of Argentina, Ecuador, Italy, Jordan, Panama, Peru, Philippines, Spain, Venezuela, The Netherlands, and Greece. He has been named Distinguished Alumnus at both the University of Texas and Johns Hopkins University and has received honorary Doctor of Humanities degrees from the Hellenic College and Holy Cross Greek Orthodox School of Theology and the Houston Baptist University.

In 1972, the Denton A. Cooley Cardiovascular Surgical Society was founded as a tribute to Dr. Cooley's contributions to cardiovascular surgery and physician education throughout the world, with goals of continuing education, professional growth, and progress. Included in the society membership are residents and fellows who have received surgical training under Dr. Cooley at the Texas Heart Institute, along with other physicians prominent in the advancement of cardiovascular medicine. In 1980, Dr. Cooley received the Theodore Roosevelt Award, the highest honor given by the National Collegiate Athletic Association to a former varsity athlete who has achieved national recognition in his profession. On March 26, 1984, Dr. Cooley received the Presidential Medal of Freedom from President Ronald Reagan. The Medal of Freedom, the nation's highest civilian honor, is awarded to persons who have

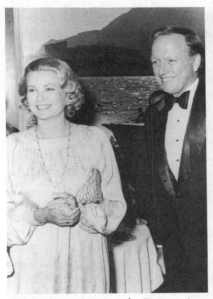

With Princess Grace at the Denton A. Cooley Cardiovascular Surgical Society Symposium in Monaco, 1979.

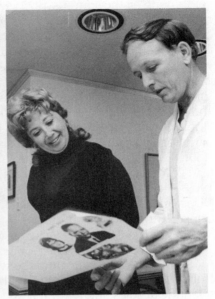

Opera personality Beverly Sills with Dr. Cooley in 1973.

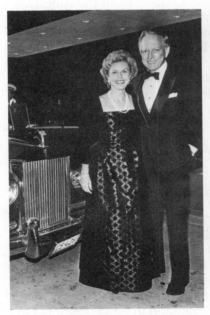

Dr. and Mrs. Cooley at a dinner for Prince Phillip, 1982; Dr. Cooley's 1962 vintage Rolls-Royce is in the background.

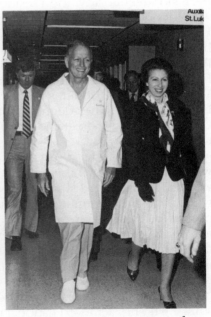

Dr. Cooley shows Princess Anne of Great Britain the Texas Heart Institute.

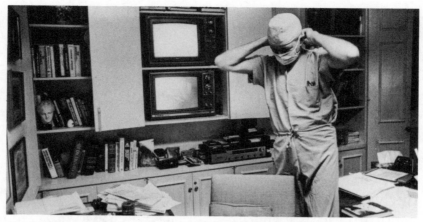

Dr. Cooley preparing for surgery. The television screens allow the physician to monitor the progress of operations in adjoining surgical suites.

made especially meritorious contributions to the security or national interests of the United States, world peace, or cultural or other significant public or private endeavors. Dr. Cooley recently received the Gifted Teacher Award of the American College of Cardiology, for having spent his life teaching others his skills.

Dr. Cooley and his wife, Louise Goldsborough Thomas Cooley, have five daughters and already six granddaughters and five grandsons. During occasional hours away from professional activities, he and the entire family enjoy their country home and ranch near Houston or their beach home in Galveston. Dr. Cooley also plays the bass viol (viola da gamba) and for a number of years participated in an all-physician orchestra called the Heart Beats.

Dr. Cooley's life truly reflects his prescription for a healthy heart: the appropriate combination of work, exercise, relaxation, and rest—all in practice with good nutrition and healthful eating habits.

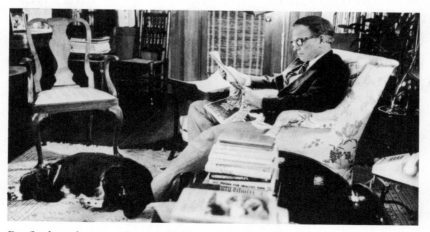

Dr. Cooley relaxing at home with his springer spaniel Atticus.

CHAPTER 1

ATHEROSCLEROSIS AND HEART DISEASE

Atherosclerosis, the underlying cause of coronary artery disease, is the accumulation of plaque—cholesterol, fat, and calcium—along the inner wall of an artery or vessel that transports blood from the heart to organs and tissues of the body. This plaque buildup causes the artery to become thick and narrowed, partially or totally blocking normal blood flow. The coronary arteries, which surround the heart and reach into the heart muscle, supply the heart with blood. When plaque accumulates in the coronary arteries, restriction of blood flow to heart muscle may cause damage or even a heart attack. Figure 1.1 shows the three major branches of the coronary artery system.

Arteries are composed of three layers: the intima, or inner layer; the media, or middle layer; and the adventitia, or outer layer (figure 1.2). The intima is the layer involved in the buildup of plaque.

Stages of Atherosclerosis

Although clinical signs of athero-sclerosis often appear later in life, the disease begins in childhood. Three stages have been identified. The first occurs between infancy and adolescence; during this time, the inner layer of the arterial wall—the intima—undergoes changes, particularly at points where blood vessels divide into branches. Local injury can occur to the endothelium, or lining of the cells (figure 1.3), resulting in exposure of the cells below the area of injury. These changes may lead to deposits of fat.

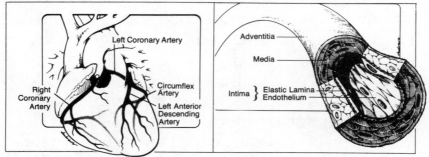

Figure 1.1.   The Heart and Coronary Arteries   Figure 1.2.   Layers of the Arterial Wall

What causes injury to blood vessels? Endothelial injury may result from high blood pressure or increased concentrations of blood fats. Thus, diets that increase blood cholesterol may cause arterial wall injury.

After a blood vessel has been injured, a series of events may occur: Sticky cells called platelets can attach to the arterial wall and release factors that promote growth. These factors increase the number of smooth muscle cells in the blood vessels (figure 1.4). Cholesterol crystals and fat may also accumulate in the smooth muscle cells. As a consequence of this plaque formation, blood flow may be obstructed (figure 1.5).

It is during the first period of atherosclerosis that fatty streaks begin to appear in blood vessels (figure 1.6). Fat carried in the blood accumulates in the blood vessel walls. As early as the first years of life, fatty streaks become visible in the aorta, the main artery that conveys blood away from the heart. By age three, nearly every-one has some fatty streaks.

The second stage of atherosclerosis occurs between adolescence and early adulthood. During this period fatty streaks begin to ap-pear in the coronary arteries that feed blood to the heart. This stage is considered to be reversible, although fatty streaks do precede the development of plaque.

It is during the final stage of atherosclerosis that the long-term effects of this process become evident. Blood flow through a coronary artery may be inadequate owing to partial blockage, even if it is not severe enough to damage the heart. The partial blockage may, however, result in discomfort, particularly in the chest, shoulder, arm, or neck. This condition is called angina pectoris (*angina* referring to pain, *pectoris* to chest).

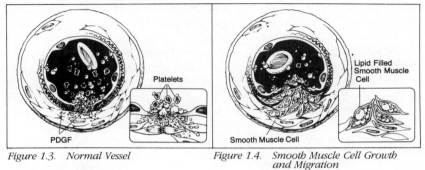

Figure 1.3.   Normal Vessel

Figure 1.4.   Smooth Muscle Cell Growth and Migration

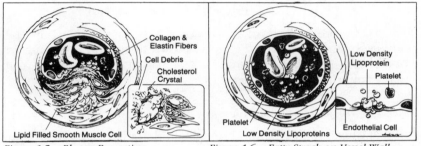

Figure 1.5.   Plaque Formation

Figure 1.6.   Fatty Streak on Vessel Wall

A more severe form of atherosclerosis occurs when extreme narrowing or obstruction of the coronary arteries causes damage by reducing the important supply of oxygen and nutrients to heart muscle. The presence of heart muscle damage is signaled by a heart attack, or myocardial infarction (figure 1.7).

Coronary Artery Disease Risk Factors

While experimental studies provide a better understanding of the origins of atherosclerosis, population studies have been useful in identifying factors that increase the likelihood of heart disease. In 1952, the small community of Framingham, Massachusetts, was selected for a study of the development of heart disease in 6,600 individuals ranging from 30 to 59 years of age. Extensive medical examinations were given periodically. As people in the study developed cardiovascular disease, certain risk factors for the disease were identified.

These factors have been divided into two categories. Primary risk factors—those that have been shown without question to contribute to the development of atherosclerosis—include elevated blood cholesterol, hypertension, and cigarette smoking (table 1.1). Secondary risk factors are not necessarily of lesser importance but need additional research before they can be classified as primary risk factors. Secondary risk factors that increase the likelihood of heart disease include elevated blood triglycerides (fat), diabetes, obesity, inactivity, stress, and possibly personality type (table 1.1).

PRIMARY	SECONDARY
Hypertension Cigarettes Elevated blood cholesterol	Elevated triglycerides Diabetes Obesity Inactivity Stress Personality type

Table 1.1 Coronary Heart Disease Risk Factors

Elevated Blood Cholesterol

Elevated blood cholesterol is a major risk factor for heart disease and may be influenced by diet. As is shown in figure 1.8, the higher your blood (plasma or serum) cholesterol level, the greater your risk of suffering a heart attack.

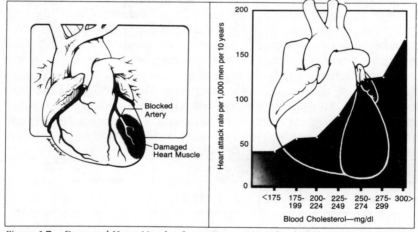

Figure 1.7. Damaged Heart Muscle of a Heart Attack

Figure 1.8. Blood Cholesterol and the Risk of Heart Attack †

The 1984 National Institutes of Health (NIH) Consensus Development Conference separated total blood cholesterol into different risk categories by age (see table 1.2). A precise definition of abnormally high blood cholesterol levels, called hypercholesterolemia (*hyper* = high, *emia* = blood), is difficult to establish. But the NIH Consensus Conference did define high-risk blood cholesterol (severe hypercholesterolemia) as values in the upper 10 percent of the population (90th percentile). This category, which includes individuals with hereditary forms of high blood cholesterol, requires the most aggressive treatment.

† Adapted from Inter-Society Commission for Heart Disease Resources. Atherosclerosis Study Group and Epidemiology Study Group. Primary Prevention of Atherosclerotic Disease. Circulation 42: A55, 1970.

The NIH Consensus Conference defined moderate-risk blood cholesterol (moderate hypercholesterolemia) as values between the 75th and 90th percentile of the population (table 1.2). The moderate-risk category includes large numbers of people whose elevated blood cholesterol is partially related to diet. The recent Lipid Research Clinic Study's distribution of total blood cholesterol according to both age and sex is provided in table D.1 on page

AGE	MODERATE RISK *(75th to 90th percentile)*	HIGH RISK *(Greater than 90th percentile)*
20–29	200 to 220 mg/dl	greater than 220 mg/dl
30–39	220 to 240 mg/dl	greater than 240 mg/dl
40 & over	240 to 260 mg/dl	greater than 260 mg/dl
mg = milligrams dl = deciliter (1 dl = 100 cubic centimeters = 100 milliliters) *Adapted from* National Institute of Health Consensus Development Conference Statement, *Volume 5(7), 1985.*		

Table 1.2 Moderate-Risk and High-Risk Blood Cholesterol Levels

373. You can compare your blood cholesterol levels with those in this table to estimate your risk of heart disease.

Lipid (fat) in the blood is transported attached to proteins called lipoproteins. Low-density lipoproteins (LDLs) transport approximately 65 percent of the blood cholesterol. LDLs are thought to be involved with the transport of cholesterol to tissues. When present in high amounts, LDLs are deposited in the tissues and make a major contribution to the buildup of plaque; consequently, LDL-cholesterol is often referred to as the "bad" form of cholesterol. A significant increase in the risk of coronary artery disease is associated with elevated LDL-cholesterol.

In contrast, the high-density lipoproteins (HDLs) may promote artery health. HDLs transport cholesterol away from tissues to the liver and so are often referred to as "good" cholesterol. In general HDLs carry about 20 percent of the total cholesterol in the blood. High levels of HDL-cholesterol may provide some degree of protection against coronary artery disease.

The ratio of total cholesterol to HDL-cholesterol has recently been used by physicians to estimate the risk of developing heart disease. An optimal ratio, for both men and women, of total cholesterol to HDL-cholesterol is less than 4 : 1. A high risk of coronary artery disease is associated with a ratio of 5 : 1 or greater.

Hypertension

High blood pressure (hypertension) is another powerful predictor of coronary artery disease. Blood pressure is the force needed to pump blood through the arteries in the body. Normal blood pressure varies from person to person and from time to time in each individual. A problem occurs, however, when high blood pressure is sustained. Hypertension may increase the workload of the heart and the risk of heart attack. It also accelerates the atherosclerotic process and contributes to the risk of stroke and kidney disease.

Although hypertension can be readily identified, repeated blood pressure measurements should be performed to confirm the diagnosis. Research indicates that reduction of elevated blood pressure with medication, restriction of dietary sodium, weight loss, and possibly calcium supplementation can lower the incidence of stroke and heart attack.

Cigarette Smoking

Cigarette smoking is another primary risk factor for coronary heart disease; it also contributes to lung and throat cancer, as well as to emphysema. Research has clearly shown that the risk and frequency of heart attacks are greater in people who smoke, and that they increase in relation to the number of cigarettes smoked. Thus, we cannot overemphasize the importance of giving up smoking.

Secondary or Contributing Risk Factors

A few unalterable factors are also associated with a greater risk of coronary artery disease. Certainly the older we become, the greater our risk of death from coronary artery disease. In addition to age, a family history of premature heart attacks increases risk. Men have an increased risk of coronary heart disease compared to premenopausal women.

Diabetes

Diabetes is a major contributor to the increased risk of coronary artery disease. Diabetic men have twice the risk of coronary artery disease when compared to nondiabetic men, and diabetic women are at three times the risk of nondiabetic women.

Obesity

Evidence for a relationship between obesity and atherosclerosis comes from population studies. The Framingham study found that obesity was a risk factor for heart disease for both men and women. Interestingly, weight gain after age 25 in both men and women increased the risk of coronary artery disease independent of initial weight. A more complete discussion concerning treatment of obesity is found in Chapter 3.

Exercise

A significant relationship exists between the incidence of coronary artery disease and physical activity. People who exercise regularly have fewer fatal heart attacks than those who are sedentary. Any continuous rhythmic exercise—such as walking, running, biking, or swimming—increases heart and lung fitness.

Stress and Personality Type

Stress is physical, mental, or emotional tension that develops as a reaction to daily situations. The incidence of heart disease has been linked to personalities more prone to stress.

Coronary Risk Profile

A Coronary Risk Profile (table 1.3) was developed from the Framingham study for use in estimating an individual's risk of coronary artery disease. The primary risk factors (hypertension, elevated blood cholesterol, and cigarette use) are totaled as follows:

Number of Risk Factors	Level of Risk
0	low risk
1	moderate risk
2 or 3	high risk

Thus, moderate risk occurs with one primary risk factor, and high risk occurs with two or three factors.

There are also a number of secondary risk factors listed on the Coronary Risk Profile; these include blood triglyceride (fat) levels, blood glucose level, body fat, stress, physical inactivity, electrocardiogram abnormalities, family history of premature heart attack, and age. They can be totaled in the following manner:

Number of Risk Factors	Level of Risk
1 or 2	low risk
3	moderate risk
4 or more	high risk

Thus, having one or two secondary risk factors would place you in a low-risk category, and having three risk factors would make your risk moderate. The presence of more than four secondary risk factors is associated with a high risk for heart disease.

You will notice that the risk factors are divided into two major categories: controllable and fixed (uncontrollable). It is important to concentrate on modifying those risk factors that can be controlled, particularly hypertension, cigarette smoking, and elevated blood cholesterol. While medical science has made significant advances in the treatment of coronary heart disease, prevention is the best treatment of all.

Risk Factor	Relative Level of Risk				
	Very Low	Low	Moderate	High	Very High
CONTROLLABLE					
Primary					
Blood Pressure(mmHg)					
Systolic	<110	120	130–140	150–160	170>
Diastolic	< 70	76	82–88	94–100	106>
Cigarettes (per day)	Never or none in one year	5	10–20	30–40	50>
Cholesterol					
—Total (mg/dl)	180	200	200–240	260–280	300>
—Ratio (mg/dl)[a]	<3.0	<4.0	<4.5	5.2	7.0>
Secondary					
Triglycerides (mg/dl)	<50	<100	130	200	300>
Glucose (mg/dl)	<80	90	100–110	120–130	140>
Body Fat (percentage)					
Men	12	16	20	25	30>
Women	16	20	25	32	40>
Stress-Tension	Never	Almost never	Occasional	Frequent	Nearly constant
Physical Activity					
Total minutes/week	240	180–120	100	80–60	30<
Minutes/week at moderate to high intensity[b]	120	90	30	0	0
ECG abnormality (ST depression-mv)[c]	0	0	0.05	0.10	0.20
FIXED					
Family history of premature heart attack (blood relative)[d]	0	0	1	2	3+
Age	<30	35	40	50	60>

Adapted with permission from Pollock, M.L., Wilmore, J.H., Fox, S.M.: Exercise in Health & Disease. *Philadelphia: W.B. Saunders Company, 1984.*

Key: *< means less than, > means greater than.*

[a]*Ratio of HDL (high-density lipoprotein) to total cholesterol.* [b]*Brisk walking is considered moderate intensity; jogging/ running is considered high-intensity exercise.* [c]*Other ECG abnormalities are also potentially dangerous and are not listed here.* [d]*Premature heart attack refers to less than 60 years of age.*

Table 1.3 Coronary Risk Profile

CHAPTER 2

THE *EAT SMART* DIET FOR A HEALTHIER HEART

Eating should be both a pleasurable and a healthful experience. Our recipes and dietary guidelines incorporate the most recent research available linking diet modification with the prevention of heart disease. We designed this diet to help you reduce your risk of heart disease while enjoying healthful food fit for a gourmet.

The 13 Steps of the *Eat Smart* Diet:

1. Achieve ideal body weight.
2. Reduce fat to 30 percent of total calories.
3. Limit saturated fat to 10 percent of total calories.
4. Increase polyunsaturated fat to 10 percent of total calories. Balance the remaining intake of fat with monounsaturated fats.
5. Reduce cholesterol intake to about 100 milligrams per 1,000 calories, with no more than 300 milligrams each day.
6. Increase the intake of fish oil.
7. Reduce the use of refined sugar without reliance on artificial sweeteners.
8. Increase the intake of complex carbohydrates (starches).
9. Include more dietary fiber.
10. Use garlic and onions frequently.
11. Restrict sodium (salt) intake to less than 3 grams per day.
12. Drink alcohol in moderation. Reduce daily alcohol intake to no more than 1½ ounces of pure alcohol (about two 12-ounce beers or two 4-ounce glasses of wine).
13. Avoid caffeine.

Nutrition and Atherosclerosis

Diet plays a major role in reducing heart disease because dietary changes can have a major impact on two of the risk factors for heart disease: elevated blood cholesterol and high blood pressure.

There is no argument regarding the importance of lowering blood cholesterol to reduce the risk of heart disease. Controversy does exist, however, concerning the significance of certain dietary factors on blood cholesterol. Research suggests that fat, carbohydrate, protein, fiber, and other nutrients may affect blood cholesterol. Furthermore, the type of dietary fat may also affect blood clotting. Recent studies have indicated that two entirely different families of fatty acids, found in vegetable and fish oils, appear to have different effects on blood clotting and fat content of blood.

Cholesterol

Cholesterol is a waxy, fatlike substance found in all animal tissues. In addition to being manufactured in the body, it is present in foods of animal origin such as meat, fish, poultry, egg yolk, and dairy products. Egg yolks and organ meats are concentrated sources of cholesterol.

To many Americans, a "low-cholesterol diet" simply means no eggs. These individuals correctly identify eggs as a cholesterol-rich food, but incorrectly assume that avoiding eggs will solve the cholesterol problem. No one benefits from such oversimplified dietary advice. Instead, we should all be concerned about our overall diet. While many Americans' average daily intake of dietary cholesterol is 500 milligrams (mg) the National Institutes of Health (NIH) Consensus Development Conference recommended that this be reduced to 300 milligrams or less per day (about 100 milligrams per 1,000 calories). The cholesterol content of some common foods is provided in table D.2 on page 373. Recipes developed for this cookbook limit cholesterol to 300 milligrams per day. The chefs have used egg whites or egg substitutes to reduce the cholesterol content of many recipes.

Shellfish and shrimp are often restricted on a low-fat, low-cholesterol diet because of their cholesterol content. The American Heart Association currently believes that two ounces of shrimp should be considered equivalent to three ounces of meat because of the shrimp's higher cholesterol content.

Shellfish and shrimp appear on several of the lunch and dinner menus. Because of their cholesterol content, other low-cholesterol items are included at the same meal. Thus, total intake of cholesterol remains below the recommended maximum of 300 milligrams per day.

Dietary Fat

Fat is a concentrated source of energy, supplying nine calories per gram—more than twice the energy provided by carbohydrates or protein. For individuals concerned with weight control, limiting fat can help control caloric intake. The amount and kinds of fat in the diet have a well-documented effect on plasma lipid levels. The NIH Consensus Conference and the American Heart Association urge all Americans to adopt a diet that reduces total fat from the current average of 40 percent to 30 percent of total calories.

Every attempt was made by our chefs to limit the fat content of lunch and dinner menus to 30 percent of their total calories. When a menu's fat content exceeds 30 percent, control of fat intake at other meals will result in an overall daily limitation of fat to the recommended level. Use of the exchange system discussed in Chapter 3 will also help control total fat intake.

More specific recommendations concerning the types of fat consumed are based on the division of fats into three classes identified by saturation and unsaturation. Many experimental and clinical studies have demonstrated that these three types of fat have different effects on blood cholesterol levels and the development of atherosclerosis.

SATURATED FATS Saturated fats raise the level of cholesterol in the blood. The current American diet is about 40 percent fat, of which 15 to 17 percent of the total calories are saturated. The NIH Consensus Conference and the American Heart Association recommend reduction of saturated fat to about 10 percent of total calories.

Saturated fats are usually solid at room temperature and are primarily found in foods of animal origin (see table 2.1)—for instance, in whole-milk dairy products (cream, milk, cheese, ice cream) and meat. There are, however, a few saturated fats of vege-

KIND OF FAT	EXAMPLES	
Saturated	Butter Beef Cheese Chocolate Coconut Coconut oil	Egg yolk Lard Milk Palm oil Poultry Vegetable shortening
Monounsaturated	Avocado Cashews Olives Olive oil	Peanuts Peanut oil Peanut butter
Polyunsaturated	Almonds Corn oil Cottonseed oil Filberts Fish Margarine	Mayonnaise Pecans Safflower oil Soybean oil Sunflower oil

Table 2.1 Types of Dietary Fat

table origin, principally coconut oil and palm oil. Saturated fats are also produced when vegetable oils are hydrogenated during the manufacture of margarine. Recipes included in this cookbook limit saturated fats through the use of nonfat milk products, skim-milk cheese, leaner cuts of meat, and the avoidance of coconut oil.

MONOUNSATURATED AND POLYUNSATURATED FATS The fatty acids of unsaturated fats can be either monounsaturated or polyunsaturated. Oleic acid is the major monounsaturated fatty acid and linoleic acid the major polyunsaturated fatty acid present in vegetable oils. Both types of fatty acids lower plasma cholesterol when substituted for saturated fat; linoleic acid, however, may be more effective in cholesterol reduction than is oleic acid. Consequently, we believe that some saturated fats should be replaced by polyunsaturated fatty acids, not to exceed 10 percent of total calories.

Usually liquid at room temperature, polyunsaturated fats are primarily of vegetable origin (table 2.1). Oils such as corn, cottonseed, sesame, soybean, and safflower are good sources of polyunsaturated fat. A comparison of the percent of saturated and polyunsaturated fats present in different fats and oils is shown in figure 2.1. Safflower oil is a particularly rich source of polyunsaturated fats; coconut and palm oils should be avoided because of their higher saturated-fat content.

Monounsaturated fats are also common in foods (table 2.1); rich sources include olive oil, peanuts, peanut butter, peanut oil, avocados, and nuts such as pecans, almonds, and cashews. Although monounsaturated fats may not reduce blood cholesterol levels as much as polyunsaturated fats, they do have potential benefit.

For the most part, our recipes call for polyunsaturated margarine or safflower oil, although other vegetable oils can be substituted. Butter, which contains more saturated fat, is not permitted (figure 2.1). Recipes in this book occasionally call for olive oil, a rich source of monounsaturated fat. Olive oil is allowed when its flavor contribution is important.

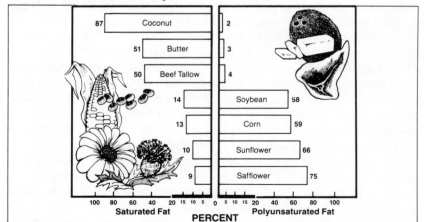

Figure 2.1. Comparison of fats and oils. Adapted from USDA Handbook 8-4. Composition of Foods: Fats and Oils, *1979.*

Exciting new studies suggest that vegetarianism may reduce the risk of coronary artery disease. In the Leiden Intervention Trial, undertaken in the Netherlands between 1978 and 1982, a vegetarian diet was shown to reduce the intake of saturated fat and cholesterol while it doubled that of polyunsaturated fat. The significance of the study is that blood cholesterol levels were lowered with dietary measures alone. The findings suggest that adding more vegetables and vegetable oils to the diet may reduce the risk of coronary artery disease.

Investigators in the Netherlands have recently found that habitual fish consumption decreases the risk of coronary heart disease. Other researchers at the University of Oregon have also concluded that eicosapentenoic acid, a fatty acid present in fish, is two to five times more effective in lowering blood cholesterol than are the fatty acids present in vegetable oils. Fish containing high levels of eicosapentenoic acid include salmon, mackerel, herring, anchovies, trout, catfish, sardines, and smelt. In addition to influencing cholesterol metabolism, fish fatty acids may affect the tendency of blood to clot by changing platelet behavior, thereby reducing the risk of a heart attack.

Fish intake equivalent to 4 to 6 ounces of fish several times a week may be of value in the prevention of coronary heart disease. We have, therefore, included creative and delicious fish recipes.

Carbohydrates

Starches and sugars, classified as carbohydrates, contain four calories per gram. When individual sugars are linked together into chains, "complex carbohydrates" or starches are formed. Sucrose, or table sugar, is an example of a simple carbohydrate common in the diet of most Americans.

Breads, cereals, potatoes, and rice are examples of complex carbohydrates. Carbohydrates currently account for 40 to 45 percent of the total calories in the American diet, with 15 to 20 percent derived from simple sugars. Studies have shown that populations receiving a major portion of their calories from complex carbohydrates (such as starchy vegetables and whole-grain cereals) have a lower incidence of coronary artery disease than those populations that consume lower-carbohydrate or higher-sugar diets (which is true of most Western countries). Therefore, our intake of complex carbohydrates should be 10 to 15 percent higher than it typically is at present. Adding these starches will balance the recommended 10- to 15-percent decrease in fat calories.

We also believe it advisable to limit simple-sugar intake to 10 percent of the total calories, with the balance of remaining carbohydrates being the complex type. Recipes in this cookbook avoid using sugar as a sweetener. Fresh fruit and natural fruit purees are often included to enhance the flavor and sweetness of desserts.

ARTIFICIAL SWEETENERS Americans eat and drink more than 7 million pounds of saccharin a year. Today more and more soft drinks are being sweetened with aspartame, the most recent sugar substitute to appear on the market; it is distributed in the United States as NutraSweet® and Equal®. The subject of controversy, aspartame has been associated with headaches, nausea, diarrhea, and menstrual problems. Although most reports on side effects have been dismissed for lack of concrete evidence, it's wise to play it safe by decreasing the intake of artificial sweeteners as much as possible. This means eliminating diet drinks and substituting fruit juices or low-sodium mineral water.

Lunch and dinner menus in this book include many naturally sweet fruit desserts. Although table sugar appears in occasional recipes, no artificial sweeteners are used.

Fiber

The absence of coronary disease in black African populations has been related to their high-fiber diets. Such diets may also protect against cancer of the colon. Replacement of fat and sugar by a large amount of dietary fiber may contribute to weight reduction and a lowering of blood cholesterol. Moreover, specific properties of fiber may also influence blood fat levels.

Dietary fiber consists of the remnants of plant cells that are not digested and that pass through the body for eventual elimination. High-fiber diets allow for easier, more regular bowel movements by producing softer, bulkier stools.

Dietary fiber is not a single entity, but a mixture of various carbohydrates and other substances associated with foods of plant origin. They include cellulose, hemicellulose, pectin, lignin, gums, and bran. Cellulose has no effect on human blood fat levels; pectin, however, has definite cholesterol-lowering properties. Bran, actually a mixture of several fibers, represents the outermost layer of a kernel. Although bran usually has no effect on blood lipid levels in man, oat bran may be an exception. Although present to some extent in all plant foods, water-soluble fibers that tend to reduce blood cholesterol are especially concentrated in fruits, beans, and legumes.

Foods particularly high in pectin are effective in lowering plasma cholesterol. Citrus fruits are especially good sources of pectin, although a major portion of the citrus pectin is found in the peel rather than the flesh of the fruit. Other good pectin sources include apples, apricots, cherries, grapes, raisins, squash, and carrots.

Recipes in this book include many fruits, vegetables, beans, and whole-grain cereals. A list of these high-fiber foods can be found in Table C.2 on page 371.

Protein

All proteins consist of amino acids linked together. Dietary protein is required to provide the essential amino acids that cannot be synthesized by the body. Containing four calories per gram, proteins also supply energy. Protein typically represents 15 to 20 percent of the total calories in the American diet.

Numerous studies with experimental animals have shown that diets containing protein from animal sources (meat, eggs, dairy products) increase plasma cholesterol when compared to diets containing vegetable proteins. Animal studies indicate that a diet supplying an equal mixture of animal and vegetable proteins will maintain comparable levels of blood cholesterol to diets containing only vegetables. In the American diet the relative ratio of animal to vegetable protein is approximately 2 : 1. This should be reduced; a shift toward a more vegetarian diet would lower blood cholesterol and reduce the risk of heart disease for most people.

Good sources of vegetable proteins are listed in table D.4 on page 374. Though Americans usually eat these vegetables as side dishes, they are good sources of amino acids. Menus in this book include many of these items.

Allicin

A high intake of garlic and onion is also thought to contribute to a lower incidence of cardiovascular disease in certain population groups. Garlic and onion contain a chemical called allicin, which may inhibit the formation of blood clots. Many of our recipes include garlic and onion as major ingredients.

Sodium

Most authorities agree that sodium is responsible for the development of high blood pressure, or hypertension. Although table salt is the chief source of sodium in the American diet, it is by no means the only source. Nearly half of our sodium intake comes from salt or sodium compounds added to foods during processing. The remaining sodium is found naturally in foods or is added during home food preparation. The average American diet provides about 5,000 milligrams of pure sodium daily, which is equivalent to 12,000 milligrams of salt. We recommend limiting your sodium intake to less than 3,000 milligrams (3 grams) per day.

To reduce the sodium content of our recipes, most of the added salt was eliminated or reduced significantly. Because spices and herbs are naturally low in sodium, recipes were developed using blends of these seasonings to add flavor. A guide for reducing sodium intake is provided in table C.1 on page 369.

Alcohol

The levels of certain blood fats increase as a result of moderate alcohol consumption. Alcohol increases high-density lipoprotein (HDL) levels, which are thought to reduce the risk of coronary heart disease. But the subfraction of HDL that increases with alcohol is not the form reported to be protective against heart disease.

Moderate but regular use of alcohol also tends to raise blood triglycerides, carried by the very-low-density lipoproteins (VLDLs)—which are fats that may slightly increase the risk of heart disease. This alcohol-induced increase in blood triglycerides may be exaggerated when a high-fat diet is consumed. Thus, alcohol should be used only in moderation and should not exceed 1½ ounces of pure alcohol per day (equivalent to about two 12-ounce beers or two 4-ounce glasses of wine).

Caffeine

Decaffeinated coffee and tea are being chosen more frequently by people concerned about the harmful effects of caffeine. In addition to acting as a stimulant to the nervous system, caffeine can increase heartbeat and basal metabolic rate (the amount of energy required to maintain life at rest). Caffeine also promotes secretion of stomach acid, increases urine production, and may cause some blood vessels to dilate or constrict.

Coffee is the largest source of caffeine in the American diet, with 50 to 150 milligrams per 5-ounce cup. Ranking second as a source of caffeine are soft drinks—ahead of tea, chocolate, and other foods and beverages. Large amounts of caffeine (200 to 500 milligrams daily) can produce an abnormally fast heartbeat, irregular heart rhythm, or extra heartbeats in susceptible people. Ideally, caffeine should be limited to 250 milligrams per day; for most Americans, restricting coffee to two or three cups daily will suffice. The caffeine content of common foods and beverages is provided in table D.3 on page 373.

CHAPTER 3

WEIGHT CONTROL AND YOUR EATING HABITS

Nobody wants to be obese. As many people know, however, it is difficult to maintain weight and especially difficult to maintain weight loss. The statistics are fairly gloomy: The failure rate in long-term treatment is estimated to be 95 percent for the extremely obese and 66 percent overall. There are methods, however, that have proved successful for achieving permanent weight loss.

Obesity is defined as an excess of body fat. As fat cells enlarge, excess fat accumulates. In the extremely obese, the number of fat cells in the body also increases. Both genetic and environmental factors play important roles in the development of obesity. Some of these factors include excessive caloric intake, inactivity, and metabolic or endocrine disorders.

Desirable Body Weight

Ｈｏｗ does your weight compare to the desirable weight range by height shown in table 3.1? These tables are based on weights associated with the lowest mortality rates among insured populations of adults and are frequently used to determine desirable body weight.

MEN 25 AND OVER				WOMEN 25 AND OVER[a]			
Height with shoes on 1" heels	Small Frame	Medium Frame	Large Frame	Height with shoes on 2" heels	Small Frame	Medium Frame	Large Frame
5'2"	112–120	118–129	126–141	4'10"	92–98	96–107	104–119
5'3"	115–123	121–133	129–144	4'11"	94–101	98–110	106–122
5'4"	118–126	124–136	132–148	5'0"	96–104	101–113	109–125
5'5"	121–129	127–139	135–152	5'1"	99–107	104–116	112–128
5'6"	124–133	130–143	138–156	5'2"	102–110	107–119	115–131
5'7"	128–137	134–147	142–161	5'3"	105–113	110–122	118–134
5'8"	132–141	138–152	147–166	5'4"	108–116	113–126	121–138
5'9"	136–145	142–156	151–170	5'5"	111–119	116–130	125–142
5'10"	140–150	146–160	155–174	5'6"	114–123	120–135	129–146
5'11"	144–154	150–165	159–179	5'7"	118–127	124–139	133–150
6'0"	148–158	154–170	164–184	5'8"	122–131	128–143	137–154
6'1"	152–162	158–175	168–189	5'9"	126–135	132–147	141–158
6'2"	156–167	162–180	173–194	5'10"	130–140	136–151	145–163
6'3"	160–171	167–185	178–199	5'11"	134–144	140–155	149–168
6'4"	164–175	172–190	182–204	6'0"	138–148	144–159	153–173

Prepared by the Metropolitan Life Insurance Company. It was derived primarily from data of the Build and Blood Pressure Study, 1959, *published by the Society of Actuaries.*

[a]For women between 18 and 25, subtract 1 pound for each year under 25.

Table 3.1 *Desirable Weights in Pounds, According to Frame (in Indoor Clothing)*

Estimation of Desirable Body Weight

Desirable body weight can be estimated using a more individualized formula. Although it is best to know the distribution of your body weight as fat and muscle, this can only be determined by sophisticated techniques such as underwater weighing or measurement of skinfold thickness. When body composition cannot be measured, we use a general rule for estimating desirable weight:

- Women are allowed 100 pounds for the first 5 feet of height, with 5 pounds added for each inch over 5 feet. Therefore, a 5'5" woman should weigh 125 pounds.

- Men are allowed 110 pounds for the first 5 feet of height, with 6 pounds added for each inch over 5 feet. Therefore, a 5'5" man should weigh 140 pounds.

To allow for differences in skeletal size, an equation that compares wrist circumference to height can be used to judge frame size. The following equation can be used to estimate your frame size, r:

$$r = \frac{height\ in\ inches}{wrist\ in\ inches}$$

Then relate (r) to the following categories:

Men
r greater than 10.4 = small frame
r between 9.6 and 10.4 = medium frame
r less than 9.6 = large frame

Women
r greater than 11.0 = small frame
r between 10.1 and 11.0 = medium frame
r less than 10.1 = large frame

Different body weight allowances are given for different body frames. Desirable body weight for a person with a small frame is about 10 percent less than for one with a medium frame. Likewise, the desirable weight for a large frame is about 10 percent greater than that for a medium frame.

Caloric Intake

You can estimate your desirable weight by using the range of weights given in table 3.1 (page 18) or by estimating with the rules just given. By comparing your weight with the recommended weight you can determine an appropriate caloric intake. If weight loss is indicated, use the following appropriate factors to calculate caloric intake to achieve a weight loss of one to two pounds per week. If a gain is indicated, the appropriate factor, determined by the following formula, can be used in the same way to achieve a weight increase of one to two pounds per week. Similarly, the number of calories needed to maintain your weight can be estimated.

To calculate your caloric intake, choose the caloric factor appropriate for your needs:

- To decrease weight—9.1
- To maintain weight—13.6
- To increase weight—18.2

Then use your caloric factor in the following equation:

$$\begin{array}{ccccc} \textit{Ideal body} & & \textit{Caloric} & & \textit{Recommended} \\ \textit{weight (lbs.)} & \times & \textit{factor} & = & \textit{caloric intake} \end{array}$$

Once you have determined the number of calories required to achieve your desired weight, you can select 1,000- to 3,000-calorie diets given on pages 357 to 361. Diets using the exchange system are adjusted to follow guidelines limiting fat intake to 30 percent of total calories.

The Exchange System

The exchange system has been developed to make diet planning easier. Though it can be used to plan any type of diet, it is most often used for weight reduction, control of diabetes, and other health problems that require therapeutic diets. Foods are grouped into six major categories: dairy, vegetable, fruit, bread and starchy vegetables, meat, and fat. Each group of food is called an exchange list. In the stated quantity, each item within an exchange group provides approximately the same amount of calories, protein, and fat. Exchange lists are given on pages 362 to 367.

The term *exchange* is used to mean "substitute." When foods are chosen in the appropriate amount, they can substitute for one another in the same exchange group without significantly changing caloric content. Thus, when using the exchange system it is important that you weigh and measure foods to ensure proper caloric intake. For example, on the fruit exchange list in the Appendix, ½ cup orange juice equals 1 fruit exchange unit. You can substitute any other product on the fruit exchange list that equals 1 unit, such as a medium orange or apple. You should not, however, substitute fruit in heavy sugar syrup, which is equal to 2 exchange units. Distribute exchanges throughout the day as individual meals and snacks. This exchange pattern will control food intake to the desired caloric level. By following your meal plan, your calories for the day will be precounted.

Our recipes have been analyzed by computer, and the number of exchanges for each serving has been calculated. By controlling other exchanges on the day a lunch or dinner menu is eaten, total caloric intake will be controlled and fat will be limited to 30 percent of all calories. If the number of exchanges in a meal or recipe exceeds the desired calories, other recipes can be substituted to adjust caloric intake.

Food Records

Keeping food records is an easy way to control food intake when using the exchange system. An example of a food record form is shown in figure 3.1. On each line, record when and where you ate and what was eaten. The number of exchanges for each item is then indicated in the exchange column by abbreviation (1 cup nonfat milk = 1 dairy exchange, or 1 D). With this form you can keep a running tally of the actual number of exchanges you have consumed throughout the day.

Food records are an excellent tool for controlling food intake. In weight control classes, it has been our experience that the greatest rate of weight loss often occurs when patients keep daily food records. Make up your own food record sheets for your personal weight management program.

NAME *Jane Doe*
DAY *Monday*
DATE *Jan. 4*
DIET *1600 Calorie, stage 1*

FOOD RECORD

Time Begin/End	Situation	Hungry Y/N	Amount & Food Item (one food per line)	Exchange
6:30	home	Y	1 cup skim milk	1 D
↓			¾ cup 40% bran flakes	1 B
6:45			4 oz. orange juice	1 FR
8:30	work, desk	N	2 cups black coffee	—
11:15	lunch area	Y	2 slices whole wheat bread	2 B
			2 oz. turkey	2 M
			1 oz. low fat swiss cheese	1 D
↓			2 tsp. mayonnaise	2 F
12:00			1 tangerine	1 Fr
4:00	tired, alone	Y	1 apple	1 Fr
6:30	home with	Y	6 oz. broiled rib eye	6 M
	husband		1 cup mashed potatoes	2 B
			2 tsp. oleo	2 F
			½ cup green beans	1 V
↓			12 oz. iced tea	—
7:00			¼ cantelope	1 Fr
			1 roll	1 B

Comments:	Pattern:	Actual:	Pattern:	Actual:
overate meat	2 Dairy	//	6 Veg.	/
Not enough	7 Bread	##/	5 Meat	### ///
vegetables & fruit	6 Fruit	////	5 Fat	////

Figure 3.1. Example of a Food Record

Weight Records

In addition to food records, weight records help patients learn to control weight. Daily, or at least weekly, weight records can serve as a positive reinforcement of weight control efforts. Weighing should be done at the same time each day, preferably in the morning upon arising. The same scale should be used to keep an accurate record of weight changes.

Behavior Modification

Behavior modification is one of the most widely used techniques for weight control and, when combined with a dietary program, it has the greatest long-term success for the treatment of obesity.

Behavior therapy is based on the belief that the majority of behaviors, including those called "self-control," are learned. If behavior is changed by environment, we should be able to cause behavior changes by altering our environment.

Awareness

One of the first lines of defense against overeating is increased awareness. To change any behavior, we must understand how often it occurs and what factors influence it. Several techniques can be used to increase awareness:

1. Keep food records.
2. Avoid other activities while eating.
3. Sit down while eating.
4. Slow down the rate of eating.
5. Limit eating to only a few appropriate places.

Food records can be especially useful for determining when, where, how much, and how often you eat. Other techniques to increase awareness are avoiding distracting activities and sitting down while eating. Become more aware of what you are eating. Avoid watching television, reading, or engaging in other activities while eating. Designate an appropriate place at home and at work where you can be seated, and eat all of your meals and snacks there. Stop eating in every room of the house, in the car, or at your desk.

Slowing your rate of eating will also increase awareness. When you eat rapidly, you may not notice that you are feeling full; when you eat slowly, you are more likely to recognize the physiological response to fullness.

Cue Elimination

Behavior modification theory is often described in terms of a chain:

Trigger or cue $\longrightarrow$ *Behavior (eating)* $\longrightarrow$ *Consequence*

The trigger, or cue, is an event, situation, or emotion that typically precedes the behavior that the person is trying to modify. The behavior—in this case, eating—is the response to thoughts or actions that typically follow the trigger. The consequence can be either a positive or negative event.

Controlling and eliminating the triggers that lead to eating are a major emphasis of behavior modification for weight control. Cue elimination involves two steps. The first is to identify cues that trigger eating; the second step is to avoid them. Some of the most common cues are listed below.

---

anger	*nervousness*
boredom	*people*
depression	*places*
fatigue	*social events*
frustration	*tension*
happiness	*time of day*
hunger	*sight*
loneliness	*smell*

Your lifestyle may expose you to food too often. The following techniques will help you decrease your exposure to food.

1. Remove temptation: Store food out of sight in opaque containers. Remove food from everywhere in the house other than the usual storage areas.
2. Remove serving dishes from the table; portion out food on plates in the kitchen. If it is absolutely necessary to have containers on the table, keep them away from you. In restaurants, have the waiter remove the bread basket and butter.
3. Let someone else clear the dishes. Do not prepare more food than is necessary for the meal. Put leftovers away immediately; don't save them unless they can be worked into your exchange pattern.
4. Use a smaller plate. You will fool yourself into thinking that you have eaten more food.
5. Keep low-calorie snack items readily available to replace the usual snack foods that are high in calories, fat, sugar, or salt.
6. Enlist support from family and friends; ask them not to give food as a gift.

CHAPTER 4

THE *EAT SMART* MENUS AND HOW THEY WORK

Recipes in this cookbook were designed using lunch and dinner formats. Our restaurant chefs designed the menus to include varied colors, textures, and flavors. Whenever possible, they used existing recipes that required no modification or only minor modification to comply with our food and preparation guidelines.

All recipes have been analyzed by computer, and the number of exchanges for each serving has been calculated. The nutrient and caloric contents of each recipe are indicated. We have provided exchanges for people concerned with weight control, management of diabetes, or strict control of fat intake.

For each menu and individual recipe, a nutrition table is provided. The number of calories per serving for each menu or recipe is indicated. When a recipe serves six, for example, you should divide the dish into six equal portions. Portion control is important if the nutrient analysis is to accurately reflect the calories per serving.

Calories

Individual lunch and dinner menus were developed by each restaurant. Caloric content of the menus is limited to approximately 800 calories for lunch and 1,000 for dinner. Although a menu's calorie count may exceed your target, elimination of a dessert or appetizer can significantly reduce your caloric intake. You can also use a lower-calorie recipe from another menu.

Exchanges

Foods are divided into six major groups called exchange lists. Within each exchange list, a serving will provide approximately the same amount of calories, carbohydrates, protein, or fat. For each recipe, we have indicated the number of Dairy, Bread, Fat, Fruit, Meat, and Vegetable (Veg.) exchanges per serving. A complete description of the exchange system can be found in Chapter 3 and on page 20.

Nutrients

Gram (g) and milligram (mg) quantities for the nutrients in each recipe are provided. We've already discussed carbohydrates and protein, but here's some tips on interpreting the remaining nutritional information.

Total Fat

We have adjusted the overall fat content of menus to approximately 30 percent of the total calories. In some instances, we recommend further modification of a recipe, such as substitution of a low-calorie salad dressing, to achieve an overall limitation of fat to 30 percent of the total calories. Another way to control fat intake is to use exchange patterns at appropriate caloric levels throughout the day. By accounting for the intake of other fat exchanges on the day a lunch or dinner menu is eaten, total fat can be limited to 30 percent or less of the day's calories.

Saturated Fat

Because saturated fat tends to increase blood cholesterol levels compared to polyunsaturated and monounsaturated fats, we recommend a limitation of saturated fat to 10 percent of total calories.

We have limited the saturated fat content of our recipes by several methods, such as substitution of low-fat or nonfat dairy products for whole milk or cream, replacement of sour cream with yogurt, and use of only lean cuts of meat.

Cholesterol

We have indicated cholesterol content of each menu and recipe. The cholesterol content of menus is limited to less than 300 milligrams per day. The recipe analysis, however, reflects the cholesterol content of the menu alone and does not control for cholesterol intake at other meals. Therefore, you should be careful not to overeat cholesterol-rich foods at other meals.

Sodium

Since an excessive intake of sodium may contribute to the development of high blood pressure, we have used a moderate sodium restriction for menus (less than three grams, or 3,000 milligrams). Individuals on lower-sodium diets should, however, pay particular attention to the recipes' sodium content. Occasionally we recommend a low-sodium substitute for an ingredient to help further limit sodium intake.

Potassium

Like sodium, potassium is a mineral that may be involved in the control of blood pressure. Potassium helps increase sodium loss in urine and may contribute to a lowering of high blood pressure. We have reported the potassium content of each recipe for your information. People taking medications for high blood pressure, which can cause loss of potassium, may choose menus that are particularly high in this mineral.

Fiber

Population studies have suggested that a low fiber intake is associated with a higher incidence of colon cancer and coronary artery disease. Because of the recent increased interest in fiber, we have provided the fiber content of recipes and menus. The typical American diet of refined foods is relatively low in fiber. We recommend that people increase their average intake of total crude fiber from the average per day of 2 to 4 grams to 7 to 10 grams. Those concerned with increasing their fiber intake may wish to select high-fiber menus.

Calcium

We have also indicated the calcium content of menus and recipes. New evidence suggests that a low intake of calcium may be related to the development of hypertension and osteoporosis (thin bones).

Women, in particular, are at a risk of developing osteoporosis. The current Recommended Dietary Allowance (RDA) for calcium is 800 milligrams per day for adults. Recipes rich in calcium may be selected by women and by people with hypertension who are concerned with increasing their daily calcium intake.

Iron

Iron, an important component of a blood protein called hemoglobin, is responsible for the transport of oxygen to tissues in the body. A low blood iron content may result in anemia, or "thin blood." Premenopausal women require more iron than men because of monthly blood loss, and they may be at increased risk of developing anemia. The RDA per day for iron is 10 milligrams for men and 18 milligrams for women. Premenopausal women and those whose RDA for iron is not being met should select recipes that are a good source of iron.

Our Nutrition Guidelines

The chefs contributing to this cookbook followed our guidelines to reduce the intake of fat, cholesterol, and sodium and to increase the intake of complex carbohydrates and fiber. These positive steps should become customary practice when you prepare meals.

To reduce your saturated fat and cholesterol intake:

1. Use a minimum of fat. Decrease the use of butter or shortening and substitute vegetable oil or margarine.
2. Substitute nonfat yogurt for sour cream.
3. Use cocoa powder in place of chocolate.
4. Minimize the use of hydrogenated fat (vegetable shortening) and lard.
5. Use low-fat, skim milk cheeses instead of aged cheeses.
6. Minimize the use of whole eggs. Use egg substitutes or egg whites.
7. Avoid nondairy substitute creamers and whipped toppings containing saturated vegetable fats such as coconut and palm oil.
8. Use low-fat or nonfat milk rather than whole milk, cream, or half and half.
9. Avoid organ meats—liver, kidney, sweetbreads.
10. Minimize the use of avocados, olives, and nuts.
11. Avoid mayonnaise, gravies, and heavy cream sauces.
12. Prepare meat by braising, broiling, roasting, or grilling without additional fat and by skimming off fat while stewing. Avoid frying foods.

To reduce your sugar intake:

1. Reduce the sugar content of recipes. Try using ⅔ to ¾ of the sugar in a recipe.
2. Avoid syrups, molasses, fructose, dextrose, glucose, sucrose (table sugar), brown sugar, honey, and corn syrup. When these are listed on a label as one of the first three ingredients, sugar content will probably be too high.
3. Avoid the use of artificial sweeteners.
4. Reduce the use of jams, jellies, and fruit preserves.

To increase your complex carbohydrate and fiber intake:

1. Include complex carbohydrates such as whole-grain cereals and starchy vegetables in your meals.
2. Eat more fruits, vegetables, whole-grain breads, and other complex carbohydrates supplying a significant quantity of dietary fiber (see table C.2 on page 371).

Food Selection Guidelines

Use the following general recommendations to comply with our dietary fat limitation. The exchange system in the Appendix on pages 362 to 367 gives a more complete listing of allowed foods.

Meat

1. Select lean cuts of meat with a minimum of marbling. Those labeled "choice" or "good" usually have less fat than those labeled "prime."
2. Trim all visible fat from meat.
3. Eat more veal, which has less fat than beef.
4. Choose lean cuts of pork and lamb with little marbling.
5. Substitute poultry; poultry contains less saturated fat than beef, lamb, and pork. Remove the skin from poultry because ⅓ of the fat is found in the skin.
6. Select game wisely. Venison, rabbit, quail, and dove are acceptable. Avoid duck and goose because of their high fat content.

Fish

Fish are rich in polyunsaturated fat. Most fish contain less fat than meat. All fish are allowed, with the exception of shrimp, lobster, oysters, mussels, and crawfish; eat these shellfish in moderation.

Stocks and Gravies

Remove as much fat as possible from meat stocks and gravies. Several recommended techniques to remove fat include hardening it in the refrigerator or adding ice cubes, then using a gravy skimmer to remove fat that collects at the surface.

Eggs and Dairy Products

1. Avoid egg yolks, which are high in cholesterol, or use egg substitutes.
2. Remember that most dairy products contain saturated fat. Use nonfat dairy products containing less than 1 percent butterfat.
3. Choose low-fat cheeses with less than 12 percent butterfat.
4. Avoid high-fat dairy products such as aged cheeses, which contain more than 30 percent butterfat.

Breads and Cereals

1. Select either whole-grain or enriched products.
2. Increase your intake of pasta, low-fat crackers, and starchy vegetables.
3. Bear in mind that cakes, cookies, and other bakery products often include saturated fat, eggs, and whole milk. When these products are prepared with recommended ingredients instead, they can be included in your diet.

Fruits and Vegetables

Nearly all vegetables are allowable, but remember to season vegetables only with allowable oils, spices, and herbs. Avoid bacon fat, salt pork, and ham hocks as seasoning agents, as they contain significant amounts of salt and saturated fat. Also avoid fruit syrups and sauces with added sugar.

Restaurant Dining Guide

Eating out can be a dilemma if you are trying to watch your intake of calories and fat. Over half of the meals in the United States are now eaten in restaurants, and every indicator suggests that this trend will increase. Furthermore, nearly 25 percent of those meals are eaten in fast-food establishments where menu selections are usually limited to high-fat, high-sugar, and salty foods.

The following recommendations will aid you in making more appropriate selections in restaurants, thus helping you control your intake of calories and fat.

1. Preplan your meal before arriving at the restaurant. Avoid changing your meal plan when you review menu selections.
2. Be the first to order whenever possible. Do not change your selection after hearing what your companions have selected.
3. Have unnecessary foods such as bread and butter removed from the table.

4. If you are not certain of a menu item's composition or how it is prepared, ask the waiter to provide this information before making your selection.
5. Order butter, margarine, salad dressing, sauces, and gravies "on the side" to limit the intake of fat.
6. Always order a "regular"-size portion, not "large."
7. Take a break in the middle of the meal to prevent overeating. If you are full, have the waiter remove the dish from the table.
8. Eat slowly and drink water frequently to extend the length of the meal and to increase the feeling of fullness.
9. When traveling and dining out frequently, abide by a regular eating schedule. Do not skip meals or eat only one large meal late in the evening. Generally, more food will be consumed in one large meal than if smaller meals had been eaten during the day.
10. Plan for a small breakfast and lunch. Save adventurous eating for the evening meal, but don't overeat.

Appetizers

Before ordering any food or an alcoholic drink, have a large low-calorie beverage to relieve hunger. If you are not extremely hungry, do not eat an appetizer. If you do order one, try to split it between two people. Stay away from crackers, bread, and other extras until the food has been served.

Good appetizer selections include broth-based soups such as minestrone, Manhattan clam chowder, or gazpacho. Fresh fruit plates, such as prosciutto (thinly sliced ham) with melon, will help limit calorie and fat intake in the first course of a restaurant meal. Seafood cocktails and vegetable salads are other good appetizer selections.

Salads

Salads and salad bars can include items that are low or high in calories and fat depending on the ingredients added. Watch for high-fat items such as eggs, cheese, avocados, and salad dressing. A small portion of any of these added to a salad is acceptable, but a large serving will transform a salad into an entire meal.

Order all dressings on the side. If the waiter brings your salad with the dressing already added, return it. Substitute oil and vinegar or lemon juice for creamy dressings. Low-calorie dressings, now often available at salad bars and in restaurants, should be chosen whenever possible.

Pasta

Pasta dishes should be judged by their sauces. If you are not certain about the composition of the sauce, don't hesitate to ask the waiter.

Generally, red sauces are the lowest in fat while white sauces are high in fat, a result of the cream added in preparation. Sauces containing large amounts of vegetables or seafood are lower in calories and fat than sauces containing meat or cheese. Stuffed pasta is especially high in calories compared to plain pasta. If pasta is one of your favorite foods, have a good pasta dish and skip the entree.

Entrees

Choosing an entree that is grilled, baked, broiled, steamed, poached, or boiled will reduce fat consumption if it is prepared correctly. Often, however, entrees prepared even by these methods have fat added. Request that the entree be prepared with little or no fat and have any sauces served on the side. To control calorie and fat intake, select dishes prepared simply and without sauces.

Generally, poultry and seafood entrees will be the leanest selections. Duck and goose are high in fat and should not be eaten frequently. If chicken is not listed on a menu, ask for it; usually it will be available upon request.

Although veal is lower in fat than prime-grade beef, it is often served with a high-fat sauce. Order accompanying sauces to be served on the side. Pork, lamb, and beef can be ordered well-trimmed or can be trimmed at the table.

If the entree serving is unusually large, do not eat all of it. Have the waiter remove your plate promptly when you are finished.

Vegetables

Restaurants generally use vegetables as a garnish rather than as part of the meal. Be sure to ask the waiter what the vegetable will be and if you have a choice. Double the order of vegetables to replace the high-fat, starchy side dishes that often accompany an entree. Request that vegetables be served without butter or margarine and, if possible, that they be cooked by steaming.

Starches

Starchy foods are a good source of complex carbohydrates, not high in calories, and usually contain very little fat. However, starchy side dishes sometimes have fat added in the preparation or at the table. If most of the fat is added at the table, you will have more control over the fat and caloric content of the final product.

Change your eating patterns to avoid high-fat, starchy food. Substitute plain bread for garlic bread, which tends to be addictive. At breakfast, choose a bran muffin instead of a Danish pastry or doughnut. At other meals, select baked potatoes instead of French fries, cottage fries, or hash browns. Substitute rice for potatoes if you do not enjoy potatoes without trimmings. Baked beans can replace fried onion rings, or a double order of the vegetable of the day can substitute for a starchy side dish.

Desserts

Try to skip the dessert course whenever possible. If everyone else at the table has ordered dessert and you feel obligated to join in, order a seasonal fruit or coffee flavored with a liqueur. When you do order dessert, try to avoid such extras as ice cream or whipped cream toppings.

Recipes

The *Eat Smart Diet* is a total dietary program designed to improve your general health and increase your lifespan. Following this diet does not mean occasionally choosing the low-calorie entree or having fruit for dessert instead of pie. The diet encourages you to adjust your eating patterns so that every meal is healthful. This means learning to plan your meals so that they stay within the dietary guidelines. The recipes in this book have been grouped into menus to make your meal planning easier. And because these menus have been planned by leading restaurants, they offer exciting combinations of dishes as well as innovative and refreshing entrees.

The menus have been grouped into three separate chapters. Luncheons, which range from quick fruit salads to delicate seafood or meat dishes, are simple menus that usually involve a small appetizer, a light entree, and a light dessert. Light Dinners, which include seafood, chicken, and meat entrees, are suitable for a more elaborate luncheon or a simple but elegant dinner. Full-course meals are complete dinners, including an appetizer, entree, side dishes, and dessert. All menus are classified according to the entree, and each includes nutritional information for the complete menu. In addition, each recipe within the menu includes a separate nutritional chart, should you wish to alter the menu or skip one of its elements. The number of servings for each recipe in a particular menu is the same (with the exception of some basic recipes such as salad dressings and some desserts that are only practical when made in a certain size), and the number of servings is given at the beginning of the menu.

Although these recipes have been grouped for you, do not feel obligated to follow them rigidly. Mix and match, and create your own menus to suit your particular needs and likes. For example, if the fat exchange pattern for a particular menu is too high for your diet, substitute another dessert or even a different entree so that your totals add up to your goals. The Recipe Quick-Reference List (pages 37–48) groups recipes in more traditional categories of soups, salads, and so on. Use it, or the recipe index at the end of the book, to find additional recipes that will round out your new menus. Remember, however, that when you make up your own menus, you must total the nutritional information for each of the recipes to determine if your menu stays within the dietary guidelines. Since individual recipes have their own nutritional charts, this is a simple matter.

The Nutritional Charts

A full explanation of the nutritional charts is included in Chapter 3, and we suggest you read that chapter before attempting the recipes. In addition, you should be aware that nutritional information for most auxiliary recipes (such as salad dressings, sauces, and garnishes) has been calculated separately and has *not* been included in the main recipe. For example, the Fruit Salad Carousel (page 51) is served with a Honey-Lime Dressing. The recipe for the dressing follows the recipe for the salad itself, with its own corresponding nutritional chart. If, for example, you wish to know the total number of calories for the salad with the dressing, you should add the two calorie figures. On the other hand, if you want to substitute your favorite low-calorie commercial dressing, then just use the figures for the salad itself and add the figures shown on the bottle of commercial dressing. We've presented the information in this way to give you maximum flexibility in determining your menu.

Other Important Items

There are a few special things to note when using these recipes: (1) all spoon and cup measurements are level unless otherwise indicated; (2) all vegetables and fruits are medium size unless otherwise indicated; (3) all margarine is unsalted; (4) all flour is sifted before measuring; (5) all eggs are large size. For greatest accuracy, measure all ingredients carefully before use. Follow recipe instructions closely for best results.

Chicken stock is used in a number of the recipes that follow. For best results and most accurate nutritional calculations, we suggest you use the following recipe for Homemade Chicken Stock. This recipe makes 2 quarts; prepare it ahead of time and freeze some so you always have it ready for use in a recipe.

Homemade Chicken Stock

1 chicken, skinned; or 2¹/₂
   pounds chicken wings,
   necks, and backs
1 onion, coarsely chopped
3 stalks celery, coarsely chopped

2 carrots, coarsely chopped
2 whole cloves garlic
1 bay leaf
¹/₄ teaspoon dried thyme
2 quarts water

- Combine all ingredients in a large pot and bring to a boil. Reduce heat and simmer for 30 minutes.

- Remove chicken, chicken bones, and vegetables from stock. Strain. Puree vegetables in a blender and return to broth. (Reserve the meat for another use.)

- Refrigerate stock overnight to allow any fat to float to surface. Skim fat. Use stock in recipe or freeze in 1-cup containers for future use. Makes about 2 quarts.

PER SERVING: 68 CALORIES		
MENU EXCHANGE PATTERN		
Dairy ..... —	Fruit ..... —	
Bread .... —	Meat ..... —	
Fat 1	Veg. 1	
NUTRITIONAL INFORMATION		
Carbohydrate 4	g	
Protein 3	g	
Total fat 5	g	
Saturated fat 1.3	g	
Cholesterol............0	mg	
Sodium 88	mg	
Potassium 164	mg	
Fiber 0.4	g	
Calcium 19	mg	
Iron .... 0.4 mg		

CHAPTER 5

RECIPE QUICK-REFERENCE LIST

The recipes in this book are grouped into menus, according to the entree. Since these menus are designed to conform to the dietary guidelines described elsewhere in the book, you will probably want to follow the menus as they are presented. However, the following lists group most of the individual recipes in the more traditional cookbook manner. Use these listings if you want ideas to design your own menus. The number in parentheses that follows the recipe name indicates the serving quantity for that recipe, when appropriate.

Appetizers

(See also Salads)

Cheese-Stuffed Tortillas (4), page 167
Crab Claws with Cocktail Sauce (6), page 312
Crab with Belgian Endive (6), page 309
Eggplant Caviar (4), page 233
Grilled Sardines with Lime (6), page 263
Mushrooms, Marinated (4), page 246
Mushrooms, Sautéed (4), page 207
Onion Timbale (4), page 355
Oysters Baccarat (6), page 321
Oysters Landry (6), page 252
Prosciutto with Melon (4), page 210
Scallop and Shrimp Ceviche (6), page 287
Scallop Ceviche (6), page 192
Scallops, Cape Cod, with Mussels (6), page 351
Scallops and Prawns Bercy (6), page 303
Shrimp Cocktail (6), page 196
Shrimp Dumplings (4), page 103
Shrimp, Hickory-Smoked (2), page 243
Shrimp, Spiked Cold (8), page 255
Smoked Salmon Appetizers (6), page 294
Spicy Squid (2), page 204
Vegetable Crudités with Crabmeat Dip (6), page 147
Vegetables, Raw, with Basil Dip (4), page 200
Vegi-Nachos (4), page 269

Soups

Cold

Chilled Romaine Lettuce Soup (4), page 72
Chilled Vegetable Puree (4), page 84
Chilled Watercress Soup with Tart Apples (6), page 297
Cold Cucumber Soup (4), page 78
Gazpacho (4), page 127
Gazpacho Andaluz (4), page 117
Gazpacho Mexicano (6), page 154
Red Pepper Soup with Cilantro Yogurt (6), page 347
Tomato-Vegetable Soup (4), page 130
Vichyssoise (4), page 75

Hot

Salads

Green Salads

Vegetable Salads

Seafood Salads

Chicken and Meat Salads

Chicken Cucumber Salad (4), page 104
Ensalada de Pollo (6), page 154
Marinated Beef Salad (4), page 170
St. Tropez Chicken Salad (4), page 164
Summer Salad with Marinated Pepper Steak (6), page 173

Pasta Dishes

Chilled Pasta Salad with Pesto and Grilled Shrimp (4), page 87
Fettuccine Alfredo (6), page 295
Fettuccine, "Buttered" (6), page 300
Fettuccine Florentine (4), page 177
Fettuccine Primavera (4), page 189
Fettuccine Salad with Tomatillo-Herb Dressing (6), page 318
Fettuccine with Fennel (4), page 96
Fettuccine with Parmesan (6), page 304
Linguini with Pesto (6), page 82
Pasta with Chicken and Broccoli (6), page 161
Spaghetti with Eggplant and Ricotta (4), page 336
Spaghetti, Thin, with Fresh Basil (4), page 210
Spicy Noodles (4), page 227
Spinach Noodles with Tomatoes (6), page 310
Vegetable Ravioli with Tomato Sauce (6), page 173

Fish and Shellfish

Baked Stuffed Fish (4), page 246
Catfish Fillets with Creole Sauce (6), page 147
Crab Cakes, Gulf of Mexico (6), page 100
Crab Leg Do-Fu (2), page 205
Crawfish Étouffée with Rice (6), page 196
Flounder Fillets, Stuffed (6), page 252
Frogs Legs, Sautéed (4), page 150
Lobster with Tomato-Tarragon Fettuccine (6), page 193
Pine Nut Fish (4), page 249
Red Snapper Brazilian Style (4), page 233
(Red) Snapper Charlotte (6), page 240
Red Snapper, Grilled, with Basil Tomato Sauce (6), page 230
Red Snapper Fillets with Tomato-Ginger Vinaigrette (4), page 238
Red Snapper, Steamed Baby (4), page 227
Redfish, Beer-Batter Fried (2), page 243
Salmon, Grilled, with Julienne of Vegetables (2), page 220

Poultry

Meat and Game

Beef

Peppered Fillet of Beef with Grilled Red Onions and Ancho
   Pepper Preserve (6), page 297
Steak Forestière (6), page 295

Veal

Grilled Veal Chops (6), page 313
Paillard of Veal with Lemon and Tarragon (6), page 318
Saltimbocca (4), page 335
Veal Chops with Mushroom Sauce (6), page 309
Veal Grillades (6), page 315
Veal Medallions à la Grecque (8), page 306
Veal Medallions with Crabmeat (6), page 303
Veal Piccata (4), page 176
Veal Scallopini with Lemon Sauce (6), page 300

Pork

Broiled Pork Chops (4), page 332
Grilled Pork Loin with Apple Butter (4), page 338
Herbed Garlic Pork Chops (2), page 182
Marinated Pork Roast (8), page 179

Lamb

Brochette of Lamb (8), page 326
Grilled Lamb Chops (2), page 329
Rack of Lamb Lafayette (6), page 321

Game

Breast of Pheasant with Mushrooms and Cognac (8), page 344
Broiled Partridge (4), page 341
Grilled Venison Chops and Medallions (6), page 351
Roasted Rabbit with Poblano Pepper Sauce (6), page 348

Vegetables

Acorn Squash, Stuffed (8), page 256
Asparagus (2), page 135
Asparagus, Chilled (6), page 304
Beans and Rice, Red (6), page 66
Beans, Refried (4), page 270
Blackeyed Peas (4), page 151
Broccoli and Carrots, Seasoned (4), page 247
Broccoli and Carrots, Steamed (4), page 124

Broccoli and Carrots with Rosemary (6), page 301
Broccoli with Lemon, Steamed (6), page 215
Cabbage, Braised (4), page 338
Carrots, Braised with Onions (4), page 208
Carrots and Onions (2), page 330
Carrots, Herbed (4), page 342
Cauliflower with Vegetable Sauce (6), page 278
Corn Relish (4), page 284
Corn and Pepper Relish (6), page 349
Eggplant and Tomatoes, Herbed (6), page 260
Eggplant, Peppercorn (4), page 115
Green and White Jade (6), page 186
Green Beans (8), page 256
Green Beans with Dill (6), page 231
Green Beans with Potatoes, Creole (6), page 253
Green Beans with Tomatoes (2), page 244
Lord Han's Vegetable Delight (4), page 228
Mixed Mexican Vegetables (4), page 291
Mustard Greens with Onion (6), page 67
Mustard Greens, Boiled (4), page 333
Okra with Caraway (4), page 93
Peas and Carrots (6), page 313
Peas and Onions (6), page 322
Peas and Pimientos (6), page 241
Peas with Water Chestnuts (4), page 127
Potato Pancakes (4), page 284
Potatoes, Baked (8), page 218
Potatoes, Baked Stuffed (2), page 329
Potatoes, Boiled (4), page 118
Potatoes, Boiled New (4), page 145
Potatoes Florentine, New (6), page 277
Potatoes, Herbed (4), page 107
Potatoes Lyonnaise (6), page 280
Potatoes, Oven-Fried (2), page 243
Potatoes Sautéed with Parsley, New (4), page 224
Potatoes, Scalloped (6), page 215
Potatoes, Tarragon (6), page 322
Potatoes with Dillseed-Yogurt Sauce, New (4), page 341
Ratatouille (4), page 201
Red Cabbage, Braised, with Cider Sauce (6), page 352
Snow Peas, Sautéed (4), page 250
Spinach, Creamed (6), page 281
Spinach, Sautéed Fresh (8), page 307
Spinach, Southern-Style (6), page 197
Squash Casserole (6), page 315
Squash, Dilled Yellow (4), page 333
Tomatillos, Grilled (4), page 285
Tomato Slices, Grilled (8), page 218
Tomatoes, Baked (4), page 151

Rice, Noodles, and Grains

Desserts

Warm Desserts

Cold Fruits and Puddings

Frozen Desserts

Cakes and Pastries

Cookies

Breads

Yeast Breads

French Bread, page 70
Poppyseed Bread, page 259
Whole Wheat Bread, page 201

Quick Breads and Muffins

Banana Nut Bread, page 52
Bran Muffins, page 60
Cornbread, page 180
Cornbread, Jalapeño, page 253
Cranberry-Nut Bread, page 79
Zucchini Nut Bread, page 73

Note: For additional and more complete recipe listings, see the recipe index on page 379.

CHAPTER 6

LUNCHEONS

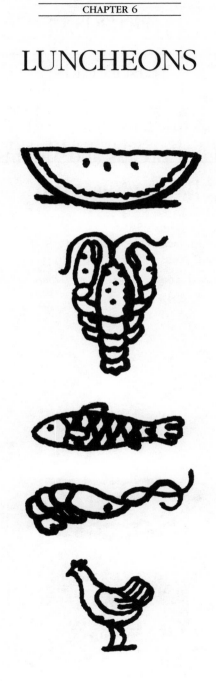

FRUIT SALADS

1

Fruit Salad Carousel
with Honey-Lime Dressing

Banana Nut Bread

Sesame Cookies

Serves 8

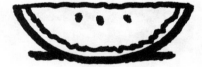

PER SERVING: 610 CALORIES			
MENU EXCHANGE PATTERN			
Dairy . . . . . —	Fruit 5		
Bread . . . 4½	Meat . . . . . —		
Fat 2	Veg. . . . . . . —		
NUTRITIONAL INFORMATION			
Carbohydrate 120	g		
Protein 11	g		
Total fat 14	g		
Saturated fat 3.3	g		
Cholesterol 35	mg		
Sodium 122	mg		
Potassium 1198	mg		
Fiber 3.3	g		
Calcium 229	mg		
Iron 2.5	mg		

Fruit Salad Carousel

16 red lettuce leaves
8 slices watermelon, sliced
   ¼ inch thick
8 slices cantaloupe, sliced
   ¼ inch thick
8 slices honeydew melon, sliced
   ¼ inch thick
4 kiwis, peeled and sliced

3 oranges, peeled and
   sectioned
8 apples, center core removed
8 scoops sherbet (⅓ cup each)
8 small bunches grapes
1 cup Honey-Lime Dressing
   (recipe follows)
8 fresh strawberries, sliced

- Place red lettuce leaves on individual salad plates and arrange the following in a pinwheel pattern: watermelon, cantaloupe, honeydew, kiwi. In the center of the pinwheel, place cored apple. Place sherbet scoop on apple. Put grapes beside the apple. Top with Honey-Lime Dressing and garnish with sliced strawberries.

PER SERVING: 390 CALORIES		
MENU EXCHANGE PATTERN		
Dairy . . . . . —	Fruit 4	
Bread 3	Meat . . . . . —	
Fat . . . . ½	Veg. . . . . . . —	
NUTRITIONAL INFORMATION		
Carbohydrate 90	g	
Protein 7	g	
Total fat 4	g	
Saturated fat 1.6	g	
Cholesterol 8	mg	
Sodium 81	mg	
Potassium 996	mg	
Fiber 2.6	g	
Calcium 209	mg	
Iron 1.4	mg	

Honey-Lime Dressing

8 ounces low-fat plain yogurt
2 tablespoons honey
2 teaspoons lime juice
Pinch of ginger

- Combine yogurt with honey, lime juice, and ginger. Whip and chill. Makes 1 cup; 1 serving = 2 tablespoons.

PER SERVING: 35 CALORIES		
MENU EXCHANGE PATTERN		
Dairy . . . . . —	Fruit . . . . . —	
Bread . . . . . ½	Meat . . . . . —	
Fat . . . . —	Veg. . . . . . . —	
NUTRITIONAL INFORMATION		
Carbohydrate 7	g	
Protein 2	g	
Total fat 1	g	
Saturated fat 0.3	g	
Cholesterol 2	mg	
Sodium 20	mg	
Potassium 73	mg	
Fiber 0	g	
Calcium 53	mg	
Iron 0.1	mg	

Banana Nut Bread

½ cup sugar
½ cup margarine
2 egg substitutes, lightly beaten
2¾ cups all-purpose flour

½ teaspoon baking soda
1½ teaspoons baking powder
1½ cups mashed ripe bananas
⅓ cup chopped pecans

- Preheat oven to 350°F. Coat a 9 × 5-inch loaf pan with non-stick vegetable spray. In a bowl, cream the sugar and margarine, then mix in beaten egg. In another bowl, sift together flour, baking soda, and baking powder. Gradually add to the egg mixture, alternating with some of the banana. Mix in chopped pecans. Transfer to loaf pan and bake for about 1 hour, or until a tester inserted in center comes out clean. Let cool for about 10 minutes, then remove from pan and let cool on a rack. Serves 20; 1 serving = one ½-inch slice.

PER SERVING: 156 CALORIES		
MENU EXCHANGE PATTERN		
Dairy ..... —	Fruit 1	
Bread 1	Meat ...... —	
Fat 1	Veg. .... —	
NUTRITIONAL INFORMATION		
Carbohydrate 22	g	
Protein 3	g	
Total fat 7	g	
Saturated fat 1.1	g	
Cholesterol 27	mg	
Sodium 9	mg	
Potassium 170	mg	
Fiber 0.5	g	
Calcium 18	mg	
Iron 0.8	mg	

Sesame Cookies

2 cups all-purpose flour
1½ teaspoons baking powder
½ teaspoon salt
⅔ cup sugar
⅔ cup margarine

2 egg substitutes, lightly beaten
1 tablespoon low-fat milk
1 teaspoon vanilla extract
2½ tablespoons sesame seeds

- Preheat oven to 375°F. Sift flour, baking powder, and salt together. In a separate bowl, cream together sugar and margarine. While mixing, add beaten egg, milk, and vanilla to sugar-margarine mixture. Gradually stir in dry ingredients and mix thoroughly. Drop cookie dough by teaspoonfuls onto ungreased cookie sheet. Flatten each with a fork dipped in water and then sprinkle each with sesame seeds. Bake for 10 to 15 minutes, or until lightly brown. Cool on a rack. Makes 40 cookies; 1 serving = 1 cookie.

PER SERVING: 65 CALORIES		
MENU EXCHANGE PATTERN		
Dairy ..... —	Fruit ..... —	
Bread .....½	Meat ..... —	
Fat ....½	Veg. .... —	
NUTRITIONAL INFORMATION		
Carbohydrate 8	g	
Protein 1	g	
Total fat 4	g	
Saturated fat 0.6	g	
Cholesterol 0	mg	
Sodium 32	mg	
Potassium 32	mg	
Fiber 0.2	g	
Calcium 6	mg	
Iron 0.3	mg	

FRUIT SALADS

2

Spicy Mussel Soup
with Ancho Pepper Preserve

Papaya and Crabmeat
with Tomato-Pepper Vinaigrette

Grapefruit-Orange Terrine

Serves 8

PER SERVING: 503 CALORIES		
MENU EXCHANGE PATTERN		
Dairy . . . . . —	Fruit 3	
Bread 2	Meat 4	
Fat . . . . —	Veg. . . . . . . ½	
NUTRITIONAL INFORMATION		
Carbohydrate 70	g	
Protein 36	g	
Total fat 5	g	
Saturated fat 0.1	g	
Cholesterol 128	mg	
Sodium 455	mg	
Potassium 1804	mg	
Fiber 3.7	g	
Calcium 206	mg	
Iron 7.4	mg	

Spicy Mussel Soup with Ancho Pepper Preserve

40 mussels, cleaned
2 cups dry white wine
2 cups fish broth or Homemade
   Chicken Stock (page 36)
2–3 tablespoons Cilantro-
   Serrano Puree (recipe
   follows)

4 teaspoons Ancho Pepper
   Preserve (page 298)
2–3 sprigs cilantro (fresh
   coriander)

- Clean mussels as described on page 259.

- Place mussels in a sauté pan with the wine and stock. Cover and bring to a boil. Steam mussels until shells open, then remove mussels from pan. Discard any that did not open. Take mussels from their shells and set aside.

- Add 1 to 2 tablespoons of the Cilantro-Serrano Puree to the mussel liquid and blend well. Add mussels and bring liquid to a boil for a few seconds, then transfer puree and mussels to soup bowls. Fill 1 mussel shell half with ½ teaspoon Ancho Pepper Preserve and float the half shell on the soup. Garnish with a few cilantro leaves. Continue for remaining soup bowls, floating a preserve-filled mussel shell half in each and garnishing each with some cilantro leaves.

Note: Nutritional analysis includes Puree.

PER SERVING: 178 CALORIES		
MENU EXCHANGE PATTERN		
Dairy ..... —	Fruit ..... —	
Bread .... —	Meat 3	
Fat .... —	Veg. .... ½	
NUTRITIONAL INFORMATION		
Carbohydrate 4	g	
Protein 20	g	
Total fat 3	g	
Saturated fat 0	g	
Cholesterol 71	mg	
Sodium 78	mg	
Potassium 387	mg	
Fiber 0	g	
Calcium 23	mg	
Iron .... 5.0 mg		

Cilantro-Serrano Puree

2 large bunches cilantro (fresh
   coriander)
1 bunch parsley
¼ red onion, chopped
2 cloves garlic, chopped

2 serrano peppers, stems
   removed
1 cup Homemade Chicken
   Stock (page 36)

- Place ingredients in a blender and puree with just enough stock to form a very thick and smooth puree. Refrigerate any unused puree. Makes 1½ cups; 1 serving = 2 tablespoons.

PER SERVING: 8 CALORIES		
MENU EXCHANGE PATTERN		
Dairy ..... —	Fruit ..... —	
Bread .... —	Meat ..... —	
Fat .... —	Veg. .... ½	
NUTRITIONAL INFORMATION		
Carbohydrate 2	g	
Protein 1	g	
Total fat 0	g	
Saturated fat 0	g	
Cholesterol 0	mg	
Sodium 7	mg	
Potassium 117	mg	
Fiber 0.3	g	
Calcium 32	mg	
Iron .... 0.9 mg		

Papaya and Crabmeat with Tomato-Pepper Vinaigrette

8 papayas, peeled and seeded
16 ounces lump crabmeat
8 sprigs watercress

Tomato-Pepper Vinaigrette

16 ripe plum tomatoes, roughly
*   chopped*
⅔ red onion, minced
1 bunch cilantro, chopped

1 jalapeño or 2 serrano chilies,
*   seeded and minced*
Juice of 1½ limes
Black pepper

- Prepare the vinaigrette. Combine ingredients in a jar and shake well. Set aside.

- Slice the papayas on the bias (at a 45° angle). Arrange the slices in a fan on each salad plate, then place some crabmeat at the base of each fan. Garnish each plate with watercress and serve with the vinaigrette.

PER SERVING: 199 CALORIES			
MENU EXCHANGE PATTERN			
Dairy	—	Fruit	2
Bread	1	Meat	1
Fat	—	Veg.	—
NUTRITIONAL INFORMATION			
Carbohydrate		37	g
Protein		13	g
Total fat		2	g
Saturated fat		0.1	g
Cholesterol		57	mg
Sodium		325	mg
Potassium		1102	mg
Fiber		3	g
Calcium		118	mg
Iron		1.4	mg

Grapefruit-Orange Terrine

2 grapefruit
4 oranges
1 package (3 ounces) lime
*   gelatin*

- Peel grapefruit and oranges and divide each into individual sections.

- Prepare gelatin according to package instructions, without chilling. In a 9 × 5-inch loaf pan, arrange a layer of the fruit sections. Pour in enough gelatin to cover the mixture. Follow with another layer of fruit and follow with more gelatin. Continue with layers until all the fruit is used. Pour enough gelatin for the last layer so that it adequately covers the fruit. Refrigerate until firm, then unmold by briefly dipping the pan in hot water and inverting mold onto a serving plate. Slice and serve.

PER SERVING: 117 CALORIES			
MENU EXCHANGE PATTERN			
Dairy	—	Fruit	1
Bread	1	Meat	—
Fat	—	Veg.	—
NUTRITIONAL INFORMATION			
Carbohydrate		28	g
Protein		2	g
Total fat		0	g
Saturated fat		0	g
Cholesterol		0	mg
Sodium		45	mg
Potassium		198	mg
Fiber		0.4	g
Calcium		32	mg
Iron		0.1	mg

FISH SOUPS AND STEWS

1

Classic Bouillabaisse

Garlic Bread

Baked Apple Crisp

Serves 6

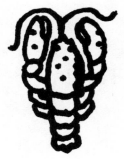

PER SERVING: 808 CALORIES

MENU EXCHANGE PATTERN

Dairy	—	Fruit	2
Bread	3	Meat	5½
Fat	4	Veg.	1

NUTRITIONAL INFORMATION

Carbohydrate	80	g
Protein	46	g
Total fat	33	g
Saturated fat	6.2	g
Cholesterol	196	mg
Sodium	655	mg
Potassium	1189	mg
Fiber	2.6	g
Calcium	310	mg
Iron	5.6	mg

Classic Bouillabaisse

½ pound lobster meat
¼ pound striped bass, cleaned
½ pound red snapper, cleaned
¼ pound trout, cleaned
¼ pound haddock, cleaned
½ pound shrimp, shelled
6 mussels (see page 259)
6 clams
¼ cup safflower oil
½ cup chopped carrot
2 leeks, chopped
½ cup chopped onion

2 cloves garlic, chopped
¼ cup chopped fresh fennel
2 fresh tomatoes, chopped
½ bay leaf
¼ teaspoon dried thyme
1½ teaspoons salt
½ teaspoon black pepper
¼ teaspoon saffron, crumbled
4 cups water
1 tablespoon chopped fresh
  parsley

- Cut up lobster; leave meat in shell. Cut all other fish into 1-inch pieces. Clean the mussels and clams (see note). Heat the safflower oil in a Dutch oven over low heat. Add carrot, leek, onion, garlic, and fennel and sauté for 5 minutes. Add tomatoes and seasonings. Add the lobster and water, bring soup to a boil, and simmer for 5 minutes. Add bass and red snapper and simmer for 5 minutes. Add trout, haddock, shrimp, mussels, and clams and simmer until clam shells open, about 15 minutes. Sprinkle with parsley and serve.

Note: To clean clams, cover clams in a large bowl of salt water (⅓ cup salt to 1 gallon water). Soak at least 30 minutes. Discard any clams that will not close when touched. Rinse clams in cold water and scrub if necessary to remove other debris.

PER SERVING: 306 CALORIES

MENU EXCHANGE PATTERN

Dairy	—	Fruit	—
Bread	—	Meat	5
Fat	—	Veg.	1

NUTRITIONAL INFORMATION

Carbohydrate	9	g
Protein	36	g
Total fat	14	g
Saturated fat	1.1	g
Cholesterol	188	mg
Sodium	221	mg
Potassium	807	mg
Fiber	0.7	g
Calcium	92	mg
Iron	3.3	mg

Garlic Bread

¹/₄ cup margarine
2 cloves garlic, crushed
1 small loaf French bread
    (6 slices)
2 ounces Parmesan cheese,
    grated (¹/₂ cup)

- Blend margarine with garlic. Spread mixture on one side of bread slices. Sprinkle with cheese and toast margarine side up in the broiler until brown. Turn slices and broil other side until golden. Serve hot.

Note: To reduce fat intake, substitute French bread for Garlic Bread. Adjusted analysis, per slice: calories = 70; exchange = 1 Bread.

PER SERVING: 186 CALORIES

MENU EXCHANGE PATTERN

Dairy	—	Fruit	—
Bread	1	Meat	¹/₂
Fat	2	Veg.	—

NUTRITIONAL INFORMATION

Carbohydrate	15	g
Protein	6	g
Total fat	11	g
Saturated fat	3.5	g
Cholesterol	8	mg
Sodium	323	mg
Potassium	42	mg
Fiber	0.6	g
Calcium	146	mg
Iron	0.7	mg

Baked Apple Crisp

8 cups thinly sliced peeled
    apples
1¹/₂ tablespoons lemon juice
1 tablespoon sugar
4 teaspoons ground cinnamon
1 cup rolled oats

¹/₄ cup instant nonfat milk
    powder
¹/₃ cup all-purpose flour
¹/₂ cup firmly packed brown
    sugar
¹/₄ cup margarine

- Preheat oven to 350°F. Arrange apple slices on bottom of a 2-quart casserole. Add lemon juice, sugar, and 2 teaspoons cinnamon and stir to coat slices.

- Combine remaining ingredients in a separate bowl. Spread topping over apples and bake until top is golden brown, about 30 minutes. Serve warm.

PER SERVING: 316 CALORIES

MENU EXCHANGE PATTERN

Dairy	—	Fruit	2
Bread	2	Meat	—
Fat	2	Veg.	—

NUTRITIONAL INFORMATION

Carbohydrate	58	g
Protein	4	g
Total fat	9	g
Saturated fat	1.6	g
Cholesterol	0	mg
Sodium	111	mg
Potassium	341	mg
Fiber	1.3	g
Calcium	72	mg
Iron	1.6	mg

FISH SOUPS AND STEWS

2

Fish Broth with Watercress and Haddock

Bran Muffins

Cantaloupe and Blueberries with Yogurt Dressing

Serves 4

PER SERVING: 401 CALORIES		
MENU EXCHANGE PATTERN		
Dairy 1	Fruit 2½	
Bread 1	Meat 1½	
Fat 1	Veg. . . . . . . ½	
NUTRITIONAL INFORMATION		
Carbohydrate 63	g	
Protein 27	g	
Total fat 8	g	
Saturated fat 1.6	g	
Cholesterol 57	mg	
Sodium 341	mg	
Potassium 1741	mg	
Fiber 3.3	g	
Calcium 261	mg	
Iron 3.1	mg	

Fish Broth with Watercress and Haddock

2 pounds fish scraps and bones
2 quarts cold water
1 onion, coarsely chopped
3 stalks celery, coarsely chopped
2 bay leaves
2 whole cloves
2 peppercorns

1 teaspoon dried thyme
2 to 3 sprigs parsley
¾ pound haddock, boned,
    skinned, and cut in
    1-inch chunks
2 bunches watercress, trimmed
    and chopped (about 1 cup)

- Cover fish scraps and bones with 2 quarts cold water and bring to a boil. Add the onion, celery, bay leaves, cloves, peppercorns, thyme, and parsley. Lower heat and simmer gently for 30 minutes. Strain broth and measure out 4 cups; reserve remainder for another use (broth can be frozen).

- Add the diced haddock to the 4 cups strained broth and simmer slowly until fish is cooked, about 5 minutes. Add watercress and allow to wilt, then serve immediately.

PER SERVING: 91 CALORIES		
MENU EXCHANGE PATTERN		
Dairy . . . . . —	Fruit . . . . . —	
Bread . . . . . —	Meat 1½	
Fat . . . . —	Veg. . . . . ½	
NUTRITIONAL INFORMATION		
Carbohydrate 5	g	
Protein 17	g	
Total fat 0	g	
Saturated fat 0.1	g	
Cholesterol 51	mg	
Sodium 99	mg	
Potassium 459	mg	
Fiber 0.5	g	
Calcium 58	mg	
Iron . . . . 1.1 mg		

Bran Muffins

1 cup whole wheat flour
1 cup raw bran
2 teaspoons baking powder
½ teaspoon salt

1 egg substitute, beaten
¼ cup molasses
1½ cups skim milk
½ cup raisins

- Preheat oven to 400°F. Combine dry ingredients in a large bowl. Blend egg substitute, molasses, and milk in a separate bowl and fold into dry ingredients just until flour is moistened. Fold in raisins. Spoon into 12 greased muffin cups and bake until a tester inserted in the center of one muffin comes out clean, about 20 minutes. Cool muffins in pan for 10 minutes, then turn out onto racks. Makes 12; 1 serving = 1 muffin.

PER SERVING: 127 CALORIES		
MENU EXCHANGE PATTERN		
Dairy . . . . . —	Fruit . . . . . —	
Bread 1	Meat . . . . . —	
Fat 1	Veg. . . . . . . —	
NUTRITIONAL INFORMATION		
Carbohydrate 18	g	
Protein 4	g	
Total fat 5	g	
Saturated fat 1	g	
Cholesterol 2	mg	
Sodium 174	mg	
Potassium 200	mg	
Fiber 1	g	
Calcium 58	mg	
Iron . . . . 1 mg		

Cantaloupe and Blueberries with Yogurt Dressing

2 cantaloupes
Juice of 2 lemons
2 cups blueberries

1 cup plain low-fat yogurt
Dash of vanilla extract
⅓ cup strawberries, hulled

- Cut each melon in half and remove seeds. To keep the cantaloupe from rolling off the dessert plate, slice a small portion from the bottom of each half. Sprinkle melons with lemon juice. Combine blueberries, yogurt, and vanilla and fill cantaloupe halves with the mixture. Top with strawberries.

PER SERVING: 183 CALORIES		
MENU EXCHANGE PATTERN		
Dairy 1	Fruit 2½	
Bread .... —	Meat ..... —	
Fat .... —	Veg. ...... —	

NUTRITIONAL INFORMATION		
Carbohydrate 40	g
Protein 6	g
Total fat 2	g
Saturated fat 0.6	g
Cholesterol 4	mg
Sodium 68	mg
Potassium 1082	mg
Fiber 2.1	g
Calcium 145	mg
Iron 1	mg

FISH SOUPS AND STEWS

3

Green Salad with Acadian Dressing

Fish Court-Bouillon with Rice

Peach-Glazed Cake

Serves 4

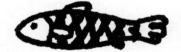

PER SERVING: 676 CALORIES			
MENU EXCHANGE PATTERN			
Dairy	—	Fruit	½
Bread	4	Meat	3
Fat	3	Veg.	3
NUTRITIONAL INFORMATION			
Carbohydrate	81	g	
Protein	30	g	
Total fat	26	g	
Saturated fat	3.1	g	
Cholesterol	66	mg	
Sodium	696	mg	
Potassium	1168	mg	
Fiber	1.9	g	
Calcium	173	mg	
Iron	4.5	mg	

Green Salad

½ head of red-leaf lettuce,
about 2 cups
½ head of green leaf lettuce,
about 2 cups

2 tomatoes, sliced
¼ cup Acadian Dressing (recipe
follows)
Black pepper

PER SERVING: 30 CALORIES			
MENU EXCHANGE PATTERN			
Dairy . . . . . —		Fruit . . . . . —	
Bread . . . . . —		Meat . . . . —	
Fat . . . . —		Veg. 1	
NUTRITIONAL INFORMATION			
Carbohydrate 6			g
Protein 2			g
Total fat 0			g
Saturated fat 0			g
Cholesterol 0			mg
Sodium 8			mg
Potassium 367			mg
Fiber 0.9			g
Calcium 49			mg
Iron 1.2			mg

- Arrange lettuce leaves and sliced tomatoes on salad plates. Top with dressing and season with pepper.

Acadian Dressing

⅔ cup safflower oil
2 cloves garlic, mashed
3 tablespoons thinly sliced
celery
3 tablespoons thinly sliced bell
pepper

3 tablespoons thinly sliced
black olives
⅓ cup white wine vinegar

PER SERVING: 84 CALORIES			
MENU EXCHANGE PATTERN			
Dairy . . . . . —		Fruit . . . . . —	
Bread . . . . . —		Meat . . . . . —	
Fat 2		Veg. . . . . . . —	
NUTRITIONAL INFORMATION			
Carbohydrate 0			g
Protein 0			g
Total fat 9			g
Saturated fat 0.8			g
Cholesterol 0			mg
Sodium 18			mg
Potassium 14			mg
Fiber 0			g
Calcium 3			mg
Iron 0.1			mg

- Mix ingredients. Makes about 1½ cups; 1 serving = 1 table-spoon.

Fish Court-Bouillon with Rice

1 pound red snapper, redfish,
or salmon, cut in serving
pieces
Cayenne pepper
1 garlic clove, minced
2 tablespoons safflower oil
¼ cup all-purpose flour
1 onion, minced
1 stalk celery, finely chopped
½ cup chopped tomato

2 tablespoons tomato sauce
1 bay leaf
½ teaspoon sugar
4 cups water
½ lemon, sliced crosswise
1 tablespoon chopped fresh
parsley
1 tablespoon chopped green
onion (green part only)
2 cups cooked rice

- Season fish generously with cayenne and garlic. Place in a covered baking dish and chill several hours before cooking.

- Heat oil in saucepan over low heat. Add flour. Cook, stirring constantly, until light brown, about 15 to 20 minutes. Remove from heat and add onion and celery. Return to heat and stir constantly for 4 to 5 minutes. Add tomato, tomato sauce, bay leaf, sugar, and water and bring to a boil. Cover, reduce heat, and simmer for 45 minutes. Add fish and lemon slices and simmer 20 minutes longer.
- Add parsley and green onion and heat through. Serve in soup plates with a scoop of cooked rice.

PER SERVING: 351 CALORIES		
MENU EXCHANGE PATTERN		
Dairy . . . . . —	Fruit . . . . . —	
Bread 2	Meat 3	
Fat . . . . —	Veg. 2	
NUTRITIONAL INFORMATION		
Carbohydrate 37		g
Protein 26		g
Total fat 11		g
Saturated fat 1.1		g
Cholesterol 65		mg
Sodium 555		mg
Potassium 682		mg
Fiber 0.8		g
Calcium 91		mg
Iron 2.9		mg

Peach-Glazed Cake

¼ cup margarine, at room temperature
½ teaspoon vanilla extract
¾ cup sugar

1¼ cups cake flour, sifted
½ teaspoon baking powder
⅔ cup buttermilk
2 egg whites

Peach Glaze

5 canned peach halves (in juice or water), thinly sliced, juice retained
1½ tablespoons sugar
1½ teaspoons cornstarch

½ cup peach liquid
1 teaspoon almond extract
1 to 2 drops yellow food coloring

- Preheat oven to 350°F. Cream margarine, vanilla, and all but 2 tablespoons sugar in a large bowl until fluffy. Sift together flour and baking powder and add to the creamed mixture alternately with buttermilk. Beat egg whites until foamy. Gradually add the remaining 2 tablespoons sugar and beat until stiff peaks form. Fold egg whites into cake batter. Pour into a 9-inch round cake pan sprayed with nonstick spray. Bake until tester inserted in center comes out clean, about 30 minutes. Cool completely on a rack.

- Prepare glaze. Arrange peach slices in two circles on top of cake. Blend sugar and cornstarch in a saucepan. Add ½ cup peach liquid and cook over low heat, stirring constantly, until thickened and smooth. Remove from heat, add almond extract and food coloring and cool for 15 minutes. Pour over peaches. Chill cake before serving. Cover leftover cake tightly and refrigerate. Makes 8 servings.

Note: Other canned fruits, such as apricots, cherries, pineapple, strawberries, raspberries, or blueberries, can be substituted.

Photo opposite page 66.

PER SERVING: 211 CALORIES		
MENU EXCHANGE PATTERN		
Dairy . . . . . —	Fruit . . . . . . ½	
Bread 2	Meat . . . . . . —	
Fat 1	Veg. . . . . . . —	
NUTRITIONAL INFORMATION		
Carbohydrate 37		g
Protein 3		g
Total fat 6		g
Saturated fat 1.2		g
Cholesterol 1		mg
Sodium 115		mg
Potassium 104		mg
Fiber 0.2		g
Calcium 30		mg
Iron 0.3		mg

FISH SOUPS AND STEWS

4

Willie's Seafood Gumbo

Red Beans and Rice

Mustard Greens with Onion

Pecan Cookies

Serves 6

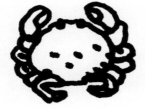

PER SERVING: 612 CALORIES		
MENU EXCHANGE PATTERN		
Dairy . . . . . —	Fruit . . . . . —	
Bread 3½	Meat 3	
Fat 2	Veg. 4	
NUTRITIONAL INFORMATION		
Carbohydrate 78	g	
Protein 30	g	
Total fat 21	g	
Saturated fat 2.4	g	
Cholesterol 90	mg	
Sodium 392	mg	
Potassium 1261	mg	
Fiber 3.7	g	
Calcium 355	mg	
Iron 10.5	mg	

Willie's Seafood Gumbo

4 cups hot water
1½ teaspoons cayenne pepper
½ lemon, sliced crosswise
½ pound shrimp, shelled and
    deveined
½ pound oysters, liquor
    reserved
3 cups (about) fish stock or
    Homemade Chicken Stock
    (page 36)

½ cup crabmeat
¼ cup safflower oil
⅓ cup all-purpose flour
1 onion, finely chopped
2 cloves garlic, minced
1 tablespoon chopped green
    onion
1 tablespoon chopped fresh
    parsley
6 teaspoons filé powder

- In a large saucepan, combine hot water with cayenne pepper and lemon slices. Add shrimp and oysters and cook over medium heat until shrimp turn pink, about 5 minutes. Turn off heat and let stand, covered, for 3 minutes; drain, reserving liquid. Add oyster liquor and enough stock to make 7 cups liquid. Add crabmeat to shrimp and oysters.

- Heat oil in a large heavy pot over low heat. Add flour and cook, stirring constantly, until roux is deep golden brown, 15 to 20 minutes. Remove from heat and add onion and garlic. Return to heat; slowly add stock mixture and bring to a boil; stir constantly until thickened. Add seafood, green onion, and parsley; heat through. Ladle into serving bowls and top each with 1 teaspoon filé.

Note: Filé powder is available in specialty food stores and gourmet shops. It is a Creole thickening agent, made from ground sassafras leaves.

PER SERVING: 187 CALORIES		
MENU EXCHANGE PATTERN		
Dairy . . . . . —	Fruit . . . . . —	
Bread . . . . —	Meat 2	
Fat 1	Veg. 1	
NUTRITIONAL INFORMATION		
Carbohydrate 9		g
Protein 13		g
Total fat 10		g
Saturated fat 0.8		g
Cholesterol 85		mg
Sodium 216		mg
Potassium 190		mg
Fiber 0.1		g
Calcium 75		mg
Iron 3.1		mg

Red Beans and Rice

1 large onion, finely chopped
1 tablespoon margarine
4 cups water
½ pound dried red or kidney
    beans, rinsed and drained
2 cloves garlic, finely minced

½ cup diced lean ham
2 large tomatoes, chopped
1 small bay leaf
¼ teaspoon cayenne pepper
½ teaspoon dried oregano
½ cup chopped green onion

Rice

1 cup rice
2 cups water
Paprika

*Peach-Glazed Cake;
recipe page 64*

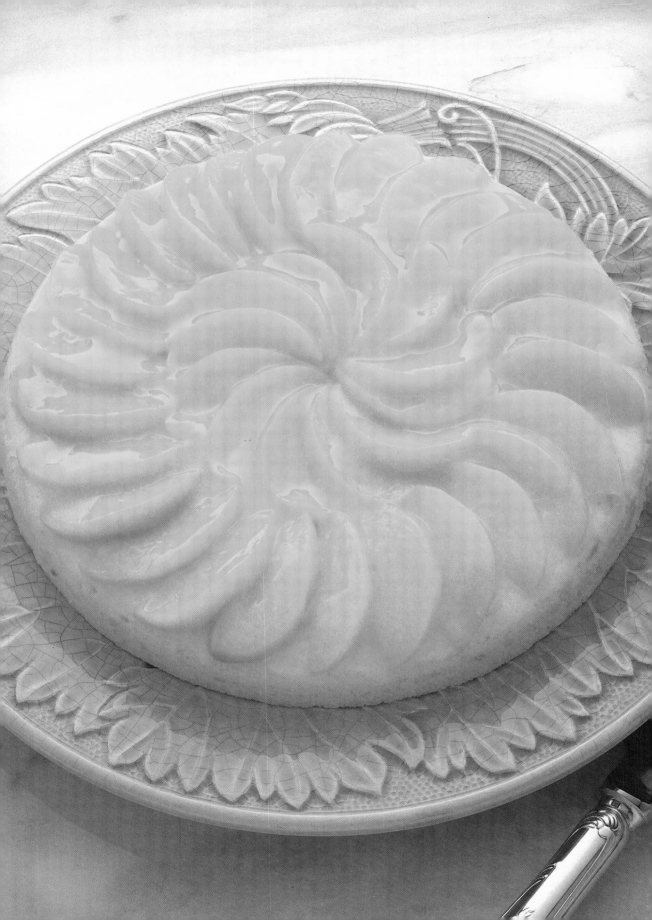

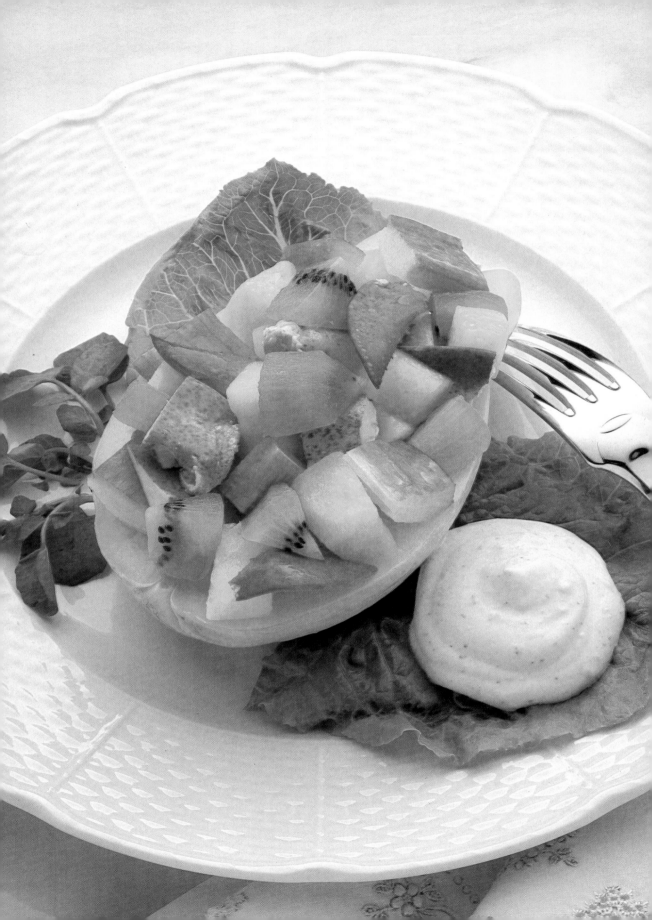

- Sauté onion in margarine in a large saucepan until translucent. Add water and bring to a boil.

- Add beans, garlic, ham, tomato, bay leaf, and cayenne pepper and cook over high heat for 15 minutes, then reduce heat and simmer until beans are tender, 2½ to 3 hours.

- Combine rice and water in a saucepan and bring to boil. Cover, reduce heat to low, and cook for 15 minutes. Remove from heat and let stand for 10 minutes without removing lid. Sprinkle with paprika. Stir oregano into beans and divide beans among soup plates. Add a scoop of rice to each plate. Sprinkle with green onion and serve.

PER SERVING: 287 CALORIES			
MENU EXCHANGE PATTERN			
Dairy .... —	Fruit .... —		
Bread 3	Meat 1		
Fat .... —	Veg. 1		
NUTRITIONAL INFORMATION			
Carbohydrate 52	g		
Protein 12	g		
Total fat 4	g		
Saturated fat 0.6	g		
Cholesterol 5	mg		
Sodium 135	mg		
Potassium 583	mg		
Fiber 2	g		
Calcium 62	mg		
Iron 3.7	mg		

Mustard Greens with Onion

1½ bunches mustard greens
3 cups water
1½ tablespoons margarine

1½ tablespoons flour
1 onion, finely chopped
Black pepper

- Boil greens in water until tender, 40 to 60 minutes. Drain, reserving 1 cup liquid. Chop greens. Melt margarine in a saucepan over low heat. Add flour and cook, stirring constantly, until light brown, about 5 to 10 minutes. Add onion and continue cooking until tender, about 5 minutes. Add greens, pepper, and reserved liquid and bring to a boil. Cover, reduce heat and simmer for 20 minutes. Serve hot.

PER SERVING: 72 CALORIES			
MENU EXCHANGE PATTERN			
Dairy .... —	Fruit .... —		
Bread .... —	Meat .... —		
Fat .... ½	Veg. 2		
NUTRITIONAL INFORMATION			
Carbohydrate 9	g		
Protein 4	g		
Total fat 3	g		
Saturated fat 0.5	g		
Cholesterol 0	mg		
Sodium 38	mg		
Potassium 452	mg		
Fiber 1.3	g		
Calcium 212	mg		
Iron 3.5	mg		

Pecan Cookies

¼ cup margarine
½ cup sugar
1 egg white, lightly beaten
1 tablespoon skim milk

½ teaspoon vanilla extract
1 cup all-purpose flour
1 teaspoon baking powder
24 pecan halves

- Cream margarine and sugar, then blend in egg white, milk, and vanilla in a large bowl. Sift flour and baking powder together and blend into creamed mixture. Chill dough thoroughly. Preheat oven to 375°F.

- Roll out small portions of dough on a lightly floured board to ¼-inch thickness. Using a 1½-inch round cookie cutter, cut out circles and top each with a pecan half. Arrange on a lightly greased cookie sheet and bake until light golden, about 10 minutes. Cool on racks. Makes 24; 1 serving = 1 cookie.

PER SERVING: 66 CALORIES			
MENU EXCHANGE PATTERN			
Dairy .... —	Fruit .... —		
Bread .... ½	Meat .... —		
Fat .... ½	Veg. .... —		
NUTRITIONAL INFORMATION			
Carbohydrate 8	g		
Protein 1	g		
Total fat 4	g		
Saturated fat 0.5	g		
Cholesterol 0	mg		
Sodium 3	mg		
Potassium 36	mg		
Fiber 0.2	g		
Calcium 5	mg		
Iron 0.2	mg		

Tropical Seafood Salad;
recipe page 78

FISH SOUPS AND STEWS

5

Spinach Salad with Herbed Honey Dressing

Shrimp and Okra Gumbo

French Bread

Lemon Cookies

Serves 4

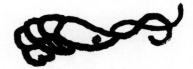

PER SERVING: 530 CALORIES		
MENU EXCHANGE PATTERN		
Dairy ..... —	Fruit ..... —	
Bread 3	Meat 1½	
Fat 3	Veg. 4½	
NUTRITIONAL INFORMATION		
Carbohydrate 67	g	
Protein 25	g	
Total fat 21	g	
Saturated fat 2.2	g	
Cholesterol 79	mg	
Sodium 404	mg	
Potassium 1190	mg	
Fiber 2.9	g	
Calcium 193	mg	
Iron 7.1	mg	

Spinach Salad

6 cups fresh spinach leaves
1 cup sliced mushrooms
¼ red onion, thinly sliced

4 tablespoons Herbed Honey
Dressing (recipe follows)

- Place spinach on individual salad plates and top with mushrooms and red onion. Drizzle each serving with 1 tablespoon dressing and serve.

PER SERVING: 34 CALORIES		
MENU EXCHANGE PATTERN		
Dairy . . . . . —	Fruit . . . . . —	
Bread . . . . —	Meat . . . . . —	
Fat . . . . . . —	Veg. 1½	
NUTRITIONAL INFORMATION		
Carbohydrate 6	g	
Protein 4	g	
Total fat 0	g	
Saturated fat 0	g	
Cholesterol 0	mg	
Sodium 63	mg	
Potassium 494	mg	
Fiber 0.8	g	
Calcium 83	mg	
Iron 2.8	mg	

Herbed Honey Dressing

1 tablespoon margarine
¼ cup chopped onion
¼ cup red wine vinegar
1 teaspoon dried thyme

1 teaspoon dried basil
1 tablespoon honey
¼ cup safflower oil

- Melt the margarine in a saucepan over medium heat, add onion, and cook until soft, about 10 minutes. Add the vinegar and herbs and simmer until reduced by half. Let cool to room temperature. Whisk in honey and oil. Makes about ¾ cup; 1 serving = 1 tablespoon.

PER SERVING: 61 CALORIES		
MENU EXCHANGE PATTERN		
Dairy . . . . . —	Fruit . . . . . —	
Bread . . . . —	Meat . . . . . —	
Fat 1	Veg. . . . . . . ½	
NUTRITIONAL INFORMATION		
Carbohydrate 3	g	
Protein 0	g	
Total fat 5	g	
Saturated fat 0.5	g	
Cholesterol 0	mg	
Sodium 0	mg	
Potassium 12	mg	
Fiber 0	g	
Calcium 2	mg	
Iron 0.1	mg	

Shrimp and Okra Gumbo

2 teaspoons safflower oil
1 tablespoon margarine
½ cup chopped onion
1 stalk celery, diced
1 small clove garlic, chopped
3 tablespoons all-purpose flour
4 cups fish stock or Homemade
*   Chicken Stock (page 36)*
½ pound shelled small shrimp

1 cup sliced okra
1 green bell pepper, cored,
*   seeded, and diced*
1 fresh tomato, peeled, seeded,
*   and diced*
1 teaspoon Worcestershire
*   sauce*
Black pepper

- Heat oil and margarine in a Dutch oven over medium heat. Add onion, celery, and garlic and sauté until soft, about 10 minutes. Add flour and stir for 2 minutes. Add stock and bring to a boil; boil for 5 minutes.

- Add the okra, shrimp, green pepper, tomato, Worcestershire sauce, and pepper to taste and simmer until shrimp are cooked, about 5 to 7 minutes.

PER SERVING: 191 CALORIES		
MENU EXCHANGE PATTERN		
Dairy . . . . . —	Fruit . . . . . —	
Bread . . . . —	Meat 1½	
Fat 1	Veg. 2½	
NUTRITIONAL INFORMATION		
Carbohydrate 13	g	
Protein 13	g	
Total fat 10	g	
Saturated fat 0.8	g	
Cholesterol 79	mg	
Sodium 116	mg	
Potassium 460	mg	
Fiber 1.1	g	
Calcium 82	mg	
Iron 1.9	mg	

French Bread

1½ envelopes active dry yeast
1 tablespoon sugar
2 cups warm water
1½ teaspoons salt

5 to 6 cups all-purpose flour
3 tablespoons yellow cornmeal
1 tablespoon egg white mixed
   with 1 tablespoon cold water

- Combine the yeast with sugar and warm water in a large bowl and let stand until bubbly, about 5 minutes. Mix the salt with the flour and blend into the yeast mixture, 1 cup at a time, until a stiff dough forms. Place on a lightly floured board and knead until dough is no longer sticky, about 10 minutes, adding flour as necessary. Transfer to an oiled bowl and turn to coat the surface with oil. Cover and let rise in a warm place until doubled in bulk, about 1½ to 2 hours.

- Punch the dough down, turn it out onto a floured board, and shape into 2 long, thin loaves. Transfer to a baking sheet that has been sprinkled with cornmeal. Slash the tops of the loaves diagonally in 2 places and brush with egg white mixture. Place in a cold oven, set the temperature to 400°F and bake until crusty and golden, about 35 minutes. Cool on racks before slicing. Makes 2 loaves, each making 8 slices; 1 serving = 1 slice.

PER SERVING: 165 CALORIES

MENU EXCHANGE PATTERN

Dairy	—	Fruit	—
Bread	2½	Meat	—
Fat	—	Veg.	—

NUTRITIONAL INFORMATION

Carbohydrate	35	g
Protein	7	g
Total fat	1	g
Saturated fat	0.2	g
Cholesterol	0	mg
Sodium	220	mg
Potassium	224	mg
Fiber	1	g
Calcium	21	mg
Iron	2.0	mg

Lemon Cookies

1 cup margarine
1 cup sugar
2 egg substitutes
1 teaspoon lemon extract

¼ cup skim milk
3 cups all-purpose flour, sifted
2 teaspoons cream of tartar
1 teaspoon baking soda

- Cream the margarine and sugar in a large bowl. Beat in egg substitutes, lemon extract, and milk. Gradually blend in the flour, cream of tartar, and baking soda. Form dough into ¾-inch balls and arrange on a greased baking sheet. Refrigerate for 2 hours. Preheat oven to 350°F. To shape the cookies, press down on each ball of dough with the bottom of a glass. Bake until edges are golden, about 10 to 12 minutes. Cool on racks. Makes 48 cookies; 1 serving = 1 cookie.

PER SERVING: 78 CALORIES

MENU EXCHANGE PATTERN

Dairy	—	Fruit	—
Bread	½	Meat	—
Fat	1	Veg.	—

NUTRITIONAL INFORMATION

Carbohydrate	10	g
Protein	1	g
Total fat	4	g
Saturated fat	0.7	g
Cholesterol	0	mg
Sodium	4	mg
Potassium	0	mg
Fiber	0	g
Calcium	4	mg
Iron	0.3	mg

SEAFOOD SALADS

1

Chilled Romaine Lettuce Soup

Grilled Fresh Tuna Salad

Zucchini Nut Bread

Grilled Pineapple Boats with Raspberries

Serves 4

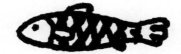

PER SERVING: 867 CALORIES		
MENU EXCHANGE PATTERN		
Dairy . . . . . —	Fruit 2½	
Bread 3	Meat 4	
Fat 4½	Veg. 5	
NUTRITIONAL INFORMATION		
Carbohydrate 97		g
Protein 47		g
Total fat 28		g
Saturated fat 3.5		g
Cholesterol 72		mg
Sodium 306		mg
Potassium 2371		mg
Fiber 6.3		g
Calcium 295		mg
Iron 8.1		mg

Chilled Romaine Lettuce Soup

½ head romaine, about 3 cups
⅔ cup Homemade Chicken
  Stock (page 36)
½ onion, finely chopped
2 tablespoons margarine

4 teaspoons all-purpose flour
1⅓ cups skim milk
¼ teaspoon white pepper
¼ teaspoon garlic powder
⅛ teaspoon cayenne

- Blanch lettuce leaves in chicken stock for about 3 to 5 minutes, or until bright green. Drain and reserve stock. Sauté onion in margarine until limp, then sprinkle in flour and mix well. With a whisk, slowly add hot stock and stir to mix in flour.

- Spin lettuce in a blender or food processor until very fine, then add ⅓ of roux mixture. Stir lettuce mixture back into soup, add milk and seasonings, and simmer for about 10 minutes. Remove from heat, let cool, then refrigerate overnight. Serve chilled.

PER SERVING: 102 CALORIES

MENU EXCHANGE PATTERN

Dairy	—	Fruit	—
Bread	—	Meat	—
Fat	1	Veg.	2

NUTRITIONAL INFORMATION

Carbohydrate	9	g
Protein	4	g
Total fat	6	g
Saturated fat	1.2	g
Cholesterol	1	mg
Sodium	48	mg
Potassium	281	mg
Fiber	0.4	g
Calcium	123	mg
Iron	1	mg

Grilled Fresh Tuna Salad

½ teaspoon black pepper
Grated zest of 1 lemon
1 pound fresh tuna steaks
4 cups red leaf lettuce
1 pound green beans, trimmed
  and blanched
2 tomatoes, cut in wedges
1½ pounds red potatoes,
  cooked and sliced

1 tablespoon capers
3 tablespoons chopped red
  onions
3 tablespoons chopped green
  onions
½ cup Red Pepper Vinaigrette
  (page 264)
4 radish roses

- Mix black pepper with lemon zest. Sprinkle pepper mixture on tuna, then grill over hot coals for about 15 minutes or broil for about 10 minutes until done. Refrigerate overnight or for several hours.

- Place lettuce on dinner plates. In center, break up tuna into chunks. Garnish with beans, tomato wedges, sliced potatoes, capers, and chopped red and green onion. Top each with 2 tablespoons Red Pepper Vinaigrette and garnish with a radish rose.

Note: Analysis does not include dressing. For analysis, see page 264.

PER SERVING: 343 CALORIES

MENU EXCHANGE PATTERN

Dairy	—	Fruit	—
Bread	1	Meat	4
Fat	—	Veg.	3

NUTRITIONAL INFORMATION

Carbohydrate	44	g
Protein	40	g
Total fat	2	g
Saturated fat	0.2	g
Cholesterol	71	mg
Sodium	70	mg
Potassium	1690	mg
Fiber	2.9	g
Calcium	132	mg
Iron	5.5	mg

Zucchini Nut Bread

4 egg substitutes
1 cup safflower oil
2/3 cup sugar
2 teaspoons vanilla extract
2 cups grated raw zucchini
2 cups drained crushed
   pineapple
1 1/2 cups all-purpose flour
1 1/2 cups whole wheat flour

2 tablespoons baking soda
1 1/2 teaspoons ground
   cinnamon
1 teaspoon ground allspice
1/2 teaspoon salt
3/4 teaspoon ground nutmeg
1/4 teaspoon baking powder
1 cup chopped dates
1 cup chopped walnuts

- Preheat oven to 350°F. Spray two 5 × 9-inch loaf pans with nonstick spray. Mix egg substitutes, oil, sugar, and vanilla until thick. Add zucchini and crushed pineapple. In a separate bowl, stir together dry ingredients and add to liquid ingredients. Stir in dates and walnuts. Mix only until all ingredients are moistened. Turn into loaf pans and bake for 1 hour, or until a toothpick comes out clean. Makes 2 loaves; 1 serving = one 1/2-inch slice.

PER SERVING: 147 CALORIES			
MENU EXCHANGE PATTERN			
Dairy ..... —	Fruit ..... —		
Bread 1	Meat ..... —		
Fat 1 1/2	Veg. ..... —		
NUTRITIONAL INFORMATION			
Carbohydrate 17		g	
Protein 2		g	
Total fat 8		g	
Saturated fat 0.7		g	
Cholesterol 0		mg	
Sodium 177		mg	
Potassium 116		mg	
Fiber 0.4		g	
Calcium 14		mg	
Iron 0.6		mg	

Grilled Pineapple Boats with Raspberries

2 ripe pineapples
4 tablespoons Chambord
   liqueur
1 pint raspberries
4 sprigs mint

- Cut each pineapple in half lengthwise. Scoop out the core and some of the flesh from the center. Dice flesh. Sprinkle liqueur over pineapple boats and diced pineapple. Let set for 10 minutes.

- Grill pineapple boats over hot coals, flesh side down, for about 2 minutes, then remove and fill with raspberries and diced pineapple. Garnish each with a sprig of mint.

PER SERVING: 177 CALORIES			
MENU EXCHANGE PATTERN			
Dairy ..... —	Fruit 2 1/2		
Bread 1	Meat ..... —		
Fat .... —	Veg. .... —		
NUTRITIONAL INFORMATION			
Carbohydrate 26		g	
Protein 1		g	
Total fat 1		g	
Saturated fat 0.1		g	
Cholesterol 0		mg	
Sodium 1		mg	
Potassium 269		mg	
Fiber 1		g	
Calcium 24		mg	
Iron 1		mg	

SEAFOOD SALADS

2

Vichyssoise

Shrimp Salad Remoulade

Apricot Bundt Cake

Serves 4

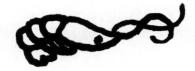

PER SERVING: 615 CALORIES		
MENU EXCHANGE PATTERN		
Dairy . . . . . . ½	Fruit . . . . . —	
Bread 3	Meat 2	
Fat 4½	Veg. 2½	
NUTRITIONAL INFORMATION		
Carbohydrate 66	g	
Protein 39	g	
Total fat 22	g	
Saturated fat 3	g	
Cholesterol 219	mg	
Sodium 872	mg	
Potassium 1242	mg	
Fiber 2.1	g	
Calcium 311	mg	
Iron 5.2	mg	

Vichyssoise

2 Idaho potatoes, washed,
    peeled, and quartered
1 leek, sliced
1 small onion, quartered
1 tablespoon chopped chives

3 cups Homemade Chicken
    Stock (page 36)
2/3 cup low-fat milk
White pepper
1/2 teaspoon salt

- Cook potatoes, leek, onion, and chives in stock for 20 minutes, then remove from heat and pour into blender or food processor. Puree mixture until smooth, then add milk and pepper to taste. Let cool, then chill in refrigerator. If desired, add additional chives as a garnish.

PER SERVING: 136 CALORIES		
MENU EXCHANGE PATTERN		
Dairy ..... —	Fruit .... —	
Bread 1	Meat ..... —	
Fat 1	Veg. 1	
NUTRITIONAL INFORMATION		
Carbohydrate 21	g	
Protein 4	g	
Total fat 4	g	
Saturated fat 0.5	g	
Cholesterol 3	mg	
Sodium 373	mg	
Potassium 509	mg	
Fiber 1	g	
Calcium 90	mg	
Iron 0.9	mg	

Shrimp Salad Remoulade

1 pound shrimp (about 5
    shrimp per person)
2 quarts water
1 tablespoon paprika
1/2 bay leaf

1 head Boston or red-leaf
    lettuce
Lemon wedges
Remoulade Sauce (recipe
    follows)

- Peel and devein shrimp. Bring water to a boil, add paprika and bay leaf, and then boil shrimp for about 5 minutes, or until tender. Immediately drain shrimp and place in ice water.

- Arrange lettuce leaves on salad plates. Top each with about 5 shrimp and garnish with lemon wedges. Serve with Remoulade sauce.

PER SERVING: 111 CALORIES		
MENU EXCHANGE PATTERN		
Dairy ..... —	Fruit .... —	
Bread .... —	Meat 2	
Fat .... —	Veg. 1	
NUTRITIONAL INFORMATION		
Carbohydrate 3	g	
Protein 21	g	
Total fat 1	g	
Saturated fat 0	g	
Cholesterol 158	mg	
Sodium 164	mg	
Potassium 394	mg	
Fiber 0.3	g	
Calcium 91	mg	
Iron 3.0	mg	

Remoulade Sauce

1 cup low-fat cottage cheese
1/2 cup plain low-fat yogurt
1 tablespoon lemon juice
1 tablespoon creole mustard or
   Dijon-style mustard

2 tablespoons capers, drained
1/4 cup chopped celery
1/4 cup chopped fresh parsley
1/4 cup chopped green onions
   (green portion only)

- Place cottage cheese, yogurt, lemon juice, mustard, and capers in a food processor or blender and mix well. Chop celery, parsley, and green onions together and combine with cottage cheese-yogurt mixture. Blend well and serve at once or chill in refrigerator for later use. Makes about 2 cups; 1 serving = 1/4 cup.

PER SERVING: 79 CALORIES

MENU EXCHANGE PATTERN

Dairy	1/2	Fruit	—
Bread	—	Meat	—
Fat	1/2	Veg.	1/2

NUTRITIONAL INFORMATION

Carbohydrate	6	g
Protein	10	g
Total fat	2	g
Saturated fat	1	g
Cholesterol	7	mg
Sodium	308	mg
Potassium	198	mg
Fiber	0.2	g
Calcium	108	mg
Iron	0.5	mg

Apricot Bundt Cake

3 egg substitutes
1 cup safflower oil
1 1/2 cups sugar
2 small jars (4 1/2 ounces each)
   strained apricot-tapioca baby
   food

2 cups whole wheat flour
   mixed with 2 teaspoons
   baking powder
1 teaspoon ground cinnamon
3/4 cups dried currants

- Preheat oven to 300°F. Generously grease and flour a 10-inch Bundt pan. Beat egg substitutes until foamy, then add oil and mix well. Slowly add sugar and mix well. Add baby food and mix; stir in flour, cinnamon, and currants. Pour into Bundt pan and bake for 1 hour, 15 minutes, or until a tester comes out clean. Let stand 15 minutes, then turn out onto a rack to cool completely. This cake will stay moist if tightly covered and actually tastes better the next day. Makes 16 servings; 1 serving = 1-inch slice.

PER SERVING: 289 CALORIES

MENU EXCHANGE PATTERN

Dairy	—	Fruit	—
Bread	2	Meat	—
Fat	3	Veg.	—

NUTRITIONAL INFORMATION

Carbohydrate	37	g
Protein	4	g
Total fat	15	g
Saturated fat	1	g
Cholesterol	0	mg
Sodium	27	mg
Potassium	141	mg
Fiber	0.5	g
Calcium	22	mg
Iron	0.3	mg

SEAFOOD SALADS

3

Cold Cucumber Soup

Tropical Seafood Salad

Cranberry-Nut Bread

Mandarin Orange Sherbet

Serves 4

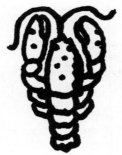

PER SERVING: 721 CALORIES		
MENU EXCHANGE PATTERN		
Dairy . . . . . ½	Fruit 5½	
Bread 2	Meat 3	
Fat 2	Veg. 2	
NUTRITIONAL INFORMATION		
Carbohydrate 102	g	
Protein 37	g	
Total fat 21	g	
Saturated fat 3.9	g	
Cholesterol 111	mg	
Sodium 625	mg	
Potassium 1680	mg	
Fiber 3.9	g	
Calcium 406	mg	
Iron 3.6	mg	

Cold Cucumber Soup

4 cucumbers, peeled, seeded,
   and diced
Juice of ½ lemon
1½ cups chilled Homemade
   Chicken Stock (page 36)
1½ cups plain low-fat yogurt

2 tablespoons sliced green
   onion
White pepper
1½ teaspoons chopped fresh dill
1 tablespoon chopped fresh
   chives

- Combine all ingredients except the chives in a blender and mix well, but not until completely smooth. Chill the soup thoroughly. Ladle into bowls, sprinkle with chives and serve.

PER SERVING: 76 CALORIES		
MENU EXCHANGE PATTERN		
Dairy . . . . . . ½	Fruit	—
Bread . . . . —	Meat	—
Fat . . . . —	Veg.	1
NUTRITIONAL INFORMATION		
Carbohydrate 11		g
Protein 6		g
Total fat 2		g
Saturated fat 0.9		g
Cholesterol 5		mg
Sodium 66		mg
Potassium 398		mg
Fiber 0.7		g
Calcium 187		mg
Iron . . . . 1.4 mg		

Tropical Seafood Salad

½ pound monkfish
2 quarts water
½ pound lobster meat
Cottage Cheese Dressing (recipe
   follows)
4 ripe papayas

2 kiwi fruit
4 sprigs watercress, stemmed
   and chopped
4 leaves romaine lettuce
Parsley sprigs (garnish)

- Poach monkfish by first dropping fish into 4 cups boiling water and then reducing heat to a simmer. Cook monkfish until firm and opaque, about 10 minutes. Drain, then cool in ice water. Simmer lobster meat in same 4 cups water until firm and opaque, 15 to 20 minutes. Drain fish and lobster and plunge into ice water to cool; drain well. Cut monkfish and lobster into bite-size pieces. Toss with dressing and refrigerate overnight.

- Shortly before serving, halve and hollow papayas, keeping shell intact. Discard seeds; cut flesh into chunks. Peel and cube kiwi. Gently toss papaya, kiwi, and watercress with lobster and monkfish. Fill the hollowed papaya shells and serve on lettuce leaf; garnish with parsley.

Photo opposite page 67.

PER SERVING: 244 CALORIES		
MENU EXCHANGE PATTERN		
Dairy . . . . . —	Fruit	2
Bread . . . . —	Meat	2½
Fat . . . . —	Veg.	1
NUTRITIONAL INFORMATION		
Carbohydrate 32		g
Protein 23		g
Total fat 3		g
Saturated fat 0.1		g
Cholesterol 97		mg
Sodium 224		mg
Potassium 995		mg
Fiber 2.8		g
Calcium 121		mg
Iron 1.3		mg

Cottage Cheese Dressing

½ cup low-fat cottage cheese
2 tablespoons white wine
2 tablespoons lemon juice
2 tablespoons safflower oil

1 teaspoon Dijon-style mustard
¼ teaspoon dried tarragon
White pepper

- Mix cottage cheese in blender until smooth. Add remaining ingredients and process until well combined. Makes about 1 cup; 1 serving = about ¼ cup.

PER SERVING: 95 CALORIES			
MENU EXCHANGE PATTERN			
Dairy ..... —	Fruit ...... ½		
Bread .... —	Meat ...... ½		
Fat 1	Veg. ...... —		
NUTRITIONAL INFORMATION			
Carbohydrate 2	g
Protein 4	g
Total fat 7	g
Saturated fat 0.9	g
Cholesterol 2	mg
Sodium 131	mg
Potassium 45	mg
Fiber 0	g
Calcium 22	mg
Iron 0.1	mg

Cranberry-Nut Bread

1 cup all-purpose flour
1 cup whole wheat flour
1 cup sugar
1½ teaspoons baking powder
1 teaspoon salt
½ teaspoon baking soda
¼ cup margarine

1 tablespoon grated orange rind
¾ cup orange juice
1 egg substitute
1 cup coarsely chopped cranberries
1 cup coarsely chopped nuts

- Preheat oven to 350°F. Sift together dry ingredients in a large bowl. Cut in margarine with a pastry blender until mixture resembles coarse meal. Blend rind, juice, and egg substitute in a separate bowl, add to flour mixture, and stir just to moisten. Fold in berries and nuts. Turn into greased 9 × 5-inch loaf pan and bake until tester inserted near center comes out clean, about 1 hour. Cool on rack in pan. One loaf makes 18 servings; 1 serving = one ½-inch slice.

PER SERVING: 156 CALORIES			
MENU EXCHANGE PATTERN			
Dairy ..... —	Fruit 1		
Bread 1	Meat ..... —		
Fat 1	Veg. ...... —		
NUTRITIONAL INFORMATION			
Carbohydrate 23	g
Protein 3	g
Total fat 6	g
Saturated fat 0.8	g
Cholesterol 0	mg
Sodium 160	mg
Potassium 89	mg
Fiber 0.3	g
Calcium 13	mg
Iron 0.6	mg

Mandarin Orange Sherbet

2 cups orange sherbet
⅔ cup mandarin orange sections
Mint sprigs (garnish)

- Scoop ½ cup sherbet into each of 4 dessert glasses. Garnish with several mandarin orange sections and a sprig of fresh mint.

PER SERVING: 149 CALORIES			
MENU EXCHANGE PATTERN			
Dairy ..... —	Fruit 2		
Bread 1	Meat ..... —		
Fat .... —	Veg. ...... —		
NUTRITIONAL INFORMATION			
Carbohydrate 33	g
Protein 2	g
Total fat 2	g
Saturated fat 1.2	g
Cholesterol 7	mg
Sodium 44	mg
Potassium 153	mg
Fiber 0.1	g
Calcium 63	mg
Iron 0.2	mg

SEAFOOD SALADS

4

Herbed Seafood Salad

Linguine with Pesto

Peaches Galliano

Serves 6

PER SERVING: 515 CALORIES			
MENU EXCHANGE PATTERN			
Dairy	—	Fruit	1
Bread	2	Meat	2½
Fat	3	Veg.	2
NUTRITIONAL INFORMATION			
Carbohydrate	45	g	
Protein	27	g	
Total fat	25	g	
Saturated fat	3	g	
Cholesterol	93	mg	
Sodium	487	mg	
Potassium	730	mg	
Fiber	1.2	g	
Calcium	231	mg	
Iron	5.5	mg	

Herbed Seafood Salad

½ pound small or medium
   shrimp
4 tablespoons vinegar
1 bay leaf
½ pound scallops
12 mussels, cleaned (see page
   259)
12 littleneck clams (the smallest
   you can find), scrubbed
6 Greek black olives, pitted and
   quartered

6 green olives, pitted and
   quartered
⅓ cup roasted sweet red pepper
   cut in ½-inch-wide strips
¼ cup lemon juice
¼ cup safflower oil
Black pepper
1 large clove garlic, lightly
   crushed
¼ teaspoon dried marjoram, or
   ½ teaspoon fresh

- Rinse the shrimp in cold water but do not shell. Bring 2 quarts water to a boil with 2 tablespoons vinegar and the bay leaf. Drop in shrimp and cook for 2 minutes after the water returns to a boil. (Very small shrimp may take 1½ minutes or less.) Drain. When cool, shell and devein shrimp and cut into rounds ½ inch thick (if very tiny, leave whole). Set aside.

- Rinse the scallops in cold water. Bring 2 cups water to a boil with 1 tablespoon vinegar. Add the scallops and cook for 2 minutes after the water returns to a boil. Drain. When cool, cut into ½-inch cubes if scallops are large (leave small scallops whole). Set aside.

- In separate covered pans, heat the mussels and clams in 1 quart of water over high heat until their shells open. Detach the mussels from their shells and set aside. Detach the clams from their shells and rinse to remove any possible sand.

- Combine all the seafood in a mixing bowl. Add the olives, red pepper, lemon juice, and oil and mix thoroughly. Add pepper, garlic, and marjoram and toss well. Let salad marinate 2 hours, then remove the garlic before serving. (Salad is best served at room temperature, but it should not remain at room temperature longer than 2 hours. If necessary, cover tightly with plastic wrap and refrigerate until 1 hour before serving.)

PER SERVING: 186 CALORIES		
MENU EXCHANGE PATTERN		
Dairy ..... —	Fruit ..... —	
Bread .... —	Meat 2	
Fat 1	Veg. 1	
NUTRITIONAL INFORMATION		
Carbohydrate 4	g	
Protein 17	g	
Total fat 11	g	
Saturated fat 0.9	g	
Cholesterol 86	mg	
Sodium 325	mg	
Potassium 323	mg	
Fiber 0.2	g	
Calcium 58	mg	
Iron 3	mg	

Linguine with Pesto

2 cups fresh basil leaves (see
   note)
1/4 cup olive or safflower oil
2 tablespoons pine nuts
4 cloves garlic, lightly crushed
1/2 cup grated Parmesan cheese

2 tablespoons grated Romano
   cheese
1/2 pound linguine, freshly
   cooked and drained (reserve
   1 tablespoon cooking water)

- Combine the basil, oil, pine nuts, and garlic in a blender and mix at high speed, stopping from time to time to scrape down the sides of the container.

- When the ingredients are evenly blended, transfer the pesto to a bowl and stir in the grated cheeses by hand (this results in better texture and flavor than when the cheese is added to the blender).

- Blend the reserved tablespoon of pasta cooking water into the pesto and toss pesto with the linguine to coat evenly.

Note: The quantity of basil in most recipes is given in terms of whole leaves. American basil, however, varies greatly in sizes. There are small, medium, and very large leaves, and they all pack differently in the measuring cup. For the sake of accurate measurement, tear all but the tiniest leaves into 2 or more small pieces. Be gentle, so as not to crush the basil; this would discolor it and waste the first fresh droplets of juice.

PER SERVING: 286 CALORIES

MENU EXCHANGE PATTERN

Dairy	—	Fruit	—
Bread	2	Meat	1/2
Fat	2	Veg.	1

NUTRITIONAL INFORMATION

Carbohydrate	31	g
Protein	10	g
Total fat	14	g
Saturated fat	2.1	g
Cholesterol	8	mg
Sodium	162	mg
Potassium	236	mg
Fiber	0.4	g
Calcium	168	mg
Iron	2.4	mg

Peaches Galliano

6 peaches, peeled, pitted, and
   sliced
1 tablespoon Galliano liqueur
Mint sprigs (garnish)

- Stir together peaches and Galliano. Serve in dessert glasses and garnish with a sprig of mint.

PER SERVING: 43 CALORIES

MENU EXCHANGE PATTERN

Dairy	—	Fruit	1
Bread	—	Meat	—
Fat	—	Veg.	—

NUTRITIONAL INFORMATION

Carbohydrate	10	g
Protein	1	g
Total fat	0	g
Saturated fat	0	g
Cholesterol	0	mg
Sodium	0	mg
Potassium	171	mg
Fiber	0.6	g
Calcium	5	mg
Iron	0.1	mg

Papaya Slices with Raspberries; recipe page 88

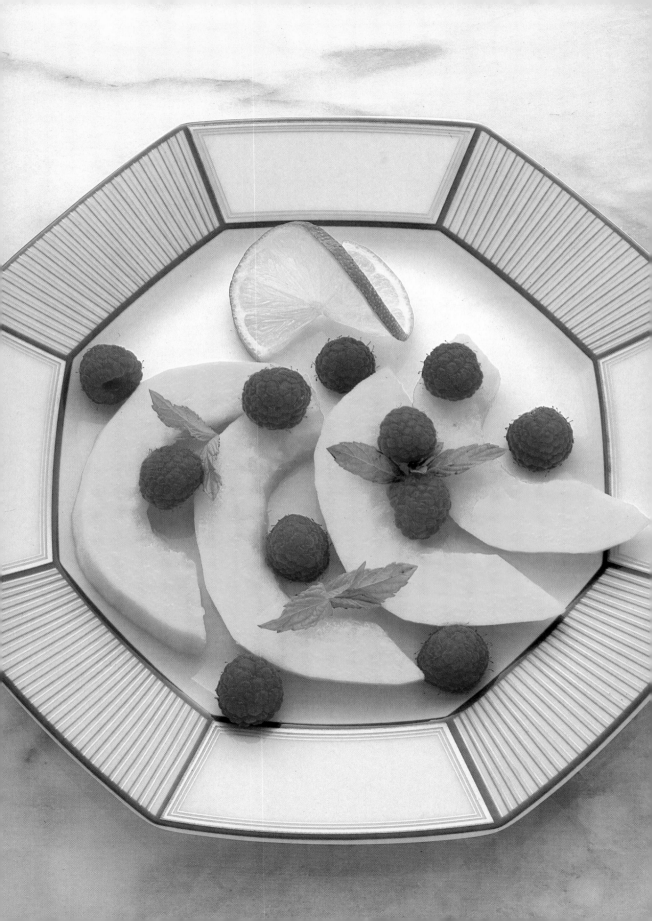

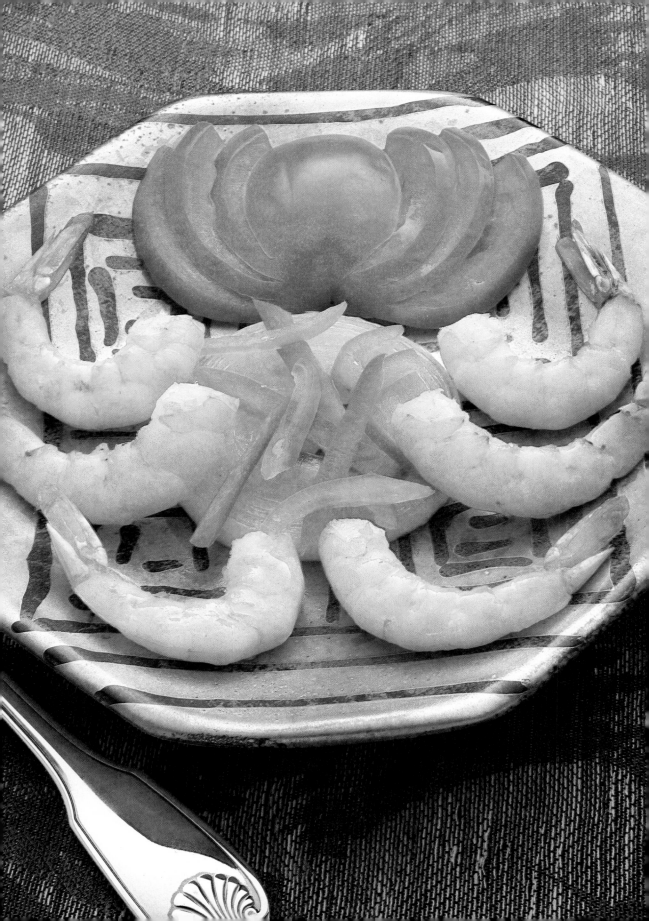

SEAFOOD SALADS

5

Chilled Vegetable Puree

Seafood Salad Basquaise

Strawberry Sorbet

Serves 4

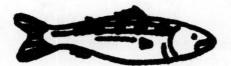

PER SERVING: 623 CALORIES		
MENU EXCHANGE PATTERN		
Dairy ..... —	Fruit 4½	
Bread ..... ½	Meat 3	
Fat 3	Veg. 4	
NUTRITIONAL INFORMATION		
Carbohydrate 89	g	
Protein 30	g	
Total fat 18	g	
Saturated fat 1.6	g	
Cholesterol 13	mg	
Sodium 377	mg	
Potassium 1298	mg	
Fiber 3.1	g	
Calcium 258	mg	
Iron 5.7	mg	

Shrimp a la Parrilla;
recipe page 90

Chilled Vegetable Puree

2 cucumbers, peeled and diced
1 large tomato, peeled and
    diced
1/2 large onion, diced
1 green pepper, diced
1 clove garlic, minced
1/4 cup fine breadcrumbs

1 1/2 cups water
3 tablespoons red wine vinegar
3 tablespoons low-sodium
    tomato juice
1/4 teaspoon black pepper
1 tablespoon safflower oil

- Combine cucumbers, tomato, onion, pepper, and garlic in a food processor or blender. Add breadcrumbs, water, vinegar, tomato juice, and pepper and puree mixture until blended but retains a coarse texture. Gradually add the oil, continuing to blend. Refrigerate at least 2 hours, and stir again before serving.

PER SERVING: 90 CALORIES		
MENU EXCHANGE PATTERN		
Dairy .... —	Fruit .... —	
Bread .... —	Meat .... —	
Fat 1	Veg. 2	
NUTRITIONAL INFORMATION		
Carbohydrate 13		g
Protein 3		g
Total fat 4		g
Saturated fat 0.4		g
Cholesterol 0		mg
Sodium 78		mg
Potassium 322		mg
Fiber 1		g
Calcium 36		mg
Iron 1.5		mg

Seafood Salad Basquaise

8 leaves escarole, washed and
    dried
8 leaves romaine lettuce,
    washed and dried
8 ounces white tuna, packed in
    water, drained
8 ounces poached boneless
    salmon
1/2 cup canned baby flageolet
    beans

2/3 cup rice, cooked with a
    pinch of saffron
1/4 Bermuda onion, cut into
    rings
1 tomato, quartered
1 cucumber, sliced
6 spinach leaves, chopped
4 tablespoons Olive Oil and
    Oregano Dressing (recipe
    follows)

- Arrange escarole and romaine leaves on individual salad plates or tear into bite-size pieces and place in a large bowl. In the center, arrange tuna and salmon. Around the fish, place baby beans and rice. Add onion rings, a tomato quarter, and cucumber slices. Garnish with chopped spinach leaves. Drizzle each plate with 1 tablespoon dressing and serve.

PER SERVING: 240 CALORIES		
MENU EXCHANGE PATTERN		
Dairy ..... —	Fruit ..... —	
Bread 1/2	Meat 3	
Fat .... —	Veg. 2	
NUTRITIONAL INFORMATION		
Carbohydrate 22		g
Protein 28		g
Total fat 5		g
Saturated fat 0		g
Cholesterol 13		mg
Sodium 297		mg
Potassium 862		mg
Fiber 1.8		g
Calcium 212		mg
Iron 3.9		mg

Olive Oil and Oregano Dressing

½ cup wine vinegar
1 tablespoon dried oregano
* leaves*
1 teaspoon finely diced shallots
1 teaspoon dried thyme

2 tablespoons chopped fresh
* parsley*
1 teaspoon sugar
1 cup olive oil

- Combine vinegar, oregano, shallots, thyme, and parsley in a saucepan. Bring to a boil, then remove from heat and stir in sugar. Whip in olive oil, then cool before serving. Makes 1½ cups; 1 serving = 1 tablespoon.

PER SERVING: 81 CALORIES		
MENU EXCHANGE PATTERN		
Dairy . . . . . —	Fruit . . . . . —	
Bread . . . . —	Meat . . . . . —	
Fat 2	Veg. . . . . . . —	
NUTRITIONAL INFORMATION		
Carbohydrate 0	g	
Protein 0	g	
Total fat 9	g	
Saturated fat 1.2	g	
Cholesterol 0	mg	
Sodium 0	mg	
Potassium 7	mg	
Fiber 0	g	
Calcium 1	mg	
Iron 0	mg	

Strawberry Sorbet

1⅓ cups strawberries, washed
* and hulled*
1 cup sugar
2 teaspoons lemon juice

3 teaspoons unflavored gelatin
4 teaspoons cold water
4 fresh strawberries

- Puree hulled strawberries in a blender or food processor to make about 1 cup puree. In a saucepan, combine puree with sugar and lemon juice, and bring to a slow boil. Dissolve gelatin in cold water, then stir into the boiling fruit mixture. Simmer for 5 minutes, then remove from heat. Let cool.

- Transfer mixture to an ice cream freezer and process according to directions. Serve in dessert glasses and garnish each serving with a fresh strawberry.

PER SERVING: 212 CALORIES		
MENU EXCHANGE PATTERN		
Dairy . . . . . —	Fruit 4½	
Bread . . . . . ½	Meat . . . . . —	
Fat . . . . —	Veg. . . . . . . —	
NUTRITIONAL INFORMATION		
Carbohydrate 54	g	
Protein 0	g	
Total fat 0	g	
Saturated fat 0	g	
Cholesterol 0	mg	
Sodium 1	mg	
Potassium 107	mg	
Fiber 0.3	g	
Calcium 9	mg	
Iron 0.3	mg	

LIGHT SEAFOOD DISHES

1

Mushroom Salad with Walnut Oil Vinaigrette

Chilled Pasta Salad with Pesto and Grilled Shrimp

Papaya Slices with Raspberries

Serves 4

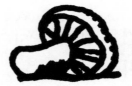

PER SERVING: 601 CALORIES		
MENU EXCHANGE PATTERN		
Dairy ..... —	Fruit 3½	
Bread 2	Meat 2	
Fat 4	Veg. 1	
NUTRITIONAL INFORMATION		
Carbohydrate 72	g	
Protein 23	g	
Total fat 30	g	
Saturated fat 2.9	g	
Cholesterol 81	mg	
Sodium 399	mg	
Potassium 1155	mg	
Fiber 4.1	g	
Calcium 137	mg	
Iron 4.7	mg	

Mushroom Salad with Walnut Oil Vinaigrette

16 large mushrooms, sliced
   into matchstick julienne
1/2 teaspoon salt
2 teaspoons chopped fresh basil
1/2 teaspoon fresh thyme

12 walnut halves
2 tablespoons red wine vinegar
4 teaspoons walnut oil
Black pepper

- Preheat oven to 400°F. Place mushrooms in a bowl and sprinkle with salt. Add basil and thyme, toss well, and set aside. Place walnuts on a cookie sheet and toast in oven for 20 minutes. Add to mushrooms and toss.

- Whisk vinegar with walnut oil in a separate bowl. Add to mushrooms and toss. Divide among individual salad plates and sprinkle with pepper.

Note: To reduce fat and sodium, eliminate salt, walnuts, vinegar, and walnut oil; substitute 3 tablespoons of a commercial low-calorie Italian dressing. Adjusted analysis: calories = 33; exchange = 1 Vegetable.

PER SERVING: 127 CALORIES		
MENU EXCHANGE PATTERN		
Dairy . . . . . —	Fruit . . . . . —	
Bread . . . . . —	Meat . . . . . —	
Fat 2	Veg. 1	
NUTRITIONAL INFORMATION		
Carbohydrate 5		g
Protein 4		g
Total fat 11		g
Saturated fat 1		g
Cholesterol 0		mg
Sodium 278		mg
Potassium 365		mg
Fiber 0.8		g
Calcium 7		mg
Iron 1.3		mg

Chilled Pasta Salad with Pesto and Grilled Shrimp

1/3 pound linguine
8 large fresh shrimp (16/20 per
   pound size), shelled and
   deveined
1 green bell pepper, cored,
   seeded, and chopped

1 red bell pepper, cored, seeded,
   and chopped
Juice of 1/2 lemon
Olive oil

Pesto

11/2 bunches fresh basil
1/2 clove garlic, halved
Juice of 1/2 lemon
31/2 tablespoons olive oil
21/2 tablespoons toasted pine
   nuts

4 teaspoons grated Parmesan
   cheese
White pepper

- First prepare pesto. Puree basil, garlic, and lemon juice in food processor. With machine running, gradually add olive oil, then pine nuts. Stir in Parmesan and season to taste with white pepper.

- Cook linguine until *al dente*. Drain in a colander and rinse with cold water. Chill pasta in large bowl. Add pesto, peppers, and lemon juice and toss. Transfer to serving plates.

- Rub shrimp lightly with olive oil. Thread on a skewer and grill or broil until pink, about 3 to 5 minutes. Top pasta with 3 shrimp per serving.

PER SERVING: 345 CALORIES			
MENU EXCHANGE PATTERN			
Dairy	—	Fruit	—
Bread	2	Meat	2
Fat	2	Veg.	—

NUTRITIONAL INFORMATION		
Carbohydrate	33	g
Protein	17	g
Total fat	16	g
Saturated fat	1.9	g
Cholesterol	81	mg
Sodium	116	mg
Potassium	307	mg
Fiber	0.7	g
Calcium	77	mg
Iron	2.7	mg

Papaya Slices with Raspberries

2 papayas
1 cup raspberries
1 lime, cut into wedges

- Peel papayas and make 1 lengthwise slice in each. Remove seeds and discard. Slice fruit lengthwise, and arrange slices in a fan shape on dessert plates. Scatter with raspberries. Set a lime wedge at the base of each fan.

Photo opposite page 82.

PER SERVING: 129 CALORIES			
MENU EXCHANGE PATTERN			
Dairy	—	Fruit	3½
Bread	—	Meat	—
Fat	—	Veg.	—

NUTRITIONAL INFORMATION		
Carbohydrate	34	g
Protein	2	g
Total fat	3	g
Saturated fat	0	g
Cholesterol	0	mg
Sodium	5	mg
Potassium	483	mg
Fiber	2.6	g
Calcium	53	mg
Iron	0.7	mg

LIGHT SEAFOOD DISHES

2

Shrimp a la Parrilla

Pico de Gallo

Mexican Rice

Baked Bananas

Serves 8

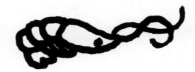

PER SERVING: 590 CALORIES		
MENU EXCHANGE PATTERN		
Dairy . . . . . —	Fruit 1½	
Bread 2½	Meat 3	
Fat 2	Veg. 3½	
NUTRITIONAL INFORMATION		
Carbohydrate 72	g	
Protein 28	g	
Total fat 21	g	
Saturated fat 3.9	g	
Cholesterol 158	mg	
Sodium 585	mg	
Potassium 1274	mg	
Fiber 2.1	g	
Calcium 137	mg	
Iron 4.6	mg	

Shrimp a la Parrilla

⅔ cup margarine
2 cloves garlic, minced
White pepper
⅓ cup low-sodium soy sauce
48 medium shrimp

1 onion, sliced
4 lemons
2 large tomatoes, sliced
2½ green bell peppers, seeded
   and sliced

- Melt margarine in a saucepan; add garlic and white pepper to taste. Toss shrimp with soy sauce in a bowl. Grill shrimp over charcoal for about 2 minutes on each side, basting frequently with margarine mixture.

- Grill onion slices over coals. Squeeze juice of 2 lemons over shrimp; slice remaining 2 lemons into 8 pinwheels for garnish. Serve with tomato slices and bell pepper.

Photo opposite page 83.

PER SERVING: 277 CALORIES
MENU EXCHANGE PATTERN

Dairy	—	Fruit	—
Bread	—	Meat	3
Fat	1	Veg.	2

NUTRITIONAL INFORMATION

Carbohydrate	10	g
Protein	23	g
Total fat	16	g
Saturated fat	3	g
Cholesterol	158	mg
Sodium	577	mg
Potassium	544	mg
Fiber	0.7	g
Calcium	99	mg
Iron	2.8	mg

Pico de Gallo

½ medium tomato, peeled and
   chopped
⅔ onion, chopped
⅔ green bell pepper, seeded
   and chopped
½ cup cold water

8 sprigs fresh coriander
   (cilantro), leaves only
1 to 8 Serrano chilies, chopped,
   or more to taste
3 tablespoons lemon juice

- Combine all ingredients and let stand for 30 minutes before serving.

PER SERVING: 16 CALORIES
MENU EXCHANGE PATTERN

Dairy	—	Fruit	—
Bread	—	Meat	—
Fat	—	Veg.	½

NUTRITIONAL INFORMATION

Carbohydrate	3	g
Protein	1	g
Total fat	0	g
Saturated fat	0	g
Cholesterol	0	mg
Sodium	3	mg
Potassium	116	mg
Fiber	0.3	g
Calcium	9	mg
Iron	0.3	mg

Mexican Rice

3 tablespoons margarine
3 tablespoons finely chopped
   onion
1 zucchini, diced (2 cups)
1 cup peeled, diced fresh
   tomato
1⅓ cups rice
1⅓ cups water
Black pepper

1⅓ cups Homemade Chicken
   Stock (see page 36 or Caldo
   de Pollo recipe, page 167)
3 sprigs fresh thyme or 1
   teaspoon dried
3 parsley sprigs
1 bay leaf
3 tablespoons chopped pimiento

- Preheat oven to 400°F. Melt margarine in a flameproof casserole over medium heat. Add the onion and sauté until wilted, about 10 minutes. Add zucchini and tomato and cook until most of the liquid evaporates. Add rice, water, pepper, and stock and bring to a boil. Add thyme, parsley, and bay leaf. Place casserole in the oven and bake until all liquid is absorbed and the rice is tender, about 18 minutes. Add the pimiento and toss to mix. Serve immediately.

PER SERVING: 164 CALORIES

MENU EXCHANGE PATTERN

Dairy	—	Fruit	—
Bread	1½	Meat	—
Fat	1	Veg.	1

NUTRITIONAL INFORMATION

Carbohydrate	28	g
Protein	3	g
Total fat	4	g
Saturated fat	0.8	g
Cholesterol	0	mg
Sodium	4	mg
Potassium	158	mg
Fiber	0.5	g
Calcium	23	mg
Iron	1.2	mg

Baked Bananas

8 bananas, peeled
2 tablespoons lemon juice
2 tablespoons sugar
¼ cup rum

- Preheat oven to 400°F. Sprinkle lemon juice and sugar over whole bananas. Transfer to a lightly oiled baking pan and bake until lightly browned, about 20 minutes. Pour rum over bananas and ignite, shaking pan gently until flames subside. Serve immediately.

PER SERVING: 135 CALORIES

MENU EXCHANGE PATTERN

Dairy	—	Fruit	1½
Bread	1	Meat	—
Fat	—	Veg.	—

NUTRITIONAL INFORMATION

Carbohydrate	30	g
Protein	1	g
Total fat	0	g
Saturated fat	0	g
Cholesterol	0	mg
Sodium	1	mg
Potassium	456	mg
Fiber	0.6	g
Calcium	7	mg
Iron	0.3	mg

LIGHT SEAFOOD DISHES

3

Shrimp Creole with Rice

Okra with Caraway

Celery Bread

Minted Fresh Fruit

Serves 4

PER SERVING: 613 CALORIES		
MENU EXCHANGE PATTERN		
Dairy 3	Fruit 2	
Bread 2½	Meat . . . . . —	
Fat 1½	Veg. 5	
NUTRITIONAL INFORMATION		
Carbohydrate 89	g	
Protein 32	g	
Total fat 16	g	
Saturated fat 2	g	
Cholesterol 158	mg	
Sodium 660	mg	
Potassium 1638	mg	
Fiber 3.3	g	
Calcium 237	mg	
Iron 6.2	mg	

Shrimp Creole with Rice

1 bay leaf
1 lemon, sliced crosswise
1 1/2 pounds shrimp, shelled and
    deveined
2 onions, chopped
3 cloves garlic, mashed
3 tablespoons safflower oil
2 cups chopped fresh tomato
1 1/2 cups low-sodium tomato
    sauce

1 green bell pepper, cored,
    seeded, and finely chopped
1 teaspoon sugar
1/8 teaspoon dried basil
1/3 teaspoon cayenne pepper
1 1/2 teaspoons cornstarch
2 tablespoons water
1 cup rice
1/2 cup chopped fresh parsley
1/2 cup chopped green onion

- Combine 1 quart water, bay leaf, lemon slices, and shrimp in a large saucepan, and bring to boil over medium heat. When water boils, cover and cook for 5 minutes. Drain shrimp, reserving 2 cups liquid.

- In a large nonstick skillet, sauté onion and garlic in oil over medium heat until tender, about 5 minutes. Add tomato, tomato sauce, reserved shrimp broth, green pepper, and sugar; reduce heat and simmer 15 minutes. Add basil and cayenne and cook 5 more minutes.

- Meanwhile, bring 2 cups water to a boil in another saucepan. Add rice, cover, and reduce heat to a simmer. Cook until water is absorbed, about 20 minutes.

- Combine cornstarch and 2 tablespoons water. Stir into sauce and cook until thickened. Add shrimp, parsley, and green onion and serve over rice.

PER SERVING: 350 CALORIES

MENU EXCHANGE PATTERN

Dairy	—	Fruit		—
Bread	1½	Meat		3
Fat	—	Veg.		3

NUTRITIONAL INFORMATION

Carbohydrate	43	g
Protein	26	g
Total fat	8	g
Saturated fat	0.6	g
Cholesterol	158	mg
Sodium	498	mg
Potassium	944	mg
Fiber	1.1	g
Calcium	124	mg
Iron	4.3	mg

Okra with Caraway

2 cups okra (¹/₂ pound), cut
   into 1-inch pieces
1 onion, finely chopped
1 tablespoon margarine
1 cup chopped fresh tomato
2 tablespoons low-sodium
   tomato paste

1 cup water
2 tablespoons finely chopped
   celery leaves
¹/₄ green bell pepper, cored,
   seeded, and finely chopped
1 clove garlic, mashed
¹/₂ teaspoon caraway seed

- Cook okra in a large quantity of boiling water until tender, about 15 minutes. Drain. In a saucepan, sauté onion in margarine over medium heat until tender, about 5 minutes. Add all remaining ingredients except okra and caraway and simmer over low heat for 20 minutes. Add okra and caraway, simmer 5 more minutes, and serve.

PER SERVING: 79 CALORIES		
MENU EXCHANGE PATTERN		
Dairy . . . . . —	Fruit . . . . . —	
Bread . . . . —	Meat . . . . . —	
Fat . . . . ½	Veg. 2	
NUTRITIONAL INFORMATION		
Carbohydrate 12	g	
Protein 3	g	
Total fat 3	g	
Saturated fat 0.5	g	
Cholesterol 0	mg	
Sodium 16	mg	
Potassium 400	mg	
Fiber 1.2	g	
Calcium 68	mg	
Iron 1.1	mg	

Celery Bread

¹/₄ cup margarine, at room
   temperature
¹/₂ teaspoon celery seed

¹/₄ teaspoon paprika
¹/₄ teaspoon cayenne pepper
1 loaf French bread

- Preheat oven to 325°F. Whip margarine with celery seed, paprika, and cayenne. Cut bread into 12 slices. Spread margarine mixture between slices. Wrap bread in foil and heat in oven for 20 minutes. Makes 12 slices; 1 serving = 1 slice.

PER SERVING: 107 CALORIES		
MENU EXCHANGE PATTERN		
Dairy . . . . . —	Fruit . . . . . —	
Bread 1	Meat . . . . . —	
Fat 1	Veg. . . . . . . —	
NUTRITIONAL INFORMATION		
Carbohydrate 14	g	
Protein 2	g	
Total fat 5	g	
Saturated fat 0.9	g	
Cholesterol 0	mg	
Sodium 145	mg	
Potassium 28	mg	
Fiber 0.1	g	
Calcium 12	mg	
Iron 0.6	mg	

Minted Fresh Fruit

2 oranges, sectioned
¹/₂ cup grapes, halved
2 peaches, peeled, pitted, and
   sliced

1 apple, cored and diced
Mint sprigs (garnish)

- Mix all ingredients and chill before serving. Garnish with mint.

PER SERVING: 77 CALORIES		
MENU EXCHANGE PATTERN		
Dairy . . . . . —	Fruit 2	
Bread . . . . —	Meat . . . . . —	
Fat . . . . —	Veg. . . . . . . —	
NUTRITIONAL INFORMATION		
Carbohydrate 20	g	
Protein 1	g	
Total fat 0	g	
Saturated fat 0	g	
Cholesterol 0	mg	
Sodium 1	mg	
Potassium 266	mg	
Fiber 0.9	g	
Calcium 3.3	mg	
Iron 0.2	mg	

LIGHT SEAFOOD DISHES

4

Fettuccine with Fennel

Stuffed Peppers with Corn and Crabmeat

Chocolate-Walnut Meringues

Serves 4

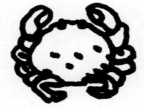

PER SERVING: 521 CALORIES		
MENU EXCHANGE PATTERN		
Dairy . . . . . —	Fruit . . . . . —	
Bread 3½	Meat 2	
Fat 2	Veg. 2	
NUTRITIONAL INFORMATION		
Carbohydrate 56	g	
Protein 28	g	
Total fat 20	g	
Saturated fat 2.8	g	
Cholesterol 75	mg	
Sodium 535	mg	
Potassium 660	mg	
Fiber 1.9	g	
Calcium 90	mg	
Iron 4.2	mg	

Fettuccine with Fennel

⅓ pound fettuccine
1 tablespoon margarine
Black pepper
1 garlic clove, minced

2 tablespoons Pernod
1 tablespoon safflower oil
1 tablespoon chopped fennel
  seed

- Cook fettuccine until *al dente*; drain. Meanwhile, melt margarine in skillet. Add pepper to taste and minced garlic and sauté until garlic is tender. Add Pernod and ignite, shaking pan gently until flames subside. Add fettuccine, oil, and fennel seed and toss. Serve on heated plates.

PER SERVING: 207 CALORIES			
MENU EXCHANGE PATTERN			
Dairy	—	Fruit	—
Bread	2	Meat	—
Fat	1½	Veg.	—
NUTRITIONAL INFORMATION			
Carbohydrate 28			g
Protein 5			g
Total fat 6			g
Saturated fat 1.1			g
Cholesterol 0			mg
Sodium 1			mg
Potassium 78			mg
Fiber 0			g
Calcium 12			mg
Iron 1.1			mg

Stuffed Peppers with Corn and Crabmeat

2 tablespoons margarine
8 ounces fresh or frozen corn
3 tablespoons finely chopped
  green bell pepper
3 tablespoons finely chopped
  red bell pepper
3 tablespoons finely chopped
  onion
3 tablespoons finely chopped
  green onion
1 clove garlic, minced

1 very small jalapeño chili,
  finely chopped
1 tablespoon all-purpose flour
1 teaspoon black pepper
⅔ pound crabmeat
Juice of 1 lemon
3 egg substitutes
4 large green or red bell
  peppers, centers hollowed
  out
3 tablespoons dry breadcrumbs

- Preheat oven to 350°F. Melt margarine in a large nonstick skillet over medium-high heat. Add corn, chopped bell peppers, onion, green onion, garlic, and jalapeño and sauté until limp, about 10 minutes. Add flour, black pepper, and crabmeat and mix well. Blend in lemon juice and egg substitutes. Divide crab mixture among bell peppers. Top with breadcrumbs. Bake until crumbs are golden, about 40 to 45 minutes. Serve hot.

PER SERVING: 252 CALORIES			
MENU EXCHANGE PATTERN			
Dairy	—	Fruit	—
Bread	1	Meat	2
Fat	½	Veg.	2
NUTRITIONAL INFORMATION			
Carbohydrate 22			g
Protein 21			g
Total fat 9			g
Saturated fat 1.4			g
Cholesterol 75			mg
Sodium 521			mg
Potassium 536			mg
Fiber 1.8			g
Calcium 76			mg
Iron 2.7			mg

Chocolate-Walnut Meringues

4 egg whites
1 teaspoon vanilla extract
Pinch of cream of tartar
*½ cup confectioners sugar,
  sifted*

*1½ tablespoons unsweetened
  cocoa powder*
1 cup chopped toasted walnuts

- Preheat oven to 225°F. Beat egg whites until foamy. Add vanilla and cream of tartar and continue to beat, adding confectioners sugar and cocoa 1 teaspoon at a time, until stiff peaks form. Fold in walnuts. Drop mixture by rounded teaspoons on cookie sheet lined with parchment paper. Bake 1 hour. Turn oven off and let cookies rest in oven for 5 minutes. Remove and let cool in a dry place. Store in an airtight container. Makes 36 cookies; 1 serving = 1 cookie.

PER SERVING: 62 CALORIES		
MENU EXCHANGE PATTERN		
Dairy ..... —	Fruit ..... —	
Bread ..... ½	Meat ..... —	
Fat .... ½	Veg. ...... —	

NUTRITIONAL INFORMATION		
Carbohydrate 5	g
Protein 2	g
Total fat 4	g
Saturated fat 0.3	g
Cholesterol 0	mg
Sodium 13	mg
Potassium 45	mg
Fiber 0.1	g
Calcium 2	mg
Iron 0.4	mg

LIGHT SEAFOOD DISHES

5

Mixed Vegetable Salad with Tomato-Champagne Vinaigrette

Gulf of Mexico Crab Cakes

Lemon Crepes

Serves 6

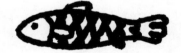

PER SERVING: 674 CALORIES			
MENU EXCHANGE PATTERN			
Dairy	1	Fruit	1
Bread	1	Meat	3
Fat	4½	Veg.	5

NUTRITIONAL INFORMATION	
Carbohydrate	62 g
Protein	39 g
Total fat	30 g
Saturated fat	5.5 g
Cholesterol	121 mg
Sodium	1034 mg
Potassium	1004 mg
Fiber	1.9 g
Calcium	265 mg
Iron	4.3 mg

Mixed Vegetable Salad with Tomato-Champagne Vinaigrette

½ ripe tomato, peeled, cored, and sliced
1 cup sliced green zucchini, ⅛ inch thick, cut lengthwise
2 carrots
1 cup green beans, ends trimmed

1 cup sliced yellow squash, ⅛ inch thick, cut lengthwise
1 cup snow peas
1 leek, sliced ½ inch thick, cut lengthwise

Tomato-Champagne Vinaigrette

½ ripe tomato
6 tablespoons commercial low-calorie Italian dressing
¼ cup Champagne

1 tablespoon chopped shallot
1 tablespoon fresh basil, or 1 teaspoon dried

- For dressing, blend all ingredients except basil. Chop basil very fine and add just before serving.

- In boiling water, separately blanch all vegetables except tomato until crisp-tender, then chill quickly in ice water, lay out in dry towels, and press with towel to remove moisture. Arrange vegetables on individual salad plates. Top each salad with 1½ tablespoons vinaigrette.

PER SERVING: 84 CALORIES		
MENU EXCHANGE PATTERN		
Dairy . . . . . —	Fruit . . . . . —	
Bread . . . . —	Meat . . . . . —	
Fat . . . . ½	Veg. 2½	
NUTRITIONAL INFORMATION		
Carbohydrate 13		g
Protein 3		g
Total fat 2		g
Saturated fat 0.2		g
Cholesterol 1		mg
Sodium 133		mg
Potassium 438		mg
Fiber 1.6		g
Calcium 52		mg
Iron 1.3		mg

Gulf of Mexico Crab Cakes

1/4 cup all-purpose flour
1 egg substitute, lightly beaten
1/2 cup breadcrumbs
1 tablespoon Parmesan cheese

Dash each of pepper and
* paprika*
1/4 cup margarine
Espazote Sauce (recipe follows)

Crab Cakes

1 pound lump crabmeat
6 ounces trout, diced 1/4 inch
* thick*
1 clove garlic, minced
1 tablespoon minced shallots
1 tablespoon margarine
1/2 teaspoon cayenne
1/2 teaspoon Tabasco sauce
1/2 tablespoon Worcestershire
* sauce*

6 slices whole wheat bread,
* toasted in oven and cubed*
1/4 teaspoon chopped chives
1/4 teaspoon chopped rosemary
1/4 teaspoon ground thyme
1/4 teaspoon dried basil
2 egg substitutes
5 tablespoons skim milk
Black pepper

- In a mixing bowl, gently toss together ingredients for crab cakes. Pat into 12 patties approximately 2 inches in diameter.

- Dredge patties with flour, then dip in egg substitute. Combine breadcrumbs, Parmesan cheese, pepper, and paprika. Dip cakes in breadcrumb mixture. Melt margarine in a nonstick skillet and sauté cakes on both sides until golden brown, about 5 minutes on each side. Serve with sauce.

Note: To reduce fat intake, serve Crab Cakes without sauce.

PER SERVING: 348 CALORIES			
MENU EXCHANGE PATTERN			
Dairy	—	Fruit	—
Bread	1	Meat	3
Fat	1½	Veg.	1½
NUTRITIONAL INFORMATION			
Carbohydrate		22	g
Protein		26	g
Total fat		16	g
Saturated fat		2.6	g
Cholesterol		92	mg
Sodium		671	mg
Potassium		375	mg
Fiber		0.1	g
Calcium		110	mg
Iron		2.4	mg

Espazote Sauce

1/4 cup chopped scallions (white
* part only)*
2 tablespoons margarine
2 cups Homemade Chicken
* Stock (page 36)*
2/3 cup evaporated skim milk

1 tablespoon chopped espazote
* (see note)*
1/2 tomato, diced
1 jalapeño chili, minced
1 tablespoon chopped chives
Black pepper

- Sauté scallions in margarine until limp, then add stock and reduce mixture to ½ cup. Add milk and reduce again to about ½ cup. Add remaining ingredients and simmer to heat through. Serve over Crab Cakes.

Note: Espazote is lamb's quarters, a wild green that grows in many parts of the United States.

PER SERVING: 53 CALORIES			
MENU EXCHANGE PATTERN			
Dairy	—	Fruit	—
Bread	—	Meat	—
Fat	1	Veg.	1
NUTRITIONAL INFORMATION			
Carbohydrate		5	g
Protein		2	g
Total fat		4	g
Saturated fat		0.9	g
Cholesterol		1	mg
Sodium		17	mg
Potassium		102	mg
Fiber		0.1	g
Calcium		48	mg
Iron		0.1	mg

Lemon Crepes

½ pound low-fat cottage cheese
⅓ cup sugar
Juice of ½ lemon
½ tablespoon light rum
½ tablespoon grated lemon
   rind

2 tablespoons brandy
2 tablespoons confectioners
   sugar, sifted

Crepes

1 egg substitute
¼ teaspoon salt
⅓ cup margarine
¾ cup skim milk
¾ teaspoon vanilla extract

3 tablespoons water
1 cup plus 1 tablespoon all-
   purpose flour
1 tablespoon safflower oil

- Make crepes. Put all ingredients except oil in a blender and blend until smooth, stirring down a couple of times if necessary. The batter should just lightly coat a spoon. If the batter is too thick, add a little more water.

- Lightly grease a small nonstick skillet with a paper towel dipped in oil. Heat skillet. When hot, thinly cover the bottom of the skillet with batter. When edge of crepe turns brown and small holes appear (about 1 minute), turn crepe and cook for about 30 seconds longer. Turn out onto a paper towel and repeat. Makes about 12. Set aside 6 for this recipe. Unused crepes can be frozen by placing wax paper between each crepe and sealing in an airtight plastic bag.

- In a blender, process cottage cheese until smooth. Gradually blend in sugar, lemon juice, rum, and lemon rind, then set aside. Spoon about 3 tablespoons of filling in a long strip down center of each crepe. Roll up, jellyroll fashion, and tuck ends under on seam side. In a nonstick chafing dish or skillet, place crepes seam side down, add brandy, swirl pan to coat the crepes, and ignite. Put 1 crepe on each dessert dish and sprinkle with confectioners sugar. Serve.

PER SERVING: 189 CALORIES		
MENU EXCHANGE PATTERN		
Dairy 1	Fruit 1	
Bread . . . . —	Meat . . . . . —	
Fat 1½	Veg. . . . . . . —	
NUTRITIONAL INFORMATION		
Carbohydrate 22		g
Protein 7		g
Total fat 8		g
Saturated fat 1.8		g
Cholesterol 27		mg
Sodium 213		mg
Potassium 89		mg
Fiber 0.1		g
Calcium 55		mg
Iron 0.5		mg

LIGHT CHICKEN DISHES

1

Shrimp Dumplings

Chicken Cucumber Salad

Steamed White Rice (page 185)

Plum Pears

Serves 4

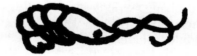

PER SERVING: 1075 CALORIES			
MENU EXCHANGE PATTERN			
Dairy	—	Fruit	4
Bread	5	Meat	5
Fat	3½	Veg.	5
NUTRITIONAL INFORMATION			
Carbohydrate	144	g	
Protein	46	g	
Total fat	37	g	
Saturated fat	6.9	g	
Cholesterol	128	mg	
Sodium	720	mg	
Potassium	1172	mg	
Fiber	4.8	g	
Calcium	157	mg	
Iron	7.8	mg	

Shrimp Dumplings

3¹/₂ cups all-purpose flour
¹/₂ cup hot water
¹/₄ cup cold water

Filling

1 cup chopped Chinese cabbage
¹/₂ pound ground lean pork
¹/₂ pound raw shrimp, chopped
2 tablespoons chopped green
   onion
1 teaspoon minced ginger

2 tablespoons Oriental sesame
   oil
¹/₂ teaspoon white pepper
2 cups shredded green cabbage
   (for steaming)

- Place 3 cups flour in a large bowl, add water, and mix until well combined. Knead dough until smooth, about 10 minutes. Let rest for 30 minutes.

- Prepare filling. Squeeze any excess moisture from chopped Chinese cabbage. Combine pork, shrimp, green onion, ginger, sesame oil, and white pepper in a large bowl. Add Chinese cabbage and mix well. Set aside.

- Cut dough in half and roll each half into a 1-inch-thick log. Pull off ½-inch pieces of dough and roll out into thin 2-inch circles with a rolling pin. (If dough becomes sticky, sprinkle work surface and hands with the additional ½ cup flour.) There should be enough dough for 24 wrappers.

- Place about 1 teaspoon filling in the center of each dumpling wrapper. Using the index finger and thumb, press opposite edges together at center. Then crimp all sides together, completely sealing dumplings.

- Line steamer with shredded cabbage. Arrange dumplings in steamer without crowding. Steam over boiling water until cooked through, 10 to 15 minutes. Serve immediately.

PER SERVING: 297 CALORIES		
MENU EXCHANGE PATTERN		
Dairy . . . . . —	Fruit . . . . . —	
Bread 2	Meat 2	
Fat . . . . . . —	Veg. 2	
NUTRITIONAL INFORMATION		
Carbohydrate 38	g	
Protein 17	g	
Total fat 10	g	
Saturated fat 2.3	g	
Cholesterol 56	mg	
Sodium 57	mg	
Potassium 355	mg	
Fiber 1.3	g	
Calcium 45	mg	
Iron 2.5	mg	

Chicken Cucumber Salad

4 chicken breasts, 5 ounces
   each
6 cucumbers, seeded and
   shredded
2 tablespoons lightly toasted
   black sesame seed
2 tablespoons black
   peppercorns

¼ cup safflower oil
1 teaspoon minced garlic
2 tablespoons sugar
1 teaspoon salt
1 cup rice vinegar
2 teaspoons hot mustard
   powder, mixed with 2
   teaspoons water

- Poach chicken breasts in barely simmering water just until firm, about 25 minutes; do not overcook. Drain and let cool. Shred meat, discarding bone and skin. Transfer to a bowl and mix in cucumber and black sesame seed.

- To prepare peppercorn oil, heat safflower oil in a small saucepan over high heat to 400°F, or extremely hot. Add peppercorns and heat, stirring, until aromatic, about 2 to 3 minutes. Strain oil to remove peppercorns.

- Combine peppercorn oil with garlic, sugar, salt, and vinegar. Whisk in mustard paste and pour dressing over chicken mixture. Transfer to individual salad plates, chill for at least 20 minutes and serve.

PER SERVING: 400 CALORIES		
MENU EXCHANGE PATTERN		
Dairy . . . . . —	Fruit . . . . . —	
Bread . . . . —	Meat 3	
Fat 3½	Veg. 3	
NUTRITIONAL INFORMATION		
Carbohydrate 16		g
Protein 26		g
Total fat 27		g
Saturated fat 4.6		g
Cholesterol 72		mg
Sodium 613		mg
Potassium 565		mg
Fiber 1.1		g
Calcium 64		mg
Iron 3.2		mg

Plum Pears

4 pears
3 tablespoons plum sauce
3 tablespoons honey

2 tablespoons white wine
1 teaspoon cornstarch

- Peel pears. Slice off top inch of pears, leaving stems intact, and reserve. Carefully hollow out core of each pear.

- Combine plum sauce, honey, wine, and cornstarch in a small saucepan and bring to a boil, stirring. Reduce heat and simmer sauce for 5 minutes. Spoon sauce into cavity of each pear. Replace top of pear and secure with toothpicks.

- Arrange pears upright in steamer and steam over boiling water for 30 minutes. Serve hot or cold.

PER SERVING: 201 CALORIES		
MENU EXCHANGE PATTERN		
Dairy . . . . . —	Fruit 4	
Bread . . . . . ½	Meat . . . . . —	
Fat . . . . —	Veg. . . . . . . —	
NUTRITIONAL INFORMATION		
Carbohydrate 51		g
Protein 1		g
Total fat 1		g
Saturated fat 0		g
Cholesterol 0		mg
Sodium 4		mg
Potassium 249		mg
Fiber 2.3		g
Calcium 36		mg
Iron 0.7		mg

LIGHT CHICKEN DISHES

2

Romaine with Dijon Herb Dressing

Chicken with Tomatoes and Fines Herbes

Herbed Potatoes

Lemon Sherbet

Serves 4

PER SERVING: 703 CALORIES		
MENU EXCHANGE PATTERN		
Dairy . . . . . —	Fruit 1½	
Bread 3	Meat 4	
Fat 3½	Veg. 3	
NUTRITIONAL INFORMATION		
Carbohydrate 74	g	
Protein 37	g	
Total fat 30	g	
Saturated fat 5	g	
Cholesterol 94	mg	
Sodium 160	mg	
Potassium 1789	mg	
Fiber 2.9	g	
Calcium 158	mg	
Iron . . . . 4.4 mg		

Romaine with Dijon Herb Dressing

1 head romaine lettuce
3 tablespoons red wine vinegar
4 teaspoons safflower oil
½ teaspoon Dijon-style mustard
½ teaspoon sugar

2 teaspoons dried basil
2 teaspoons finely chopped
    green onion
½ clove garlic, minced
¼ teaspoon black pepper

- Rinse romaine leaves and tear into bite-size pieces.

- Combine all remaining ingredients in a jar and shake well. Toss with romaine and serve.

PER SERVING: 55 CALORIES			
MENU EXCHANGE PATTERN			
Dairy	—	Fruit	—
Bread	—	Meat	—
Fat	1	Veg.	1
NUTRITIONAL INFORMATION			
Carbohydrate		3	g
Protein		1	g
Total fat		5	g
Saturated fat		0.4	g
Cholesterol		0	mg
Sodium		13	mg
Potassium		162	mg
Fiber		0.4	g
Calcium		39	mg
Iron		0.9	mg

Chicken with Tomatoes and Fines Herbes

½ large onion, sliced
2 tablespoons safflower oil
1 green bell pepper, cut in
    1-inch squares
1 red bell pepper, cut in 1-inch
    squares
1 small zucchini, cut in 1-inch
    cubes

4 tomatoes, peeled, seeded, and
    quartered
Pinch of fresh thyme
Chopped fresh basil
2 cloves garlic, chopped
½ teaspoon freshly ground
    black pepper
1 chicken, about 1½ pounds

- In large nonstick skillet, sauté the onion in 1 tablespoon oil over medium heat until tender, about 5 minutes. Add the peppers and zucchini and sauté for a few more minutes. Add the tomatoes and cook until vegetables are tender, about 10 minutes. Stir in seasonings and garlic and set aside.

- Preheat the oven to 375°F. Remove the breast and leg meat from the chicken; cut into 2-inch strips. Sauté in remaining oil in a nonstick skillet until lightly browned. Drain off the fat. Preheat the oven to 375°F. Place half the vegetables in the bottom of a 1½-quart casserole, arrange the chicken over the top, and cover with the remaining vegetables. Cover and bake for 30 minutes.

PER SERVING: 350 CALORIES			
MENU EXCHANGE PATTERN			
Dairy	—	Fruit	—
Bread	—	Meat	4
Fat	1½	Veg.	2
NUTRITIONAL INFORMATION			
Carbohydrate		12	g
Protein		31	g
Total fat		19	g
Saturated fat		3.9	g
Cholesterol		87	mg
Sodium		97	mg
Potassium		824	mg
Fiber		1.6	g
Calcium		52	mg
Iron		2.2	mg

Herbed Potatoes

1½ pounds new potatoes
4 teaspoons margarine
1 tablespoon minced fresh
*   parsley*

1 tablespoon minced fresh
*   chives*
1 teaspoon dried tarragon
Black pepper

PER SERVING: 164 CALORIES		
MENU EXCHANGE PATTERN		
Dairy . . . . . —	Fruit . . . . . —	
Bread 2	Meat . . . . . —	
Fat 1	Veg. . . . . . . —	
NUTRITIONAL INFORMATION		
Carbohydrate 29	g	
Protein 4	g	
Total fat 4	g	
Saturated fat 0.7	g	
Cholesterol 0	mg	
Sodium 6	mg	
Potassium 705	mg	
Fiber 0.9	g	
Calcium 16	mg	
Iron 1.1	mg	

- Peel potatoes and slice diagonally 1½ inches thick. Melt the margarine in a nonstick skillet over moderately high heat, then add potatoes and sauté until pale golden brown, about 4 to 5 minutes. Lower heat, cover skillet, and cook for about 15 minutes, shaking skillet periodically to prevent sticking. Remove from heat and add herbs and pepper.

Lemon Sherbet

2 cups lemon sherbet
Mint sprigs

PER SERVING: 134 CALORIES		
MENU EXCHANGE PATTERN		
Dairy . . . . . —	Fruit 1½	
Bread 1	Meat . . . . . —	
Fat . . . . —	Veg. . . . . . . —	
NUTRITIONAL INFORMATION		
Carbohydrate 29	g	
Protein 1	g	
Total fat 2	g	
Saturated fat 0	g	
Cholesterol 7	mg	
Sodium 44	mg	
Potassium 98	mg	
Fiber 0	g	
Calcium 51	mg	
Iron 0.2	mg	

- Spoon ½ cup lemon sherbet into each of 4 saucer Champagne glasses. Garnish with a sprig of mint.

LIGHT CHICKEN DISHES

3

Tomato Salad with Red Onion Marmalade

Grilled Chicken Breasts with
Honey Mustard Glaze

Vegetable Brochettes

Orange Slices in Tequila

Serves 2

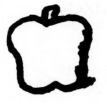

PER SERVING: 733 CALORIES		
MENU EXCHANGE PATTERN		
Dairy . . . . . . ½	Fruit 2½	
Bread 1½	Meat 4	
Fat 3½	Veg. 3½	
NUTRITIONAL INFORMATION		
Carbohydrate 73	g	
Protein 38	g	
Total fat 31	g	
Saturated fat 7	g	
Cholesterol 96	mg	
Sodium 759	mg	
Potassium 1545	mg	
Fiber 3.2	g	
Calcium 497	mg	
Iron 4.9	mg	

Tomato Salad with Red Onion Marmalade

2 tomatoes
2 teaspoons olive oil
2 teaspoons lemon juice
1/2 bunch watercress

Red Onion Marmalade

1 small red onion
1/8 teaspoon salt
2 teaspoons safflower oil

1/4 cup dry red wine
1/4 cup red wine vinegar
2 tablespoons sugar

- Prepare marmalade. Halve onion, then slice in strips. Sprinkle with salt. Sauté onion in oil in a small saucepan over medium heat until wilted and tender, about 5 minutes. Add wine, vinegar, and sugar and bring to a boil. Reduce heat and simmer, reducing liquid to jam consistency, about 10 minutes. Let cool before serving.

- Slice tomatoes crosswise and arrange slices in pinwheel fashion on salad plates. Drizzle 1 teaspoon olive oil over tomatoes. Drizzle with a few drops of lemon juice. Garnish center of pinwheel with watercress. Serve with marmalade on the side.

PER SERVING: 188 CALORIES		
MENU EXCHANGE PATTERN		
Dairy . . . . . —	Fruit 1½	
Bread . . . . . —	Meat . . . . . —	
Fat 2	Veg. 2	
NUTRITIONAL INFORMATION		
Carbohydrate 27	g	
Protein 3	g	
Total fat 10	g	
Saturated fat 1	g	
Cholesterol 0	mg	
Sodium 229	mg	
Potassium 591	mg	
Fiber 1.2	g	
Calcium 62	mg	
Iron 1.7	mg	

Grilled Chicken Breasts with Honey Mustard Glaze

1 whole chicken breast, about
*   12 ounces*
2 teaspoons virgin olive oil

Honey Mustard Glaze

2½ tablespoons coarse-grained
*   mustard*
4 teaspoons Dijon-style mustard
2 teaspoons honey

- Bone chicken breasts and lightly pound meat flat. Grill over charcoal fire for about 15 to 20 minutes, or broil in oven for about 15 minutes (begin cooking skin side down if grilling, skin side up if broiling). Prepare sauce by combining ingredients. When chicken is about half cooked, turn over and brush with sauce. Finish cooking and cut breast in half. Transfer to serving plates. Drizzle each serving with 1 teaspoon olive oil.

PER SERVING: 326 CALORIES		
MENU EXCHANGE PATTERN		
Dairy . . . . . —	Fruit . . . . . . ½	
Bread . . . . . ½	Meat 4	
Fat 1	Veg. . . . . . . —	
NUTRITIONAL INFORMATION		
Carbohydrate 8	g	
Protein 30	g	
Total fat 18	g	
Saturated fat 4.2	g	
Cholesterol 87	mg	
Sodium 463	mg	
Potassium 345	mg	
Fiber 0.3	g	
Calcium 39	mg	
Iron 1.7	mg	

Vegetable Brochettes

1 red bell pepper, cored and
   seeded
1 green bell pepper, cored and
   seeded
1 red onion
6 fresh mushrooms

- Cut each pepper and onion into 6 pieces; leave mushrooms whole. Thread vegetables alternately onto skewers. Grill or broil until vegetables are cooked but still crisp, about 10 minutes. Serve hot.

PER SERVING: 36 CALORIES		
MENU EXCHANGE PATTERN		
Dairy ..... —	Fruit ..... —	
Bread .... —	Meat ..... —	
Fat .... —	Veg. 1½	
NUTRITIONAL INFORMATION		
Carbohydrate 8	g	
Protein 2	g	
Total fat 0	g	
Saturated fat 0	g	
Cholesterol 0	mg	
Sodium 14	mg	
Potassium 239	mg	
Fiber 1.1	g	
Calcium 20	mg	
Iron 0.8	mg	

Orange Slices in Tequila

2 oranges
4 teaspoons tequila
1 teaspoon grenadine

1 cup low-fat frozen vanilla
   yogurt
Pomegranate seeds (garnish)

- Peel and slice oranges crosswise. Sprinkle with tequila and grenadine. Marinate for 1 hour.

- Transfer ½ cup each of frozen yogurt to 2 dessert dishes. Top with orange slices and garnish with pomegranate seeds.

PER SERVING: 183 CALORIES		
MENU EXCHANGE PATTERN		
Dairy ...... ½	Fruit 1	
Bread 1	Meat ..... —	
Fat .... ½	Veg. ...... —	
NUTRITIONAL INFORMATION		
Carbohydrate 30	g	
Protein 4	g	
Total fat 3	g	
Saturated fat 1.8	g	
Cholesterol 9	mg	
Sodium 53	mg	
Potassium 370	mg	
Fiber 0.6	g	
Calcium 376	mg	
Iron 0.2	mg	

LIGHT CHICKEN DISHES

4

Sliced Tomatoes

Chicken with Mushrooms and Artichokes

White and Wild Rice Pilaf

Raspberries with Sweetened Yogurt

Serves 8

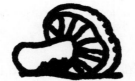

PER SERVING: 610 CALORIES		
MENU EXCHANGE PATTERN		
Dairy . . . . . . ½	Fruit 1½	
Bread 2½	Meat 3	
Fat 3	Veg. 1	
NUTRITIONAL INFORMATION		
Carbohydrate 61	g	
Protein 29	g	
Total fat 27	g	
Saturated fat 5.4	g	
Cholesterol 62	mg	
Sodium 120	mg	
Potassium 1064	mg	
Fiber 2.7	g	
Calcium 192	mg	
Iron . . . . 3.9 mg		

Sliced Tomatoes

8 leaves Bibb lettuce, washed
   and dried
8 tomatoes, sliced

Dressing
¼ cup safflower oil
¼ cup red wine vinegar
1½ teaspoons dried basil
White pepper

- Combine dressing ingredients, adding pepper to taste. 1 serving = 1 tablespoon.

- Place a lettuce leaf on each individual salad plate. Arrange 1 sliced tomato on each lettuce leaf. Serve with dressing.

Note: To reduce fat intake, substitute a commercial low-calorie Italian dressing. Adjusted analysis: calories = 47; exchanges = 1 Vegetable, ½ Fat.

PER SERVING: 92 CALORIES			
MENU EXCHANGE PATTERN			
Dairy	—	Fruit	—
Bread	—	Meat	—
Fat	1½	Veg.	1
NUTRITIONAL INFORMATION			
Carbohydrate	7		g
Protein	2		g
Total fat	7		g
Saturated fat	0.6		g
Cholesterol	0		mg
Sodium	4		mg
Potassium	358		mg
Fiber	0.8		g
Calcium	21		mg
Iron	0.9		mg

Chicken with Mushrooms and Artichokes

8 chicken breasts, boned and
   skinned (4 ounces each)
⅓ cup (about) all-purpose flour
4 tablespoons margarine
4 teaspoons safflower oil
½ pound fresh mushrooms,
   sliced

8 artichoke hearts, cut in
   quarters
⅓ cup dry white wine
Juice of 1 lemon
2 tablespoons finely chopped
   fresh parsley

- Dredge chicken breasts lightly in flour. Sauté chicken in 3 tablespoons margarine and the safflower oil over medium-high heat until firm and cooked through, about 7 minutes on each side. Add mushrooms and artichokes and cook over medium heat for 2 minutes. Transfer chicken, mushrooms, and artichokes to a warm serving platter and drain oil from skillet. Return pan to heat. Add remaining margarine, wine, lemon juice, and parsley to skillet and cook over medium-high heat for 2 minutes. Pour sauce over chicken and serve.

PER SERVING: 262 CALORIES			
MENU EXCHANGE PATTERN			
Dairy	—	Fruit	—
Bread	½	Meat	3
Fat	1½	Veg.	—
NUTRITIONAL INFORMATION			
Carbohydrate	6		g
Protein	21		g
Total fat	16		g
Saturated fat	3.7		g
Cholesterol	58		mg
Sodium	62		mg
Potassium	363		mg
Fiber	0.4		g
Calcium	20		mg
Iron	1.2		mg

White and Wild Rice Pilaf

⅓ cup wild rice
4 teaspoons margarine
2 cups unsweetened apple juice

3⅓ cups Homemade Chicken
Stock (page 36)
1⅓ cups white rice

- In a large nonstick skillet, sauté wild rice in margarine over medium-high heat for about 2 minutes. Add apple juice and chicken stock and bring to a boil. Cover and simmer for 15 minutes. Add white rice and continue to simmer until water is absorbed, about 25 more minutes. Fluff rice with fork and serve.

PER SERVING: 187 CALORIES

MENU EXCHANGE PATTERN

Dairy	—	Fruit	1
Bread	2	Meat	—
Fat	—	Veg.	—

NUTRITIONAL INFORMATION

Carbohydrate	38	g
Protein	3	g
Total fat	2	g
Saturated fat	0.4	g
Cholesterol	0	mg
Sodium	4	mg
Potassium	119	mg
Fiber	0.3	g
Calcium	13	mg
Iron	1.5	mg

Raspberries with Sweetened Yogurt

2½ cups fresh raspberries
2½ cups plain low-fat yogurt
1 tablespoon raspberry liqueur

- Wash raspberries and drain well; set several aside for garnish. Combine yogurt with liqueur. Add to raspberries and mix well. Transfer mixture to dessert glasses and garnish with reserved raspberries.

PER SERVING: 68 CALORIES

MENU EXCHANGE PATTERN

Dairy	½	Fruit	½
Bread	—	Meat	—
Fat	—	Veg.	—

NUTRITIONAL INFORMATION

Carbohydrate	9	g
Protein	4	g
Total fat	1	g
Saturated fat	0.7	g
Cholesterol	4	mg
Sodium	50	mg
Potassium	224	mg
Fiber	1.2	g
Calcium	138	mg
Iron	0.3	mg

LIGHT CHICKEN DISHES

5

Dong An Chicken

Steamed White Rice (page 185)

Peppercorn Eggplant

Frozen Ginger

Serves 4

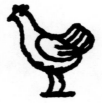

PER SERVING: 711 CALORIES		
MENU EXCHANGE PATTERN		
Dairy . . . . . . ½	Fruit 2	
Bread 3	Meat 3½	
Fat 2½	Veg. 3	
NUTRITIONAL INFORMATION		
Carbohydrate 91	g	
Protein 33	g	
Total fat 24	g	
Saturated fat 5	g	
Cholesterol 81	mg	
Sodium 394	mg	
Potassium 950	mg	
Fiber 2.3	g	
Calcium 158	mg	
Iron 4.7	mg	

Dong An Chicken

4 chicken breasts (5 ounces
    each), boned and skinned
1/4 cup cornstarch
1/2 cup water
3 tablespoons safflower oil
4 green onions, shredded
8 slices ginger, shredded

3 jalapeño chilies, minced
1 tablespoon low-sodium soy
    sauce
2 tablespoons red wine vinegar
1 teaspoon sugar
1/2 teaspoon white pepper

- Shred chicken meat. Mix cornstarch with water and 2 tea-spoons safflower oil in a large bowl. Add chicken and marinate for 20 minutes. Drain.

- Heat 2 tablespoons safflower oil in a wok or large skillet over high heat. Add chicken and stir-fry until no longer pink, about 2 to 3 minutes. Remove chicken and set aside.

- Add the remaining 1 tablespoon oil to the wok. Add green onion, ginger, and chilies and stir-fry for 1 minute. Stir in cooked chicken, soy sauce, vinegar, sugar, and white pepper; heat through and serve.

PER SERVING: 344 CALORIES		
MENU EXCHANGE PATTERN		
Dairy ..... —	Fruit ..... —	
Bread 1/2	Meat 31/2	
Fat 2	Veg. 1	
NUTRITIONAL INFORMATION		
Carbohydrate 13	g	
Protein 25	g	
Total fat 21	g	
Saturated fat 3.9	g	
Cholesterol 72	mg	
Sodium 331	mg	
Potassium 397	mg	
Fiber 0.6	g	
Calcium 32	mg	
Iron ....1.8 mg		

Peppercorn Eggplant

1 1/2 pounds Japanese eggplant
3 tablespoons minced green
    onion

1 teaspoon ground peppercorns
3/4 cup Homemade Chicken
    Stock (page 36)

- Cut off ends of eggplants. Cut remainder into 3-inch cross-wise pieces, then cut each piece in half lengthwise. Place eggplant in a steamer, cover, and steam over boiling water until tender, about 25 minutes. Transfer to a serving plate.

- Mix green onion, peppercorns, and stock and pour over eggplant. Refrigerate for at least 30 minutes before serving.

PER SERVING: 44 CALORIES		
MENU EXCHANGE PATTERN		
Dairy ..... —	Fruit ..... —	
Bread ..... —	Meat ..... —	
Fat .... —	Veg. 2	
NUTRITIONAL INFORMATION		
Carbohydrate 10	g	
Protein 2	g	
Total fat 0	g	
Saturated fat 0	g	
Cholesterol 0	mg	
Sodium 4	mg	
Potassium 375	mg	
Fiber 1.6	g	
Calcium 23	mg	
Iron ....1.2 mg		

Frozen Ginger

2 cups low-fat frozen vanilla
    yogurt
1 teaspoon ground ginger
2 tablespoons minced candied
    ginger

- Soften frozen yogurt slightly at room temperature. Add ground ginger and mix well. Return yogurt to freezer to harden. Scoop 1/2 cup yogurt into each of 4 serving dishes and sprinkle with candied ginger.

PER SERVING: 147 CALORIES		
MENU EXCHANGE PATTERN		
Dairy 1/2	Fruit 2	
Bread .... —	Meat ..... —	
Fat 1/2	Veg. .... —	
NUTRITIONAL INFORMATION		
Carbohydrate 28	g	
Protein 3	g	
Total fat 3	g	
Saturated fat 1.1	g	
Cholesterol 9	mg	
Sodium 57	mg	
Potassium 133	mg	
Fiber 0	g	
Calcium 91	mg	
Iron ....0.3 mg		

LIGHT CHICKEN DISHES

6

Gazpacho Andaluz

Chicken Breast Esterhazy with
Julienne of Vegetables

Boiled Potatoes

Rosewater Melon Cup

Serves 4

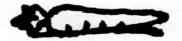

PER SERVING: 691 CALORIES			
MENU EXCHANGE PATTERN			
Dairy	—	Fruit	4
Bread	2½	Meat	3½
Fat	3	Veg.	1
NUTRITIONAL INFORMATION			
Carbohydrate	86	g	
Protein	35	g	
Total fat	26	g	
Saturated fat	4.6	g	
Cholesterol	72	mg	
Sodium	294	mg	
Potassium	2525	mg	
Fiber	4.8	g	
Calcium	138	mg	
Iron	5.2	mg	

Gazpacho Andaluz

3 large tomatoes, peeled, seeded, and finely chopped
2 cucumbers, peeled, seeded, and chopped
1 green bell pepper, seeded and chopped
1 clove garlic, chopped
1/3 cup roasted sliced almonds
1 1/4 cups Homemade Chicken Stock (page 36)
1 1/4 cups low-sodium tomato juice
Black pepper
Juice of 1 lemon
Dash of Tabasco sauce
Pinch of ground cumin
Cucumber slices (garnish)

- Combine ingredients in a bowl and chill for 2 to 3 hours. Check seasoning, then serve in chilled cups. Garnish with cucumber slices.

PER SERVING: 126 CALORIES			
MENU EXCHANGE PATTERN			
Dairy ..... —		Fruit ..... —	
Bread 1		Meat ..... —	
Fat 1		Veg. ...... —	
NUTRITIONAL INFORMATION			
Carbohydrate 16			g
Protein 5			g
Total fat 6			g
Saturated fat 0.5			g
Cholesterol 0			mg
Sodium 162			mg
Potassium 738			mg
Fiber 1.8			g
Calcium 67			mg
Iron 2.7			mg

Chicken Breast Esterhazy with Julienne of Vegetables

4 boned and skinned chicken breasts, about 5 ounces each
Black pepper
4 teaspoons safflower oil
4 teaspoons margarine
1 clove garlic, minced
1 onion, thinly sliced
1 carrot, thinly sliced
1 red bell pepper, seeded and thinly sliced
1 stalk celery, thinly sliced
3 tablespoons dry white wine
2/3 cup Homemade Chicken Stock (page 36)

- Season chicken with pepper to taste. Heat oil and margarine in a large nonstick skillet over medium-high heat. Add chicken and sauté until cooked through, about 8 minutes on each side. Remove from skillet and keep warm.

- Reduce heat to medium and, in the same pan, sauté garlic and onion until translucent. Add remaining ingredients and simmer for 5 minutes. Pour sauce over the chicken and serve.

Photo opposite page 146.

PER SERVING: 310 CALORIES			
MENU EXCHANGE PATTERN			
Dairy ..... —		Fruit ..... —	
Bread .... —		Meat 3½	
Fat 2		Veg. 1	
NUTRITIONAL INFORMATION			
Carbohydrate 8			g
Protein 25			g
Total fat 19			g
Saturated fat 4.1			g
Cholesterol 72			mg
Sodium 106			mg
Potassium 487			mg
Fiber 0.8			g
Calcium 41			mg
Iron 1.4			mg

Boiled Potatoes

4 medium-size new potatoes
2 quarts water

- Peel a strip from the middle of each potato, leaving the skin on both ends. Bring water to a boil and add potatoes. Cook until easily pierced with a skewer, about 10 to 15 minutes.

PER SERVING: 104 CALORIES		
MENU EXCHANGE PATTERN		
Dairy . . . . . —	Fruit . . . . . —	
Bread 1½	Meat . . . . . —	
Fat . . . . —	Veg. . . . . . . —	
NUTRITIONAL INFORMATION		
Carbohydrate 23		g
Protein 3		g
Total fat 0		g
Saturated fat 0		g
Cholesterol 0		mg
Sodium 4		mg
Potassium 556		mg
Fiber 0.7		g
Calcium 10		mg
Iron 0.8		mg

Rosewater Melon Cup

½ cantaloupe
½ honeydew melon
2 ripe peaches
2 tablespoons rosewater

3 tablespoons lemon juice
¼ cup sugar
Mint sprigs (garnish)

- Cut balls from cantaloupe and honeydew with a small scoop, or dice flesh into ½-inch cubes. Peel and slice peaches. Combine fruit in a large nonaluminum bowl. Mix rosewater, lemon juice, and sugar in a small bowl and pour over melon and peaches. Stir well to thoroughly coat fruit, then serve in dessert glasses garnished with a sprig of mint.

Note: Rosewater is available in gourmet and Middle Eastern food shops.

PER SERVING: 151 CALORIES		
MENU EXCHANGE PATTERN		
Dairy . . . . . —	Fruit 4	
Bread . . . . —	Meat . . . . . —	
Fat . . . . —	Veg. . . . . . . —	
NUTRITIONAL INFORMATION		
Carbohydrate 39		g
Protein 2		g
Total fat 0		g
Saturated fat 0		g
Cholesterol 0		mg
Sodium 22		mg
Potassium 744		mg
Fiber 1.5		g
Calcium 20		mg
Iron 0.3		mg

LIGHT CHICKEN DISHES

7

Green Onion Soup with Vermicelli

Grilled Marinated Chicken on Oriental Salad

Cinnamon-Poached Pears with Blueberries

Serves 4

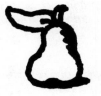

PER SERVING: 694 CALORIES			
MENU EXCHANGE PATTERN			
Dairy	—	Fruit	3
Bread	3	Meat	3
Fat	2½	Veg.	3
NUTRITIONAL INFORMATION			
Carbohydrate	69	g	
Protein	32	g	
Total fat	24	g	
Saturated fat	3.5	g	
Cholesterol	57	mg	
Sodium	486	mg	
Potassium	1117	mg	
Fiber	4.3	g	
Calcium	107	mg	
Iron	6.5	mg	

Green Onion Soup with Vermicelli

4 green onions
1/4 yellow onion
1 tablespoon margarine
1 quart Homemade Chicken
   Stock (page 36)
1 teaspoon chopped fresh
   oregano

1 bay leaf
1/2 cup uncooked and broken
   up vermicelli
White pepper

- Coarsely chop both types of onions. Melt margarine in a large saucepan over medium heat and sauté yellow onion until translucent. Add green onions and sauté until tender. Add chicken stock, oregano, and bay leaf and simmer for 25 to 30 minutes. Remove bay leaf and puree soup in a blender. Return to saucepan and reheat. Add vermicelli and cook in soup until tender, about 5 to 10 minutes. Season to taste with white pepper and serve hot.

PER SERVING: 138 CALORIES		
MENU EXCHANGE PATTERN		
Dairy . . . . . —	Fruit . . . . . —	
Bread 1/2	Meat . . . . . —	
Fat 1 1/2	Veg. 1	
NUTRITIONAL INFORMATION		
Carbohydrate 14	g
Protein 2	g
Total fat 8	g
Saturated fat 0.5	g
Cholesterol 0	mg
Sodium 103	mg
Potassium 119	mg
Fiber 0.4	g
Calcium 23	mg
Iron 0.8	mg

Grilled Marinated Chicken on Oriental Salad

4 chicken breasts, about 4
   ounces each, boned and
   skinned
1 1/3 cups bean sprouts

1 cup snow peas
1/3 cup water chestnuts
1 cup daikon sprouts

Marinade

2 tablespoons chopped garlic
2 tablespoons low-sodium soy
   sauce
2 tablespoons Oriental sesame
   oil

4 tablespoons rice vinegar
Black pepper

- Prepare marinade. Marinate chicken breasts in 3/4 of marinade for 24 hours. Remove chicken and grill for about 15 minutes over mesquite charcoal until cooked through, turning several times.

- While chicken is cooking, mix bean sprouts, snow peas, water chestnuts, and daikon sprouts. Lightly toss salad with remaining 1/4 of marinade. Arrange on plates and serve chicken breasts on top of salad.

PER SERVING: 333 CALORIES		
MENU EXCHANGE PATTERN		
Dairy . . . . . —	Fruit . . . . . —	
Bread 1	Meat 3	
Fat 1	Veg. 2	
NUTRITIONAL INFORMATION		
Carbohydrate 19	g
Protein 28	g
Total fat 15	g
Saturated fat 3	g
Cholesterol 57	mg
Sodium 375	mg
Potassium 630	mg
Fiber 1	g
Calcium 47	mg
Iron 5	mg

Cinnamon-Poached Pears
with Blueberries

4 whole fresh pears
2 cups (one 750-mL bottle) full-
*   bodied red wine such as*
*   Zinfandel, Barolo, or Rioja*

2 cinnamon sticks
Juice of 1 lemon
1 cup blueberries
Mint leaves (garnish)

- Halve pears lengthwise; core and peel. Bring wine and cinnamon sticks to a boil in a large enameled saucepan. Add lemon juice and return to boil. Remove from heat, add pear halves and allow to steep until cool.

- Place 2 pear halves, round side down, on individual dessert plates. Fill centers of pear halves with fresh blueberries and garnish with a mint leaf.

PER SERVING: 223 CALORIES		
MENU EXCHANGE PATTERN		
Dairy . . . . . —	Fruit 3	
Bread 1½	Meat . . . . . —	
Fat . . . . —	Veg. . . . . . . —	
NUTRITIONAL INFORMATION		
Carbohydrate 36	g	
Protein 1	g	
Total fat 1	g	
Saturated fat 0	g	
Cholesterol 0	mg	
Sodium 8	mg	
Potassium 368	mg	
Fiber 2.8	g	
Calcium 37	mg	
Iron 1	mg	

LIGHT CHICKEN DISHES

8

Vegetable Soup

Tossed Green Salad

Chicken Lucia

Steamed Broccoli and Carrots

Almond Pound Cake

Serves 4

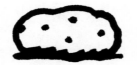

PER SERVING: 688 CALORIES
MENU EXCHANGE PATTERN

Dairy	—	Fruit	—
Bread	3	Meat	2½
Fat	3½	Veg.	6½

NUTRITIONAL INFORMATION

Carbohydrate	81	g
Protein	36	g
Total fat	27	g
Saturated fat	5.4	g
Cholesterol	58	mg
Sodium	323	mg
Potassium	2377	mg
Fiber	6.9	g
Calcium	310	mg
Iron	7.4	mg

Vegetable Soup

3 cups Homemade Chicken
   Stock (page 36)
1 boiling potato, diced
2 large carrots, diced
1/2 cup fresh or frozen peas

1/2 large onion, diced
1 rutabaga, peeled and diced
1 1/2 cups canned low-sodium
   tomatoes

- Heat stock in a large stockpot. Add vegetables except tomatoes. Bring to a boil, then simmer about 20 minutes. Add tomatoes and simmer 1 hour.

PER SERVING: 176 CALORIES		
MENU EXCHANGE PATTERN		
Dairy . . . . . —	Fruit . . . . . —	
Bread 1½	Meat . . . . . —	
Fat . . . . ½	Veg. 2	
NUTRITIONAL INFORMATION		
Carbohydrate 30		g
Protein 7		g
Total fat 4		g
Saturated fat 0.8		g
Cholesterol 0		mg
Sodium 142		mg
Potassium 817		mg
Fiber 3		g
Calcium 74		mg
Iron 2.6		mg

Tossed Green Salad

1/2 head Bibb lettuce, about
   2 cups, washed and dried
1/2 head red-leaf lettuce, about
   2 cups, washed and dried
4 tomatoes, cut in wedges
4 tablespoons Vinaigrette
   Dressing (recipe follows)

- Tear lettuces into bite-size pieces. Mix in a bowl, then arrange on salad plates. Place wedges of 1 tomato on each plate. Top with dressing.

PER SERVING: 48 CALORIES		
MENU EXCHANGE PATTERN		
Dairy . . . . . —	Fruit . . . . . —	
Bread . . . . —	Meat . . . . . —	
Fat . . . . —	Veg. 2	
NUTRITIONAL INFORMATION		
Carbohydrate 10		g
Protein 3		g
Total fat 0		g
Saturated fat 0		g
Cholesterol 0		mg
Sodium 10		mg
Potassium 588		mg
Fiber 1.3		g
Calcium 51		mg
Iron 1.8		mg

Vinaigrette Dressing

1/2 cup red wine vinegar
1/4 cup safflower oil
1 clove garlic, minced
1/2 teaspoon black pepper

- Combine ingredients in a jar and shake well. Makes 3/4 cup; 1 serving = 1 tablespoon.

PER SERVING: 42 CALORIES		
MENU EXCHANGE PATTERN		
Dairy . . . . . —	Fruit . . . . . —	
Bread . . . . —	Meat . . . . . —	
Fat 1	Veg. . . . . . . —	
NUTRITIONAL INFORMATION		
Carbohydrate 1		g
Protein 0		g
Total fat 4		g
Saturated fat 0.4		g
Cholesterol 0		mg
Sodium 0		mg
Potassium 12		mg
Fiber 0		g
Calcium 1		mg
Iron 0.1		mg

Chicken Lucia

*4 chicken breasts, about
    4 ounces each, boned
    and skinned*
4 teaspoons margarine
2 teaspoons dried oregano
¼ teaspoon garlic powder

- Spray a broiler pan with nonstick spray. Place chicken in pan and place ½ teaspoon margarine on top of each piece. Sprinkle with some of the oregano and garlic powder, then broil about 5 minutes. Turn chicken. Top each piece with ½ teaspoon margarine and remaining oregano and garlic powder. Continue to broil until chicken is done, about 5 to 10 minutes.

PER SERVING: 173 CALORIES		
MENU EXCHANGE PATTERN		
Dairy . . . . . —	Fruit . . . . . —	
Bread . . . . . —	Meat 2½	
Fat . . . . ½	Veg. . . . . . . —	
NUTRITIONAL INFORMATION		
Carbohydrate 0	g	
Protein 19	g	
Total fat 10	g	
Saturated fat 2.7	g	
Cholesterol 57	mg	
Sodium 57	mg	
Potassium 200	mg	
Fiber 0	g	
Calcium 10	mg	
Iron 0.6	mg	

Steamed Broccoli and Carrots

2 cups sliced broccoli
4 carrots, diced
1 clove garlic, minced

- In a large saucepan steam broccoli, carrots, and garlic over boiling water about 5 minutes, or until vegetables are crisp-tender. Serve hot.

PER SERVING: 69 CALORIES		
MENU EXCHANGE PATTERN		
Dairy . . . . . —	Fruit . . . . . —	
Bread . . . . . —	Meat . . . . . —	
Fat . . . . —	Veg. 2½	
NUTRITIONAL INFORMATION		
Carbohydrate 14	g	
Protein 5	g	
Total fat 0	g	
Saturated fat 0	g	
Cholesterol 0	mg	
Sodium 52	mg	
Potassium 706	mg	
Fiber 2.6	g	
Calcium 150	mg	
Iron 1.8	mg	

Almond Pound Cake

2½ cups all-purpose flour
2 cups sugar
½ teaspoon salt
½ teaspoon baking soda
*1 cup margarine, at room
    temperature*

1 teaspoon almond extract
1 cup plain low-fat yogurt
3 egg substitutes

- Preheat oven to 350°F. Mix ingredients in a large bowl and beat for 3 minutes at medium to high speed of electric mixer. Pour batter into a 10-inch nonstick-coated Bundt pan and bake until cake is springy and lightly brown, about 60 to 70 minutes. Let cool upright for at least 15 minutes, then invert pan and turn out cake. Let cool completely on a rack. Cut in 1-inch slices to serve.

PER SERVING: 181 CALORIES		
MENU EXCHANGE PATTERN		
Dairy . . . . . —	Fruit . . . . . —	
Bread 1½	Meat . . . . . —	
Fat 1½	Veg. . . . . . . —	
NUTRITIONAL INFORMATION		
Carbohydrate 25	g	
Protein 2	g	
Total fat 8	g	
Saturated fat 1.5	g	
Cholesterol 0	mg	
Sodium 62	mg	
Potassium 54	mg	
Fiber 0	g	
Calcium 24	mg	
Iron 0.4	mg	

CHAPTER 7

LIGHT DINNERS

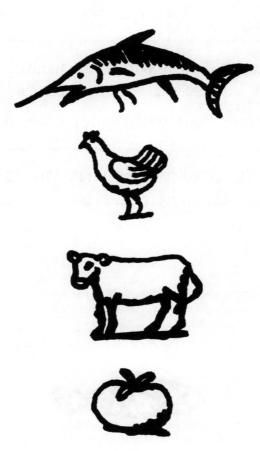

SEAFOOD ENTREES

1

Gazpacho

Rainbow Trout with Lemon and Basil

Green Peas with Water Chestnuts

Raspberry-Blueberry Parfait

Serves 4

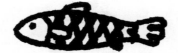

PER SERVING: 720 CALORIES		
MENU EXCHANGE PATTERN		
Dairy . . . . . . ½	Fruit 2	
Bread 1	Meat 5	
Fat 2½	Veg. 5½	
NUTRITIONAL INFORMATION		
Carbohydrate 63	g	
Protein 50	g	
Total fat 31	g	
Saturated fat 4	g	
Cholesterol 100	mg	
Sodium 444	mg	
Potassium 2507	mg	
Fiber 5.7	g	
Calcium 258	mg	
Iron 7	mg	

Gazpacho

4 very ripe tomatoes, peeled
and seeded
1 green bell pepper, cored and
seeded
1 cucumber, seeded
2 stalks celery
1 onion
1 can (12-ounces) low-sodium
tomato juice

2 cloves garlic, chopped
1/4 cup tomato puree
1 teaspoon dried thyme
1 teaspoon dried basil
Black pepper
2 tablespoons vinegar
Dash of Tabasco sauce

- Wash the vegetables well, chop coarsely, and place in a blender with enough tomato juice to partially cover. Add the garlic, tomato puree, seasonings, vinegar, and Tabasco sauce and puree until smooth. Pour mixture into a bowl and stir in the remaining tomato juice. Chill until ready to serve.

PER SERVING: 99 CALORIES		
MENU EXCHANGE PATTERN		
Dairy .... —	Fruit .... —	
Bread .... —	Meat .... —	
Fat ...... —	Veg. 4	
NUTRITIONAL INFORMATION		
Carbohydrate 22	g	
Protein 5	g	
Total fat 1	g	
Saturated fat 0	g	
Cholesterol 0	mg	
Sodium 188	mg	
Potassium 1037	mg	
Fiber 2.2	g	
Calcium 71	mg	
Iron 2.9	mg	

Rainbow Trout with Lemon and Basil

4 trout, 6 ounces each, cleaned
and dressed
1/2 teaspoon paprika
1/2 cup chopped fresh basil, or 1
tablespoon dried

Juice of 1 lemon
2 tablespoons margarine,
melted
Parsley sprigs (garnish)

- Wash the trout under cold running water and pat dry with paper towels. Place the fish next to each other on a cookie sheet. Sprinkle with paprika, basil, and lemon juice. Drizzle with melted margarine. Broil for 20 minutes, or until trout are done. Garnish with parsley sprigs.

PER SERVING: 387 CALORIES		
MENU EXCHANGE PATTERN		
Dairy .... —	Fruit .... —	
Bread .... —	Meat 5	
Fat 2	Veg. 1/2	
NUTRITIONAL INFORMATION		
Carbohydrate 1	g	
Protein 37	g	
Total fat 25	g	
Saturated fat 2.8	g	
Cholesterol 94	mg	
Sodium 67	mg	
Potassium 821	mg	
Fiber 0.1	g	
Calcium 37	mg	
Iron 1.8	mg	

Green Peas with Water Chestnuts

2 green onions, trimmed and
chopped
1 cup shredded iceberg lettuce
1 tablespoon safflower oil
1 tablespoon all-purpose flour
3 tablespoons water

1 package frozen green peas,
cooked
1 can (5 ounces) sliced water
chestnuts
Black pepper

- In nonstick skillet, sauté green onions and shredded lettuce in oil until wilted, about 3 minutes. Combine flour with water in a cup and add to onion mixture; stir until thickened. Add peas, water chestnuts, and pepper. Heat thoroughly and serve.

PER SERVING: 125 CALORIES		
MENU EXCHANGE PATTERN		
Dairy ..... —	Fruit ..... —	
Bread 1	Meat ..... —	
Fat 1/2	Veg. 1	
NUTRITIONAL INFORMATION		
Carbohydrate 18	g	
Protein 5	g	
Total fat 4	g	
Saturated fat 0.3	g	
Cholesterol 0	mg	
Sodium 9	mg	
Potassium 433	mg	
Fiber 2	g	
Calcium 36	mg	
Iron 1.9	mg	

Raspberry-Blueberry Parfait

1 cup fresh blueberries
1 cup low-fat vanilla frozen
* yogurt*
1 cup fresh raspberries
½ cup Low-Fat Whipped
* Topping (recipe follows)*

PER SERVING: 111 CALORIES			
MENU EXCHANGE PATTERN			
Dairy . . . . . . ½		Fruit	2
Bread . . . . —		Meat	—
Fat . . . . —		Veg.	—
NUTRITIONAL INFORMATION			
Carbohydrate 22			g
Protein 3			g
Total fat 2			g
Saturated fat 0.9			g
Cholesterol 6			mg
Sodium 53			mg
Potassium 216			mg
Fiber 1.4			g
Calcium 114			mg
Iron . . . . 0.4 mg			

• In each of 4 parfait glasses, layer blueberries, yogurt, and raspberries. Top each serving with whipped topping.

Note: Analysis includes topping.

Low-Fat Whipped Topping

⅓ cup evaporated skim milk   *1 tablespoon sugar*
½ teaspoon unflavored gelatin   *½ teaspoon vanilla extract*
1 tablespoon cold water   *1 teaspoon lemon juice*

PER SERVING: 29 CALORIES			
MENU EXCHANGE PATTERN			
Dairy . . . . . —		Fruit	1
Bread . . . . —		Meat	—
Fat . . . . —		Veg.	—
NUTRITIONAL INFORMATION			
Carbohydrate 6			g
Protein 2			g
Total fat 0			g
Saturated fat 0			g
Cholesterol 1			mg
Sodium 24			mg
Potassium 71			mg
Fiber 0			g
Calcium 61			mg
Iron . . . . 0.1 mg			

• Chill evaporated milk in a small bowl. Sprinkle gelatin over cold water in small saucepan, then stir over low heat until dissolved. Add to milk and beat until stiff. Add sugar, vanilla, and lemon juice. Use immediately or chill and beat again before serving. Makes about ½ cup. 1 serving = 2 table-spoons.

SEAFOOD ENTREES

2

Tomato-Vegetable Soup

Fillet of Sole

Brown Rice

Spinach Salad with Tomato and Onion

Raisin Cookies

Serves 4

PER SERVING: 715 CALORIES		
MENU EXCHANGE PATTERN		
Dairy . . . . . —	Fruit . . . . . —	
Bread 3	Meat 4	
Fat 3	Veg. 5½	
NUTRITIONAL INFORMATION		
Carbohydrate 78	g	
Protein 42	g	
Total fat 28	g	
Saturated fat 2.6	g	
Cholesterol 85	mg	
Sodium 451	mg	
Potassium 1838	mg	
Fiber 3.1	g	
Calcium 178	mg	
Iron 7.4	mg	

Tomato-Vegetable Soup

1 clove garlic
1 small onion, sliced
1 cucumber, sliced
2 tomatoes, sliced
1 green bell pepper, seeded
1 stalk celery, sliced
1/8 teaspoon cayenne pepper

3 tablespoons red wine vinegar
1 tablespoon safflower oil
3/4 cup low-sodium tomato juice
1 teaspoon chopped fresh
    parsley
1/4 teaspoon freshly ground
    pepper

Garnish

1/2 cup fresh bread cubes
2 teaspoons safflower oil
1 clove garlic, minced

1/4 cucumber, diced
1/4 onion, chopped
1/4 green bell pepper, chopped

- Chop the first six ingredients in a blender or food processor. Add cayenne pepper, vinegar, oil, and tomato juice and process briefly. Chill at least 2 hours before serving.

- For the garnish, brown the bread cubes with the garlic in the oil over medium-high heat in a nonstick skillet for about 5 minutes. Garnish soup with croutons, cucumber, onion, and green pepper just before serving.

PER SERVING: 157 CALORIES			
MENU EXCHANGE PATTERN			
Dairy	—	Fruit	—
Bread	—	Meat	—
Fat	1	Veg.	4
NUTRITIONAL INFORMATION			
Carbohydrate	22		g
Protein	4		g
Total fat	7		g
Saturated fat	0.6		g
Cholesterol	0		mg
Sodium	213		mg
Potassium	573		mg
Fiber	1.5		g
Calcium	57		mg
Iron	2.2		mg

Fillet of Sole

4 fillets of sole, 6 ounces each
2 tablespoons safflower oil
Juice of 2 lemons
Black pepper

- Sauté sole fillets in safflower oil in nonstick skillet over medium-high heat, turning at least once, for about 10 minutes (or until fish flakes easily with a fork). Add lemon juice and black pepper to taste. Serve on brown rice.

PER SERVING: 219 CALORIES			
MENU EXCHANGE PATTERN			
Dairy	—	Fruit	—
Bread	—	Meat	4
Fat	—	Veg.	—
NUTRITIONAL INFORMATION			
Carbohydrate	2		g
Protein	29		g
Total fat	10		g
Saturated fat	1		g
Cholesterol	85		mg
Sodium	133		mg
Potassium	607		mg
Fiber	0		g
Calcium	25		mg
Iron	1.4		mg

Brown Rice

2 1/2 cups water
1 cup brown rice

- Bring water to boil in medium-large saucepan. Stir in rice and return to boil. Cover, reduce heat to low, and cook until all water is absorbed, about 45 to 50 minutes.

PER SERVING: 180 CALORIES			
MENU EXCHANGE PATTERN			
Dairy	—	Fruit	—
Bread	2 1/2	Meat	—
Fat	—	Veg.	—
NUTRITIONAL INFORMATION			
Carbohydrate	37		g
Protein	4		g
Total fat	1		g
Saturated fat	0		g
Cholesterol	0		mg
Sodium	5		mg
Potassium	107		mg
Fiber	0.5		g
Calcium	16		mg
Iron	0.8		mg

Spinach Salad with Tomato and Onion

12 ounces raw spinach
1 clove garlic, peeled and split in half
4 teaspoons lemon juice
4 teaspoons safflower oil

Freshly ground black pepper
1 small ripe tomato, cut in wedges
1/4 red onion, thinly sliced

- Wash the spinach in several changes of cold water. Discard tough stems. Drain spinach leaves and chill in a damp cloth. Tear into bite-sized pieces. Rub bottom of salad bowl with garlic. Add lemon juice and oil. Chill the seasoned bowl. Just before serving, add spinach leaves and sprinkle with pepper, and toss lightly. Garnish with tomato wedges and onion rings.

Note: To reduce fat intake, eliminate lemon juice and safflower oil and substitute 3 tablespoons of a commercial low-calorie Italian dressing. Adjusted analysis: calories = 48; exchanges = 1 Vegetable, 1 Fat.

PER SERVING: 77 CALORIES		
MENU EXCHANGE PATTERN		
Dairy ..... —	Fruit ..... —	
Bread ..... —	Meat ..... —	
Fat 1	Veg. 1½	
NUTRITIONAL INFORMATION		
Carbohydrate 7	g	
Protein 3	g	
Total fat 5	g	
Saturated fat 0.4	g	
Cholesterol 0	mg	
Sodium 56	mg	
Potassium 480	mg	
Fiber 0.8	g	
Calcium 80	mg	
Iron 2.6	mg	

Raisin Cookies

1/2 cup water
1 cup raisins
1/2 cup safflower oil
3/4 cup honey
1 egg substitute
1/2 teaspoon vanilla extract
2 cups whole wheat pastry flour

1/2 teaspoon baking powder
1/2 teaspoon ground cinnamon
1/8 teaspoon ground nutmeg
1/8 teaspoon ground allspice
1/2 teaspoon salt
1/2 cup chopped nuts
1/2 cup (about) wheat germ

- Preheat oven to 400°F.

- Combine water and raisins in a small saucepan and simmer for 5 minutes. Cool. Mix oil, honey, egg substitute, and vanilla and beat well. Add cooled raisin mixture. Combine all dry ingredients and add to liquid mixture. Add enough wheat germ to form a soft dough that will hold its shape.

- Drop dough by tablespoonfuls onto greased and floured baking sheets. Bake until golden brown, about 12 to 15 minutes. Cool on racks. Makes 3 dozen; 1 serving = 1 cookie.

PER SERVING: 82 CALORIES		
MENU EXCHANGE PATTERN		
Dairy ..... —	Fruit ..... —	
Bread ..... ½	Meat ..... —	
Fat 1	Veg. ...... —	
NUTRITIONAL INFORMATION		
Carbohydrate 9	g	
Protein 2	g	
Total fat 5	g	
Saturated fat 0.3	g	
Cholesterol 0	mg	
Sodium 44	mg	
Potassium 71	mg	
Fiber 0.3	g	
Calcium 0	mg	
Iron 0.4	mg	

SEAFOOD ENTREES

3

Hearts of Palm

Grilled Swordfish with Pink and
Green Peppercorns

Baked Rice

Asparagus

Amaretti

Serves 2

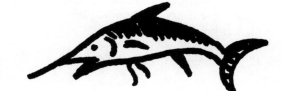

PER SERVING: 822 CALORIES		
MENU EXCHANGE PATTERN		
Dairy . . . . . —	Fruit 1½	
Bread 3	Meat 5	
Fat 4½	Veg. 5½	
NUTRITIONAL INFORMATION		
Carbohydrate 86	g	
Protein 41	g	
Total fat 36	g	
Saturated fat 3.3	g	
Cholesterol. 38	mg	
Sodium 349	mg	
Potassium 915	mg	
Fiber 3.1	g	
Calcium 174	mg	
Iron . . . . 7.4 mg		

Hearts of Palm

6 hearts of palm
2 tablespoons Onion
    Vinaigrette (recipe follows)
2 leaves romaine lettuce,
    washed and dried

1 large tomato, cut in wedges
2 black olives
1/2 lemon, cut in wedges
Parsley sprigs

- Cut hearts of palm in half crosswise and marinate in dressing overnight in refrigerator.

- Arrange lettuce leaves on individual salad plates. Top with hearts of palm. Garnish with tomatoes, olives, lemon wedges, and parsley.

Note: Hearts of palm are available in cans in the gourmet section of most supermarkets.
    To reduce fat intake, substitute 2 tablespoons of a commercial low-calorie Italian dressing for the Vinaigrette. Adjusted analysis: calories = 74; exchanges = 2 1/2 Vegetable, 1/2 Fat.

PER SERVING: 142 CALORIES

MENU EXCHANGE PATTERN

Dairy . . . . . —	Fruit . . . . . —	
Bread . . . . . —	Meat . . . . . —	
Fat 2	Veg. 2 1/2	

NUTRITIONAL INFORMATION

Carbohydrate 11	g
Protein 4	g
Total fat 10	g
Saturated fat 0.9	g
Cholesterol 0	mg
Sodium 331	mg
Potassium 497	mg
Fiber 1.7	g
Calcium 70	mg
Iron 3.4	mg

Onion Vinaigrette Dressing

1 teaspoon Dijon-style mustard
1/2 cup red wine vinegar
1/4 teaspoon black pepper
1 cup safflower oil
1 purple onion, sliced

1/2 clove garlic, minced
2 tablespoons chopped fresh
    parsley
2 tablespoons diced pimiento
Juice of 1 lemon

- Mix mustard, vinegar, and pepper in a small bowl. Slowly pour in oil, beating until smooth. Add remaining ingredients and chill. Makes 1 1/2 cups; 1 serving = 1 tablespoon.

PER SERVING: 84 CALORIES

MENU EXCHANGE PATTERN

Dairy . . . . . —	Fruit . . . . . —	
Bread . . . . . —	Meat . . . . . —	
Fat 2	Veg. . . . . . . —	

NUTRITIONAL INFORMATION

Carbohydrate 1	g
Protein 0	g
Total fat 9	g
Saturated fat 0.8	g
Cholesterol 0	mg
Sodium 3	mg
Potassium 17	mg
Fiber 0	g
Calcium 3	mg
Iron 0.1	mg

Grilled Swordfish with Pink and Green Peppercorns

2 swordfish steaks, 5 ounces
  each
Black pepper
2 teaspoons safflower oil
3 tablespoons dry white wine
Juice of ½ lemon
1 teaspoon finely chopped
  shallot

2 teaspoons margarine,
  softened
1 teaspoon pink peppercorns
1 teaspoon green peppercorns
Chopped fresh parsley

- Season swordfish with pepper. Baste with oil, then broil or grill just until firm and opaque, about 10 to 15 minutes (turn over when half-cooked). Transfer to a warm platter and keep warm.

- Combine wine, lemon juice, and shallot in a skillet. Bring to a boil, then continue boiling until reduced in volume by ½. Stir in margarine and peppercorns, then pour over swordfish. Sprinkle with parsley and serve.

Note: The cooking time for the fish will depend on the heat of the charcoal and the thickness of the fish. Be careful not to overcook.

PER SERVING: 265 CALORIES

MENU EXCHANGE PATTERN

Dairy	—	Fruit	—
Bread	—	Meat	4
Fat	½	Veg.	1

NUTRITIONAL INFORMATION

Carbohydrate	3	g
Protein	27	g
Total fat	14	g
Saturated fat	1.1	g
Cholesterol	38	mg
Sodium	1	mg
Potassium	47	mg
Fiber	0.1	g
Calcium	34	mg
Iron	1.5	mg

Baked Rice

2 teaspoons margarine
¼ cup chopped onion
½ cup white rice

1¼ cups hot Homemade
  Chicken Stock (page 36)
1 bay leaf

- Preheat oven to 350°F. Melt margarine in a heavy large skillet. Add onion and sauté over low heat until soft, about 5 minutes. Add rice and mix with a wooden spatula. Cover with the hot broth and add bay leaf. Bring to a boil, cover, and place in oven for 20 minutes. Before serving, discard bay leaf and fluff the rice with a fork.

PER SERVING: 219 CALORIES

MENU EXCHANGE PATTERN

Dairy	—	Fruit	—
Bread	2	Meat	—
Fat	1	Veg.	1

NUTRITIONAL INFORMATION

Carbohydrate	41	g
Protein	4	g
Total fat	4	g
Saturated fat	0.7	g
Cholesterol	0	mg
Sodium	5	mg
Potassium	79	mg
Fiber	0.3	g
Calcium	18	mg
Iron	1.5	mg

Asparagus

8 jumbo asparagus
1 quart water

- Trim 1 inch from the bottom of each asparagus stalk. In a large pot, bring water to a boil. Drop in asparagus and boil for 3 to 4 minutes. Drain and serve.

PER SERVING: 20 CALORIES			
MENU EXCHANGE PATTERN			
Dairy . . . . . —		Fruit . . . . . —	
Bread . . . . . —		Meat . . . . . —	
Fat . . . . —		Veg. 1	
NUTRITIONAL INFORMATION			
Carbohydrate 4			g
Protein 2			g
Total fat 0			g
Saturated fat 0			g
Cholesterol 0			mg
Sodium 1			mg
Potassium 183			mg
Fiber 0.7			g
Calcium 21			mg
Iron 0.6			mg

Amaretti

2¼ cups (9 ounces) finely
ground almonds
1 pound confectioners sugar

½ teaspoon grated lemon rind
4 egg whites
¼ cup coarse sugar

- Preheat oven to 250°F. Combine ground almonds, confectioners sugar, and lemon rind in a large bowl. Add the unbeaten egg whites and blend well. Whip slowly until foamy. Place mixture in a pastry tube and pipe dough in small mounds onto a cookie sheet lined with parchment paper. Moisten the mounds with a drop of water and sprinkle with coarse sugar. Bake for 15 minutes, then increase the heat to 300°F and continue baking until golden brown, about 15 minutes longer. Makes 60 cookies; 1 serving = 1 cookie.

Note: Coarse sugar is available in gourmet shops. It is sometimes called pearl sugar.

PER SERVING: 177 CALORIES			
MENU EXCHANGE PATTERN			
Dairy . . . . . —		Fruit 1½	
Bread 1		Meat . . . . . —	
Fat 1		Veg. . . . . —	
NUTRITIONAL INFORMATION			
Carbohydrate 28			g
Protein 3			g
Total fat 7			g
Saturated fat 0.6			g
Cholesterol 0			mg
Sodium 11			mg
Potassium 109			mg
Fiber 0.3			g
Calcium 31			mg
Iron 0.6			mg

SEAFOOD ENTREES

4

Fresh Mushroom Salad

Poached Salmon with Green Sauce

Lemon Spiced Rice

Strawberries with Raspberry Sauce

Serves 4

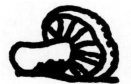

PER SERVING: 894 CALORIES		
MENU EXCHANGE PATTERN		
Dairy...... ½	Fruit 2½	
Bread 3	Meat 5½	
Fat 3	Veg. 3	
NUTRITIONAL INFORMATION		
Carbohydrate 74	g	
Protein 50	g	
Total fat 34	g	
Saturated fat 8.6	g	
Cholesterol 63	mg	
Sodium 277	mg	
Potassium 1795	mg	
Fiber 5.6	g	
Calcium 325	mg	
Iron 5.4	mg	

Fresh Mushroom Salad

⅓ cup chopped green onions
2 cloves garlic, minced
¼ cup chopped fresh parsley
1 teaspoon dry mustard
1 teaspoon Worcestershire
sauce

2 tablespoons dry red wine
2 tablespoons safflower oil
2 tablespoons red wine vinegar
⅛ teaspoon black pepper
2 cups sliced fresh mushrooms
1 head lettuce

PER SERVING: 97 CALORIES			
MENU EXCHANGE PATTERN			
Dairy	—	Fruit	—
Bread	—	Meat	—
Fat	1½	Veg.	1
NUTRITIONAL INFORMATION			
Carbohydrate	6	g	
Protein	2	g	
Total fat	7	g	
Saturated fat	0.6	g	
Cholesterol	0	mg	
Sodium	27	mg	
Potassium	372	mg	
Fiber	0.8	g	
Calcium	53	mg	
Iron	0.6	mg	

- Blend all ingredients except mushrooms and lettuce in a large nonaluminum bowl. Add sliced mushrooms and toss very well. Arrange lettuce on individual serving plates and place mushroom salad in center.

Poached Salmon

1 whole dressed salmon, about
1½ pounds
1 lemon, sliced
1 large onion, sliced

1 tablespoon whole pickling
spice
1½ cups (about) dry white wine
Green Sauce (recipe follows)

Garnishes (if serving cold)
1 lime, sliced
Cucumber slices
Dill sprigs

- You can poach on top of the stove or in the oven. If using the oven, preheat to 325°F.

- Wash the fish under cold water and pat dry. Put the fish on a double layer of cheesecloth large enough to wrap around it comfortably and leave ends for lifting. Arrange the lemon and onion slices across the top of the fish and sprinkle it with the pickling spice. Wrap up the cheesecloth; then, using the ends as handles, pick up the fish and place it in a fish poacher or a foil-lined roasting pan.

- Add enough wine to half cover the salmon. Cover the pan with a lid or seal with foil. Poach in the oven for 25 to 30 minutes, or until the fish feels firm to the touch. On top of the stove, simmer it, covered, over low heat for 20 to 30 minutes. While the fish cooks, prepare the green sauce.

- To serve hot, lift the salmon by the cheesecloth ends to a warm platter and unwrap. Serve the meat on top of the skeleton first, then remove the backbone and ribs in a single piece, starting at the tail. Serve the sauce from a separate bowl.

- To serve cold, let the fish cool, uncovered, in the poaching liquid. Lift by the cheesecloth ends and transfer the salmon to a serving board or platter. Unwrap the top of the fish and carefully peel away the skin on the exposed side, scraping off the layer of dark meat. Turn the fish over using the cheesecloth. Discard the cloth and peel and scrape the second side. Cover the fish with a damp cloth and chill for at least 2 hours. Garnish with slices of lime and cucumber and sprigs of dill. Serve with the sauce.

Note: A whole large cooked fish is a dramatic dish; it seems to mark a special occasion. The basic technique for poaching fish remains the same no matter what the variety or size. The guidelines are simple: Poach 6 to 8 minutes per pound, and never let the stock boil, just simmer. This dish can be served hot or cold.

PER SERVING: 473 CALORIES		
MENU EXCHANGE PATTERN		
Dairy . . . . . —	Fruit . . . . . —	
Bread 1	Meat 5½	
Fat 1	Veg. 2	
NUTRITIONAL INFORMATION		
Carbohydrate 11	g	
Protein 40	g	
Total fat 23	g	
Saturated fat 7.1	g	
Cholesterol 60	mg	
Sodium 91	mg	
Potassium 892	mg	
Fiber 0.5	g	
Calcium 171	mg	
Iron . . . . 2.5 mg		

Green Sauce

1 cup low-fat cottage cheese
1 tablespoon grated Parmesan
   cheese
1 clove garlic, minced
2 tablespoons minced
   watercress
1 tablespoon minced spinach
   leaves

2 teaspoons chopped fresh
   chives
2 teaspoons chopped fresh
   parsley
2 teaspoons chopped fresh dill

- Place cottage cheese in blender or food processor and blend until smooth. Add remaining ingredients and blend. Makes about 1 cup; 1 serving = ¼ cup.

PER SERVING: 34 CALORIES		
MENU EXCHANGE PATTERN		
Dairy . . . . . . ½	Fruit . . . . . —	
Bread . . . . —	Meat . . . . . —	
Fat . . . . —	Veg. . . . . . —	
NUTRITIONAL INFORMATION		
Carbohydrate 2	g	
Protein 5	g	
Total fat 1	g	
Saturated fat 0.6	g	
Cholesterol 3	mg	
Sodium 140	mg	
Potassium 51	mg	
Fiber 0.1	g	
Calcium 42	mg	
Iron . . . . 0.2 mg		

Lemon Spiced Rice

2 teaspoons margarine
1/3 cup chopped celery
1/3 cup chopped onion
2/3 cup rice
3 tablespoons lemon juice

1 1/3 cups water or Homemade
   Chicken Stock (page 36)
1/4 teaspoon dried thyme
Rind of 1/2 lemon, grated

- Melt margarine in large nonstick skillet. Add celery and onion and sauté over low heat until soft, about 5 minutes. Add rice and cook over medium heat for about 5 minutes, stirring constantly. Add lemon juice, stock, thyme, and lemon rind and bring to a boil. Cover, reduce heat, and cook until water is absorbed, about 20 to 25 minutes. Fluff with fork before serving.

PER SERVING: 144 CALORIES		
MENU EXCHANGE PATTERN		
Dairy . . . . . —	Fruit . . . . . —	
Bread 1½	Meat —	
Fat . . . . ½	Veg. 1	
NUTRITIONAL INFORMATION		
Carbohydrate 28	g	
Protein 3	g	
Total fat 2	g	
Saturated fat 0.3	g	
Cholesterol 0	mg	
Sodium 16	mg	
Potassium 99	mg	
Fiber 0.2	g	
Calcium 16	mg	
Iron 1	mg	

Strawberries with Raspberry Sauce

2 tablespoons cornstarch
1/2 cup raspberry liqueur or Port
1 pound fresh raspberries
3 cups fresh strawberries, hulled
   and sliced

- Combine the cornstarch and liqueur in a small saucepan. Stir over low heat until the mixture simmers and thickens.

- Puree the raspberries until smooth in a blender or food processor. Pour through a strainer to remove seeds and add to the liqueur mixture; heat through.

- When ready to serve, spoon the hot sauce over the strawberries.

Note: Don't feel limited to strawberries and raspberries here; do experiment with melon, banana, papaya, and other fruits. Serve the fruit puree over other whole fruits or sherbet.

PER SERVING: 146 CALORIES		
MENU EXCHANGE PATTERN		
Dairy . . . . . —	Fruit 2½	
Bread . . . . . ½	Meat . . . . . —	
Fat . . . . —	Veg. . . . . . . —	
NUTRITIONAL INFORMATION		
Carbohydrate 27	g	
Protein 2	g	
Total fat 1	g	
Saturated fat 0	g	
Cholesterol 0	mg	
Sodium 3	mg	
Potassium 381	mg	
Fiber 4	g	
Calcium 43	mg	
Iron 1.1	mg	

SEAFOOD ENTREES

5

Remington Salad with Tomato Vinaigrette

Grilled Swordfish Steaks with Sautéed Shiitake Mushrooms

Mango Sorbet with Mixed Berries

Serves 8

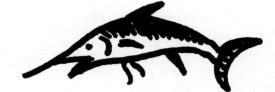

PER SERVING: 571 CALORIES			
MENU EXCHANGE PATTERN			
Dairy	—	Fruit	3
Bread	1	Meat	4½
Fat	2	Veg.	2
NUTRITIONAL INFORMATION			
Carbohydrate	47	g	
Protein	38	g	
Total fat	20	g	
Saturated fat	1.2	g	
Cholesterol	46	mg	
Sodium	423	mg	
Potassium	835	mg	
Fiber	4.7	g	
Calcium	118	mg	
Iron	3.6	mg	

Remington Salad

1 bunch watercress
1/2 head radicchio
1/2 head curly endive
5 ounces enoki mushrooms
    (2 cups)

1 cup Tomato Vinaigrette
    (recipe follows)
1/4 basket alfalfa sprouts
16 spears cooked asparagus

- Coarsely chop watercress, radicchio, curly endive, and mushrooms. Toss with vinaigrette. Serve in center of each salad plate topped with alfalfa sprouts and 2 crossed asparagus spears.

PER SERVING: 23 CALORIES		
MENU EXCHANGE PATTERN		
Dairy . . . . . —	Fruit . . . . . —	
Bread . . . . —	Meat . . . . . —	
Fat . . . . —	Veg. 1	
NUTRITIONAL INFORMATION		
Carbohydrate 4		g
Protein 2		g
Total fat 0		g
Saturated fat 0		g
Cholesterol 0		mg
Sodium 14		mg
Potassium 250		mg
Fiber 0.7		g
Calcium 43		mg
Iron 1.1		mg

Tomato Vinaigrette

1/4 cup sherry vinegar
1 teaspoon Pommery or other
    coarse-grained Dijon-style
    mustard
1/4 cup safflower oil
1/2 shallot, chopped

1/2 large tomato, peeled, seeded,
    and chopped
1 teaspoon chopped fresh
    parsley
Freshly ground black pepper

- Mix vinegar and mustard. Gradually whisk in oil. Add shallot, tomato, and parsley. Add pepper to taste and stir before serving. Makes about 1 cup; 1 serving = 2 tablespoons.

PER SERVING: 86 CALORIES		
MENU EXCHANGE PATTERN		
Dairy . . . . . —	Fruit . . . . . —	
Bread . . . . —	Meat . . . . . —	
Fat 2	Veg. . . . . . . —	
NUTRITIONAL INFORMATION		
Carbohydrate 1		g
Protein 1		g
Total fat 9		g
Saturated fat 0.7		g
Cholesterol 0		mg
Sodium 11		mg
Potassium 52		mg
Fiber 0.1		g
Calcium 4		mg
Iron 0.1		mg

Grilled Swordfish Steaks

2 teaspoons safflower oil
2 tablespoons chopped shallot
2 cups sherry
1 teaspoon sugar
1 cup veal broth or Homemade
    Chicken Stock (page 36)
3 tablespoons low-sodium soy
    sauce

Black pepper
4 tablespoons arrowroot mixed
    with 4 tablespoons water
8 swordfish steaks, 6 ounces
    each
Sautéed Shiitake Mushrooms
    (recipe follows)

- Prepare barbecue grill with mesquite charcoal. While grill is heating, heat oil in a large nonstick skillet over low heat. Add shallot and sauté until soft, about 5 minutes. Add sherry, increase heat to high, and boil until volume is reduced by ½. Add sugar and stock and cook for an additional 5 minutes. Add soy sauce and pepper to taste. Lower heat to medium-high and add arrowroot mixture and cook about 2 more minutes, stirring constantly, until sauce thickens slightly and becomes translucent.

- Grill swordfish steaks over mesquite, about 10 to 15 minutes, turning at least once. Serve with sauce. Accompany with mushrooms.

PER SERVING: 315 CALORIES			
MENU EXCHANGE PATTERN			
Dairy	—	Fruit	—
Bread	1	Meat	4½
Fat	—	Veg.	—
NUTRITIONAL INFORMATION			
Carbohydrate	10		g
Protein	33		g
Total fat	8		g
Saturated fat	0.1		g
Cholesterol	46		mg
Sodium	388		mg
Potassium	78		mg
Fiber	0		g
Calcium	38		mg
Iron	1.7		mg

Sautéed Shiitake Mushrooms

4 teaspoons margarine
10 ounces shiitake mushrooms

- Melt margarine in a small nonstick skillet. Sauté whole mushrooms over medium heat until softened, about 5–10 minutes. Serve with swordfish.

PER SERVING: 26 CALORIES			
MENU EXCHANGE PATTERN			
Dairy	—	Fruit	—
Bread	—	Meat	—
Fat	—	Veg.	1
NUTRITIONAL INFORMATION			
Carbohydrate	2		g
Protein	1		g
Total fat	2		g
Saturated fat	0.3		g
Cholesterol	0		mg
Sodium	5		mg
Potassium	145		mg
Fiber	0.2		g
Calcium	2		mg
Iron	0.2		mg

Mango Sorbet with Mixed Berries

Flesh of 4 very ripe mangos
1 cup hot water
2 cups fresh raspberries
2 cups fresh blackberries
2 cups fresh blueberries

- Puree mango in blender or processor and pass through sieve. Mix well with hot water. Churn in an ice cream maker or freeze in an ice cube tray, stirring periodically until frozen.

- Scoop sorbet onto dessert plates and surround with berries.

PER SERVING: 121 CALORIES			
MENU EXCHANGE PATTERN			
Dairy	—	Fruit	3
Bread	—	Meat	—
Fat	—	Veg.	—
NUTRITIONAL INFORMATION			
Carbohydrate	30		g
Protein	1		g
Total fat	1		g
Saturated fat	0.1		g
Cholesterol	0		mg
Sodium	4		mg
Potassium	310		mg
Fiber	4		g
Calcium	31		mg
Iron	0.5		mg

SEAFOOD ENTREES

6

Cream of Asparagus and Leek Soup

Hot Zucchini and Tomato Salad

Poached Salmon

Boiled New Potatoes

Strawberries and Grand Marnier

Serves 4

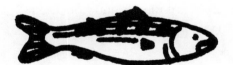

PER SERVING: 641 CALORIES		
MENU EXCHANGE PATTERN		
Dairy . . . . . . ½	Fruit 1½	
Bread 1½	Meat 4½	
Fat 2½	Veg. 3	
NUTRITIONAL INFORMATION		
Carbohydrate 53	g	
Protein 41	g	
Total fat 28	g	
Saturated fat 6.9	g	
Cholesterol 51	mg	
Sodium 170	mg	
Potassium 2053	mg	
Fiber 3.3	g	
Calcium 307	mg	
Iron 4.2	mg	

Cream of Asparagus and Leek Soup

*1 bunch asparagus spears
(about 8)
4 teaspoons margarine
1½ cups chopped leeks (white
portion only)
1 tablespoon all-purpose flour*

*2 cups Homemade Chicken
Stock (page 36)
½ cup evaporated skim milk
⅛ teaspoon white pepper
Pinch of nutmeg*

- Trim bottoms from asparagus. Steam asparagus until cooked, about 5 minutes. Cut off and reserve tips. Puree stems in blender or food processor until smooth.

- Melt margarine in saucepan, add leeks. Sauté over medium-high heat until soft, about 8 minutes. Whisk in flour; gradually stir in stock. Add pureed asparagus and simmer 10 minutes, then add milk, asparagus tips, and seasonings. Heat soup through, but do not boil, and serve.

PER SERVING: 108 CALORIES

MENU EXCHANGE PATTERN

Dairy . . . . . ½	Fruit . . . . . —
Bread . . . . —	Meat . . . . . —
Fat 1	Veg. 1

NUTRITIONAL INFORMATION

Carbohydrate	 10	g
Protein	 4	g
Total fat	 6	g
Saturated fat	. . . . 0.7	g
Cholesterol	 1	mg
Sodium	 89	mg
Potassium	 292	mg
Fiber	. . . . 0.7	g
Calcium	 117	mg
Iron	. . . . 0.7	mg

Hot Zucchini and Tomato Salad

*2 teaspoons margarine
½ onion, chopped
3 cups thinly sliced zucchini*

*2 small tomatoes, diced
½ teaspoon dried basil*

- Melt margarine in a large nonstick skillet over medium-high heat. Add onion and sauté 2 minutes. Add zucchini and continue to sauté for 2 to 3 minutes. Add tomatoes and basil, cover, and cook until vegetables are tender and hot, about 2 more minutes.

PER SERVING: 63 CALORIES

MENU EXCHANGE PATTERN

Dairy . . . . . —	Fruit . . . . . —
Bread . . . . —	Meat . . . . . —
Fat . . . . ½	Veg. 2

NUTRITIONAL INFORMATION

Carbohydrate	 10	g
Protein	 2	g
Total fat	 2	g
Saturated fat	. . . . 0.3	g
Cholesterol	 0	mg
Sodium	 6	mg
Potassium	 414	mg
Fiber	. . . . 1.1	g
Calcium	 45	mg
Iron	. . . . 0.9	mg

Poached Salmon

*1 pound salmon fillets
½ cup water
1 tablespoon lemon juice*

*2 bay leaves
Boiled New Potatoes (recipe
follows)*

- Preheat oven to 375°F.

- Place salmon fillets in shallow pan with water, lemon juice, and bay leaves. Cover and bake for 15 to 20 minutes, depending on thickness of salmon (approximately 10 minutes per inch). When salmon is just firm and opaque, remove from liquid and serve with potatoes.

PER SERVING: 308 CALORIES

MENU EXCHANGE PATTERN

Dairy . . . . . —	Fruit . . . . . —
Bread . . . . —	Meat 4½
Fat 1	Veg. . . . . —

NUTRITIONAL INFORMATION

Carbohydrate	 0	g
Protein	 31	g
Total fat	 19	g
Saturated fat	. . . . 5.9	g
Cholesterol	 50	mg
Sodium	 68	mg
Potassium	 557	mg
Fiber	 0	g
Calcium	 112	mg
Iron	. . . . 1.2	mg

Boiled New Potatoes

1 pound new potatoes
2 tablespoons chopped fresh
*   parsley*

- Place potatoes in large saucepan and cover with water.
  Cover pan and bring to boil, then simmer for 20 minutes or
  until potatoes are tender. Drain and peel if desired. Sprinkle
  with parsley and serve.

PER SERVING: 105 CALORIES

MENU EXCHANGE PATTERN

Dairy	—	Fruit	—
Bread	1½	Meat	—
Fat	—	Veg.	—

NUTRITIONAL INFORMATION

Carbohydrate	23	g
Protein	3	g
Total fat	0	g
Saturated fat	0	g
Cholesterol	0	mg
Sodium	5	mg
Potassium	574	mg
Fiber	0.8	g
Calcium	15	mg
Iron	0.9	mg

Strawberries and Grand Marnier

3½ cups sliced strawberries
1 ounce (2 tablespoons) Grand
*   Marnier*

- Mix strawberries with liqueur and let stand 30 minutes.
  Serve in dessert dishes.

PER SERVING: 57 CALORIES

MENU EXCHANGE PATTERN

Dairy	—	Fruit	1½
Bread	—	Meat	—
Fat	—	Veg.	—

NUTRITIONAL INFORMATION

Carbohydrate	9	g
Protein	1	g
Total fat	1	g
Saturated fat	0	g
Cholesterol	0	mg
Sodium	2	mg
Potassium	216	mg
Fiber	0.7	g
Calcium	1.8	mg
Iron	0.5	mg

SEAFOOD ENTREES

7

Vegetable Crudités with Crabmeat Dip

Catfish Fillets with Creole Sauce

Green Rice

Chocolate Aspic

Serves 6

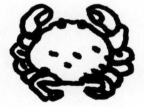

PER SERVING: 593 CALORIES			
MENU EXCHANGE PATTERN			
Dairy	½	Fruit	1
Bread	1½	Meat	4½
Fat	2	Veg.	2
NUTRITIONAL INFORMATION			
Carbohydrate	53	g	
Protein	44	g	
Total fat	24	g	
Saturated fat	3.7	g	
Cholesterol	123	mg	
Sodium	677	mg	
Potassium	1292	mg	
Fiber	1.8	g	
Calcium	196	mg	
Iron	3.7	mg	

Chicken Esterhazy with Julienne of Vegetables; recipe page 117

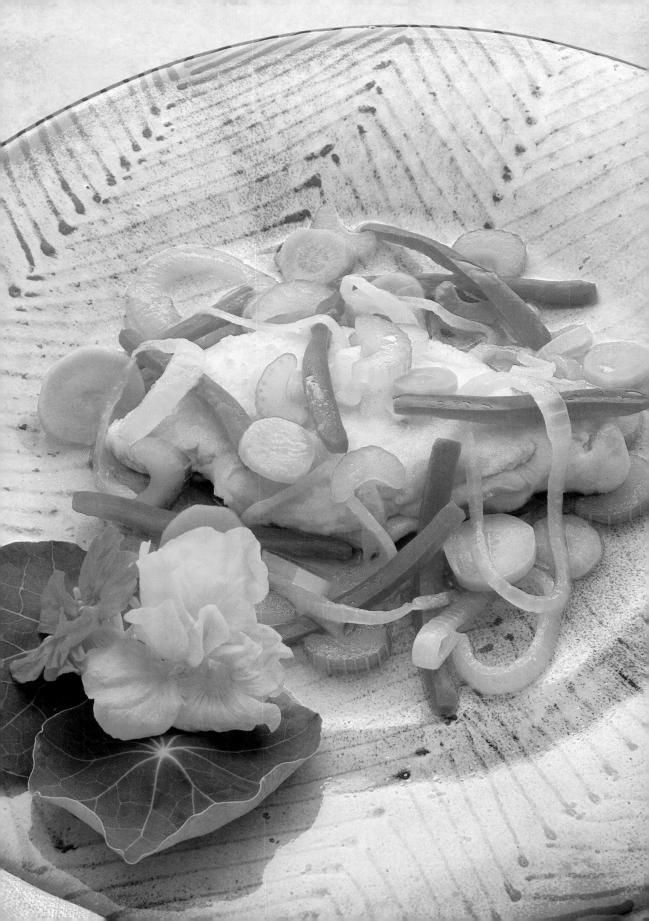

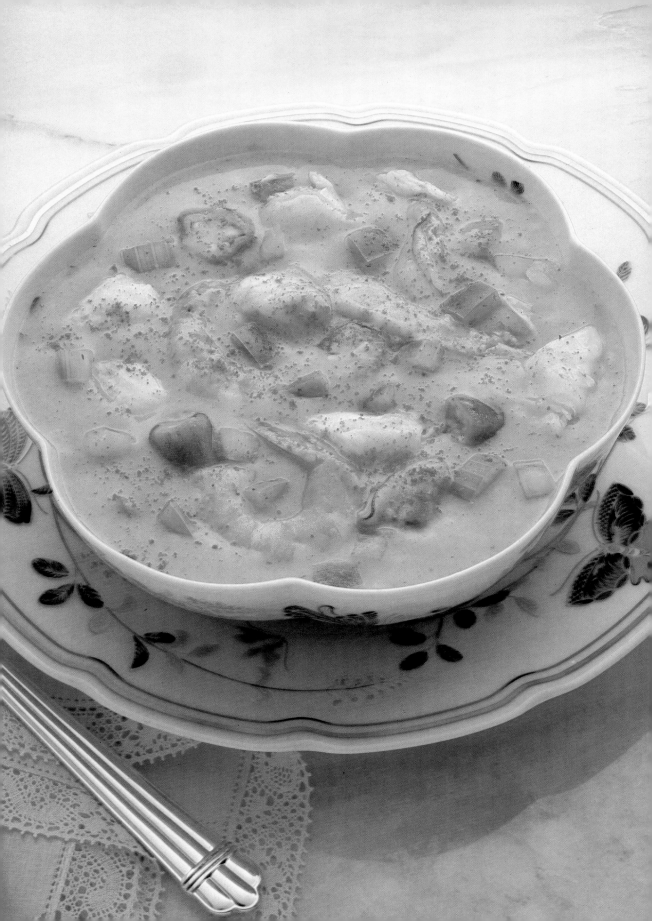

Vegetable Crudités with Crabmeat Dip

1 tablespoon low-sodium soy sauce
6 tablespoons regular mayonnaise
2 tablespoons chopped chives
1/2 cup water chestnuts, drained and sliced

1 can (6 1/2 ounces) crabmeat, drained and flaked
3 carrots, peeled and sliced into 2-inch sticks
2 cups sliced celery, in 2-inch sticks

- Blend first 3 ingredients; stir in water chestnuts and crabmeat. Chill for at least 30 minutes. Serve with carrot and celery sticks. Makes about 1 1/2 cups; 1 serving of dip = 1/4 cup, 1 serving of carrots = 1/2 carrot, 1 serving of celery = 1/2 stalk.

PER SERVING: 154 CALORIES		
MENU EXCHANGE PATTERN		
Dairy . . . . . —	Fruit . . . . . —	
Bread . . . . . —	Meat 1/2	
Fat 1 1/2	Veg. 2	
NUTRITIONAL INFORMATION		
Carbohydrate 9	g	
Protein 5	g	
Total fat 12	g	
Saturated fat 1.2	g	
Cholesterol 20	mg	
Sodium 520	mg	
Potassium 370	mg	
Fiber 0.8	g	
Calcium 41	mg	
Iron 0.8	mg	

Catfish Fillets with Creole Sauce

4 tablespoons margarine
1/2 cup chopped onion
3/4 cup chopped green bell pepper

1 1/2 cups chopped tomato
2 teaspoons drained capers
Cayenne pepper
6 catfish fillets, 6 ounces each

- Melt 2 tablespoons margarine in a small nonstick saucepan over medium-high heat. Add onion and green pepper and cook until onion is translucent, about 5 minutes. Add tomatoes and cook another 5 to 10 minutes, until tomatoes are soft. Stir in capers and season with cayenne to taste. Simmer for several minutes over medium heat to concentrate sauce.

- Meanwhile, in a nonstick skillet, lightly sauté catfish fillets in remaining 2 tablespoons margarine over medium-high heat until cooked through, about 10 minutes. Top with sauce and serve.

PER SERVING: 221 CALORIES		
MENU EXCHANGE PATTERN		
Dairy . . . . . —	Fruit . . . . . —	
Bread . . . . . —	Meat 4	
Fat . . . . —	Veg. . . . . . . —	
NUTRITIONAL INFORMATION		
Carbohydrate 4	g	
Protein 32	g	
Total fat 8	g	
Saturated fat 1.6	g	
Cholesterol 102	mg	
Sodium 108	mg	
Potassium 700	mg	
Fiber 0.5	g	
Calcium 53	mg	
Iron 1.6	mg	

Seafood Okra Gumbo;
recipe page 150

Green Rice

2 cups water
Pinch of black pepper
1 cup rice
1 tablespoon margarine

1/2 cup chopped green onion
1/2 cup chopped celery
1/2 cup finely chopped fresh
    parsley

- Bring water and pepper to a boil. Add rice and reduce heat to very low. Cover and cook rice until tender, about 20 minutes. Melt margarine in a nonstick skillet over medium heat. Add green onion, celery, and parsley and sauté until tender, about 5 minutes. Add cooked rice to vegetable mixture, heat through and serve.

PER SERVING: 141 CALORIES		
MENU EXCHANGE PATTERN		
Dairy ..... —	Fruit ..... —	
Bread 1½	Meat ..... —	
Fat ....½	Veg. ...... —	
NUTRITIONAL INFORMATION		
Carbohydrate 28		g
Protein 3		g
Total fat 2		g
Saturated fat 0		g
Cholesterol 0		mg
Sodium 17		mg
Potassium 120		mg
Fiber 0.3		g
Calcium 27		mg
Iron 1.3		mg

Chocolate Aspic

¾ cup skim milk, scalded
1½ envelopes unflavored
    gelatin
4½ tablespoons unsweetened
    cocoa powder

2 teaspoons vanilla extract
¾ cup skim milk, ice cold
4½ tablespoons sugar
1½ cups crushed ice

- Pour scalded milk into blender and sprinkle gelatin over. Blend at high speed for 30 seconds. Add next 4 ingredients and blend for 30 seconds. Add ice and blend at low speed for 20 seconds, then high speed for 20 seconds. Pour mixture into sherbet glasses and refrigerate. Aspic will set in about 20 minutes.

PER SERVING: 77 CALORIES		
MENU EXCHANGE PATTERN		
Dairy ...... ½	Fruit 1	
Bread .... —	Meat ..... —	
Fat .... —	Veg. ...... —	
NUTRITIONAL INFORMATION		
Carbohydrate 13		g
Protein 5		g
Total fat 2		g
Saturated fat 0.5		g
Cholesterol 1		mg
Sodium 32		mg
Potassium 102		mg
Fiber 0.2		g
Calcium 76		mg
Iron 0		mg

SEAFOOD ENTREES

8

Seafood Okra Gumbo

Sautéed Frogs Legs

Blackeyed Peas

Baked Tomatoes

Poppyseed Fruit Compote

Serves 4

PER SERVING: 723 CALORIES		
MENU EXCHANGE PATTERN		
Dairy . . . . . —	Fruit 3	
Bread 2½	Meat 5	
Fat 3½	Veg. 1	
NUTRITIONAL INFORMATION		
Carbohydrate 61	g	
Protein 49	g	
Total fat 34	g	
Saturated fat 5.3	g	
Cholesterol 202	mg	
Sodium 531	mg	
Potassium 1580	mg	
Fiber 3.7	g	
Calcium 242	mg	
Iron 7.7	mg	

Seafood Okra Gumbo

*½ cup chopped green bell
   pepper*
⅔ cup chopped celery
⅔ cup chopped tomato
4 tablespoons margarine
*⅔ pound shrimp, shelled and
   deveined (size 26/30 per
   pound)*
10 raw oysters
*1 quart fish stock or
   Homemade Chicken Stock
   (page 36)*

3 tablespoons all-purpose flour
4 teaspoons filé powder
¼ pound okra, sliced
3 ounces lump crabmeat
½ clove garlic, finely chopped
¼ onion, chopped
Cayenne pepper

- In a large saucepan sauté green pepper, celery, and tomato in 1 tablespoon margarine until soft, about 5 minutes. Add shrimp and oysters and simmer uncovered for 15 minutes, stirring often. Add stock and boil, covered, for 20 to 30 minutes.

- Meanwhile, combine flour and filé powder in a cup. Melt 3 tablespoons margarine in a small saucepan over low heat. Whisk in filé mixture and cook the roux for 2 to 3 minutes. Gradually add 1 cup of stock from simmering soup, stirring constantly, and bring to a boil. Transfer thickened stock to the saucepan containing the shrimp and oysters. Add okra, crab, garlic, onion, and cayenne to taste and simmer over low heat for 30 minutes. Serve hot.

Photo opposite page 147.

PER SERVING: 258 CALORIES		
MENU EXCHANGE PATTERN		
Dairy . . . . . —	Fruit . . . . . —	
Bread 1	Meat 3	
Fat . . . . ½	Veg. . . . . . . —	
NUTRITIONAL INFORMATION		
Carbohydrate 12	g	
Protein 22	g	
Total fat 13	g	
Saturated fat 2.1	g	
Cholesterol 145	mg	
Sodium 278	mg	
Potassium 473	mg	
Fiber 0.7	g	
Calcium 135	mg	
Iron . . . . 3.9 mg		

Sautéed Frogs Legs

2½ tablespoons margarine
*16 large (not jumbo) frogs legs
   (about 1 pound)*
1 teaspoon black pepper
*3 tablespoons chopped fresh
   parsley*

- Melt margarine in a large nonstick skillet over medium heat. Season frogs legs with pepper and sauté for 15 minutes, or until no longer pink. Sprinkle with chopped parsley.

PER SERVING: 142 CALORIES		
MENU EXCHANGE PATTERN		
Dairy . . . . . —	Fruit . . . . . —	
Bread . . . . —	Meat 2	
Fat 1	Veg. . . . . . . —	
NUTRITIONAL INFORMATION		
Carbohydrate 0	g	
Protein 17	g	
Total fat 8	g	
Saturated fat 1	g	
Cholesterol 49	mg	
Sodium 2	mg	
Potassium 27	mg	
Fiber 0	g	
Calcium 30	mg	
Iron . . . . 1.7 mg		

Blackeyed Peas

⅔ cup dried blackeyed peas
2 cups water
2 ounces Canadian bacon,
  chopped

1 small onion, chopped
1 clove garlic, chopped
⅛ teaspoon cayenne pepper
1 bay leaf

- Rinse peas and soak in 3 cups water for 45 minutes. Drain peas, place in large saucepan, and add enough water to just cover. Stir in the remaining ingredients and bring to a boil. Reduce heat and simmer until peas are tender, 2 to 3 hours.

PER SERVING: 79 CALORIES			
MENU EXCHANGE PATTERN			
Dairy ..... —	Fruit ..... —		
Bread 1	Meat ..... —		
Fat .... —	Veg. ...... —		
NUTRITIONAL INFORMATION			
Carbohydrate 10	g		
Protein 7	g		
Total fat 1	g		
Saturated fat 0.3	g		
Cholesterol 7	mg		
Sodium 203	mg		
Potassium 253	mg		
Fiber 0.9	g		
Calcium 19	mg		
Iron 1.1	mg		

Baked Tomatoes

2 tomatoes
4 teaspoons margarine, melted
4 teaspoons grated Parmesan
  cheese

PER SERVING: 44 CALORIES		
MENU EXCHANGE PATTERN		
Dairy ..... —	Fruit ..... —	
Bread ..... —	Meat ..... —	
Fat .... ½	Veg. 1	
NUTRITIONAL INFORMATION		
Carbohydrate 4	g	
Protein 2	g	
Total fat 2	g	
Saturated fat 1	g	
Cholesterol 1	mg	
Sodium 33	mg	
Potassium 225	mg	
Fiber 0.5	g	
Calcium 36	mg	
Iron .... 0.5 mg		

- Preheat oven to 350°F. Halve tomatoes crosswise and set in a shallow baking pan. Drizzle 1 teaspoon margarine over each tomato half. Sprinkle 1 teaspoon Parmesan over each tomato half. Bake 15 to 20 minutes, or until cheese has melted and tomato has softened.

- If desired, brown tomatoes under the broiler for 1 to 2 minutes, watching carefully to avoid burning.

Note: To further reduce fat intake, serve sliced fresh tomatoes instead of Baked Tomatoes. Adjusted analysis: calories = 25; exchange = 1 Vegetable.

Poppyseed Fruit Compote

1/4 *honeydew melon, cubed*
1/2 *cantaloupe, cubed*
1/2 *cup strawberries, hulled and*
sliced
1/2 *cup grapes, halved*

1 *pear, cored and diced*
1 *small banana, peeled and*
sliced
6 *tablespoons Poppyseed*
Dressing (recipe follows)

- Mix fruits in a large bowl. Add 6 tablespoons dressing and transfer to dessert dishes.

  Note: To further reduce fat, serve compote without dressing.

PER SERVING: 110 CALORIES		
MENU EXCHANGE PATTERN		
Dairy ..... —	Fruit	3
Bread .... —	Meat	—
Fat .... —	Veg.	—
NUTRITIONAL INFORMATION		
Carbohydrate 28		g
Protein 2		g
Total fat 1		g
Saturated fat 0.1		g
Cholesterol 0		mg
Sodium 13		mg
Potassium 598		mg
Fiber 1.5		g
Calcium 22		mg
Iron 0.5		mg

Poppyseed Dressing

2/3 *cup sugar*
1 *teaspoon dry mustard*
2/3 *cup cider vinegar*

2/3 *cup safflower oil*
4 *teaspoons poppyseed*

- For dressing, combine sugar, mustard, and vinegar in a blender and mix for a few minutes. With machine running, gradually add oil and blend until mixture thickens. Add poppyseed and blend 3 minutes. Store in a covered jar in the refrigerator. Makes about 2 cups; 1 serving = 1 tablespoon.

PER SERVING: 73 CALORIES		
MENU EXCHANGE PATTERN		
Dairy ..... —	Fruit	—
Bread 1/2	Meat	—
Fat 2	Veg.	—
NUTRITIONAL INFORMATION		
Carbohydrate 6		g
Protein 0		g
Total fat 6		g
Saturated fat 0		g
Cholesterol 0		mg
Sodium 0		mg
Potassium 4		mg
Fiber 0		g
Calcium 0		mg
Iron 0		mg

CHICKEN ENTREES

1

Gazpacho Mexicano

Ensalada de Pollo

Piña Colada Freeze

Serves 6

PER SERVING: 690 CALORIES			
MENU EXCHANGE PATTERN			
Dairy	2	Fruit	1½
Bread	1	Meat	5
Fat	1	Veg.	2
NUTRITIONAL INFORMATION			
Carbohydrate	68	g	
Protein	55	g	
Total fat	23	g	
Saturated fat	3.6	g	
Cholesterol	102	mg	
Sodium	1030	mg	
Potassium	1926	mg	
Fiber	3.5	g	
Calcium	549	mg	
Iron	5.6	mg	

Gazpacho Mexicano

3 tomatoes, seeded and cut in
   wedges
1 onion, cut in wedges
1 green bell pepper, seeded and
   coarsely chopped
1 cucumber, seeded and
   coarsely chopped

2 cloves garlic, minced
2½ cups low-sodium tomato
   juice
Tabasco sauce
2 tablespoons safflower oil
3 tablespoons red wine vinegar
Pinch of black pepper

Garnish

½ cup seeded, diced tomato
½ cup seeded, diced green bell
   pepper
½ cup seeded, diced cucumber

- Combine all ingredients in a blender in 2 batches and blend
  until well mixed but not completely smooth. Adjust seasoning and refrigerate until very cold. Garnish each serving
  with diced tomato, green pepper, and cucumber.

PER SERVING: 100 CALORIES

MENU EXCHANGE PATTERN

Dairy	—	Fruit	—
Bread	—	Meat	—
Fat	1	Veg.	2

NUTRITIONAL INFORMATION

Carbohydrate	13	g
Protein	3	g
Total fat	5	g
Saturated fat	0.3	g
Cholesterol	0	mg
Sodium	211	mg
Potassium	631	mg
Fiber	1.3	g
Calcium	36	mg
Iron	2	mg

Ensalada de Pollo

6 corn tortillas
1½ pounds chicken breast,
   grilled or broiled
1 head romaine lettuce
2 tomatoes, sliced
2 white onions, sliced
1 avocado, peeled and pitted

6 ounces low-fat Monterey Jack
   cheese, shredded
1 cup plus 2 tablespoons Pico
   de Gallo (page 90)
¾ cup commercial low-calorie
   Italian dressing

- Preheat oven to 400°F. Cut each tortilla into 6 wedges. Arrange on ungreased baking sheet and bake until crisp, 5 to
  7 minutes. Discard bones and skin from chicken; shred meat
  into bite-size pieces. Arrange lettuce leaves on salad plates
  and circle with tortilla chips. Top each serving with tomato,
  onion, ⅙ avocado, 1 ounce cheese, 3 tablespoons Pico de
  Gallo, and 2 tablespoons Italian dressing.

Note: Recipe analysis includes dressing.

PER SERVING: 442 CALORIES

MENU EXCHANGE PATTERN

Dairy	1	Fruit	—
Bread	1	Meat	5
Fat	—	Veg.	—

NUTRITIONAL INFORMATION

Carbohydrate	27	g
Protein	46	g
Total fat	16	g
Saturated fat	2.7	g
Cholesterol	98	mg
Sodium	737	mg
Potassium	872	mg
Fiber	1.8	g
Calcium	289	mg
Iron	3.2	mg

Piña Colada Freeze

3 cups plain low-fat yogurt
3 cups unsweetened canned
    crushed pineapple
2 tablespoons lemon juice
½ teaspoon coconut extract
    (optional)

- Reserve ½ cup crushed pineapple. Combine all remaining ingredients in a blender and mix thoroughly. Transfer to a shallow 2½-quart casserole and freeze for 3 to 4 hours, stirring every 30 minutes to prevent formation of ice crystals. Remove from freezer 10 to 15 minutes before serving. Top with the reserved crushed pineapple and cut into squares to serve.

PER SERVING: 148 CALORIES		
MENU EXCHANGE PATTERN		
Dairy 1	Fruit 1½	
Bread . . . . —	Meat . . . . . —	
Fat . . . . —	Veg. . . . . . . —	

NUTRITIONAL INFORMATION		
Carbohydrate 28	g
Protein 6	g
Total fat 2	g
Saturated fat 1.1	g
Cholesterol 7	mg
Sodium 82	mg
Potassium 423	mg
Fiber 0.4	g
Calcium 224	mg
Iron 0.4	mg

CHICKEN ENTREES

2

Artichokes with Hilltop Herb Dressing

Hot Chicken Salad Oreganato

Marinated Green Beans

Mixed Berry Meringues

Serves 6

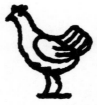

PER SERVING: 664 CALORIES		
MENU EXCHANGE PATTERN		
Dairy . . . . . —	Fruit . . . . . —	
Bread 2	Meat 5	
Fat 4	Veg. 3	
NUTRITIONAL INFORMATION		
Carbohydrate 39	g	
Protein 43	g	
Total fat 33	g	
Saturated fat 3.8	g	
Cholesterol 96	mg	
Sodium 139	mg	
Potassium 1300	mg	
Fiber 4.5	g	
Calcium 160	mg	
Iron 4.1	mg	

Artichokes with Hilltop Herb Dressing

6 whole artichokes, tips of
*   leaves trimmed*
3 cloves garlic
1 tablespoon coriander seed
¾ cup Hilltop Herb Dressing
*   (recipe follows)*

PER SERVING: 46 CALORIES		
MENU EXCHANGE PATTERN		
Dairy ..... —	Fruit ..... —	
Bread .... —	Meat ..... —	
Fat .... —	Veg. 2	
NUTRITIONAL INFORMATION		
Carbohydrate 10	g	
Protein 3	g	
Total fat 0	g	
Saturated fat 0	g	
Cholesterol 0	mg	
Sodium 30	mg	
Potassium 308	mg	
Fiber 2	g	
Calcium 51	mg	
Iron 1	mg	

- Trim bottom stems from artichokes. In a large, deep saucepan, bring 2 quarts of water to boil with garlic and coriander seed. Add artichokes and cook until bases are easily pierced with knife, about 25 to 30 minutes. Let artichokes cool in the water for 10 minutes. Lift artichokes out of water and turn upside down to drain. Let cool. Serve with dressing.

Note: To reduce fat intake, substitute a commercial low-calorie Italian dressing. Adjusted analysis for dressing: calories = 24; exchange = ½ Fat.

Hilltop Herb Dressing

1 cup safflower oil
¼ cup red wine vinegar or
*   lemon juice*
¼ cup water
1 clove garlic
½ cup chopped fresh parsley

1 tablespoon chopped fresh
*   oregano*
1 tablespoon chopped fresh
*   tarragon*
2 teaspoons Dijon-style mustard

PER SERVING: 81 CALORIES		
MENU EXCHANGE PATTERN		
Dairy ..... —	Fruit ..... —	
Bread .... —	Meat ..... —	
Fat 2	Veg. .... —	
NUTRITIONAL INFORMATION		
Carbohydrate 0	g	
Protein 0	g	
Total fat 9	g	
Saturated fat 0.8	g	
Cholesterol 0	mg	
Sodium 6	mg	
Potassium 13	mg	
Fiber 0	g	
Calcium 3	mg	
Iron 0.1	mg	

- Combine all ingredients in a blender or food processor and blend at high speed. Use for salad greens or for marinating vegetables. Makes about 1¾ cups; 1 serving = 1½ tablespoons.

Hot Chicken Salad Oreganato

1 chicken, 2½ to 3 pounds,
    skinned and cut in serving
    pieces
3 tablespoons chopped fresh
    oregano, or 2 teaspoons
    dried
¼ cup chopped fresh parsley

¼ cup safflower oil
¼ cup lemon juice
2 cloves garlic, halved
1 pound new potatoes
    (unpeeled), quartered
1 bunch watercress

- Cook chicken in water to cover (about 1 quart) until tender, about 25 minutes. Remove chicken and reserve broth. Discard bones and cut chicken into chunks.

- For dressing, combine oregano, parsley, oil, lemon juice, and garlic in a blender.

- Simmer potatoes in chicken broth until tender, about 20 minutes. Add chicken and dressing and cook uncovered over low heat for 1 hour, stirring frequently, to marinate flavors and reduce liquid. Garnish with watercress.

PER SERVING: 339 CALORIES

MENU EXCHANGE PATTERN

Dairy	—	Fruit	—
Bread	1	Meat	5
Fat	—	Veg.	—

NUTRITIONAL INFORMATION

Carbohydrate	14	g
Protein	37	g
Total fat	14	g
Saturated fat	2	g
Cholesterol	96	mg
Sodium	94	mg
Potassium	638	mg
Fiber	0.5	g
Calcium	37	mg
Iron	1.9	mg

Marinated Green Beans

½ cup water
2 cloves garlic
2 tablespoons fresh savory, or
    2 teaspoons dried
6 cups green beans, ends
    trimmed

½ cup safflower oil
¼ cup red or white wine
    vinegar

- Bring water to boil in a large saucepan with half of garlic and half of savory. Add beans, cover, and boil until beans are crisp-tender, about 5 minutes. Uncover and boil off any remaining liquid. Cool.

- Combine oil, vinegar, and remaining garlic and savory in a blender and mix at high speed until smooth. Pour over green beans. Toss lightly and refrigerate until ready to use.

Note: To reduce fat intake, substitute ¾ cup of a commercial low-calorie Italian dressing for marinade. Adjusted analysis: calories = 67; exchanges = ½ Fruit, 1 Vegetable, ½ Fat.

PER SERVING: 118 CALORIES

MENU EXCHANGE PATTERN

Dairy	—	Fruit	1
Bread	—	Meat	—
Fat	2	Veg.	1

NUTRITIONAL INFORMATION

Carbohydrate	9	g
Protein	2	g
Total fat	9	g
Saturated fat	0.8	g
Cholesterol	0	mg
Sodium	8	mg
Potassium	282	mg
Fiber	1.1	g
Calcium	63	mg
Iron	1	mg

Mixed Berry Meringues

1/2 cup sliced strawberries
1/2 cup blueberries
1/2 cup raspberries
2 tablespoons Grand Marnier

Meringue Shells

3 egg whites, at room
*   temperature*
1/8 teaspoon cream of tartar
3/4 cup sugar
1 teaspoon vanilla extract

- For meringue shells, combine egg whites and cream of tartar in a large bowl and beat with electric mixer until frothy. Add sugar 2 tablespoons at a time, beating for about 2 minutes after each addition (mixture should be thick and glossy, and form stiff peaks when beaters are raised). Beat in vanilla.

- Preheat oven to 275°F. Drop 1/4 to 1/3 cup of meringue on ungreased brown or parchment paper; spread in a 3-inch circle, hollowing out the center and building up sides. (Meringue can also be put through a pastry bag, working in circles until a 1- to 2-inch-high shell is formed; spread a little into the center to form the bottom.) Repeat with remaining meringue to form 12 shells. Bake until pale golden, about 1 hour, lowering the oven temperature to 200°F after 45 minutes if meringues begin to brown too much. Let cool on the paper, then place in an airtight container or plastic bag with crumpled waxed paper, plastic wrap, or tissue between the meringues. (Recipe makes 12 shells. Set aside 6 for the filling. Extras may be stored at room temperature for several days or frozen; do not refrigerate because meringues will become sticky.)

- For filling, combine berries and liqueur. Fill meringue shells with fruit.

Note: Substitute almond extract for vanilla in meringues.

Photo opposite page 162.

PER SERVING: 80 CALORIES			
MENU EXCHANGE PATTERN			
Dairy	—	Fruit	—
Bread	1	Meat	—
Fat	—	Veg.	—
NUTRITIONAL INFORMATION			
Carbohydrate	16		g
Protein	1		g
Total fat	0		g
Saturated fat	0		g
Cholesterol	0		mg
Sodium	1		mg
Potassium	59		mg
Fiber	0.5		g
Calcium	6		mg
Iron	0.1		mg

CHICKEN ENTREES

3

Potato Leek Soup

Pasta with Chicken and Broccoli

Carrot-Raisin Salad

Oatmeal Cookies

Serves 6

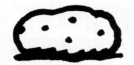

PER SERVING: 767 CALORIES		
MENU EXCHANGE PATTERN		
Dairy . . . . . —	Fruit 1½	
Bread 4	Meat 4	
Fat 3	Veg. 2	
NUTRITIONAL INFORMATION		
Carbohydrate 92	g	
Protein 35	g	
Total fat 30	g	
Saturated fat 5.3	g	
Cholesterol 57	mg	
Sodium 154	mg	
Potassium 1681	mg	
Fiber 3.7	g	
Calcium 230	mg	
Iron 5.6	mg	

Potato Leek Soup

4 large Idaho potatoes, peeled
   and cut in small chunks
2 leeks, chopped
1 carrot, chopped
Black pepper

1 quart water
1/4 cup margarine
1/4 cup all-purpose flour
Pinch of paprika

- Slowly boil potatoes, leeks, carrot, and pepper to taste in 1 quart water for 45 minutes. Melt margarine in a skillet over low heat. Add flour and stir until browned but not burned, about 3 to 5 minutes. Remove from heat and gradually whisk in 1 cup soup liquid. Return flour mixture to soup and season with paprika. Bring to a boil and serve hot.

PER SERVING: 177 CALORIES
MENU EXCHANGE PATTERN

Dairy .... —	Fruit ..... —
Bread 1½	Meat .... —
Fat 1½	Veg. ...... —

NUTRITIONAL INFORMATION

Carbohydrate	 24	g
Protein	 3	g
Total fat	 8	g
Saturated fat	 1	g
Cholesterol	 0	mg
Sodium	 12	mg
Potassium	 535	mg
Fiber	 1	g
Calcium	 32	mg
Iron	 1	mg

Pasta with Chicken and Broccoli

1/2 pound spaghetti
1/4 cup safflower oil
6 small cloves garlic, minced
2 bunches broccoli, cut into
   small pieces (3 cups)

3 whole chicken breasts, boned,
   skinned, halved, and cut in
   strips (1½ pounds)
3/4 cup chopped fresh parsley
Black pepper

- Boil spaghetti until *al dente*; drain. Heat oil in a skillet over medium-high heat. Add garlic and stir for 1 minute. Add broccoli and sauté for 2 minutes, then transfer to a heated dish. Add chicken to the skillet and sauté until no longer pink, about 5 minutes. Toss pasta with broccoli and chicken. Garnish with parsley, sprinkle with pepper and serve.

Photo opposite page 163.

PER SERVING: 421 CALORIES
MENU EXCHANGE PATTERN

Dairy ..... —	Fruit ..... —
Bread 2	Meat 4
Fat .... ½	Veg. 1

NUTRITIONAL INFORMATION

Carbohydrate	 37	g
Protein	 28	g
Total fat	 18	g
Saturated fat	 3	g
Cholesterol	 57	mg
Sodium	 79	mg
Potassium	 802	mg
Fiber	 2	g
Calcium	 159	mg
Iron	.... 3.5	mg

Carrot-Raisin Salad

3 large carrots, finely grated
3 tablespoons finely chopped
   onion
3/4 cup raisins
6 tablespoons lemon juice

- Combine all ingredients and chill for at least 30 minutes before serving.

PER SERVING: 82 CALORIES
MENU EXCHANGE PATTERN

Dairy ..... —	Fruit 1½
Bread ..... —	Meat ..... —
Fat .... —	Veg. 1

NUTRITIONAL INFORMATION

Carbohydrate	 21	g
Protein	 1	g
Total fat	 0	g
Saturated fat	 0	g
Cholesterol	 0	mg
Sodium	 20	mg
Potassium	 305	mg
Fiber	 1	g
Calcium	 28	mg
Iron	.... 0.7	mg

Oatmeal Cookies

½ cup margarine
¾ cup firmly packed brown
   sugar
1 egg substitute, lightly beaten
1½ teaspoons vanilla extract
½ teaspoon salt

½ cup whole wheat flour
¾ teaspoon baking powder
1 cup wheat germ
1½ cups rolled oats
½ cup toasted sunflower seeds

- Preheat oven to 375°F. Cream margarine and brown sugar in a large bowl. Add egg, vanilla, and salt and beat well. In a separate bowl, thoroughly combine flour, baking powder, wheat germ, and rolled oats. Blend dry ingredients into margarine mixture, adding a tablespoon or more of water if necessary to hold the mixture together.

- Drop dough by tablespoonfuls onto a greased cookie sheet and flatten lightly. Bake until golden, about 10 to 12 minutes. Makes 3 dozen; 1 serving = 1 cookie.

PER SERVING: 87 CALORIES		
MENU EXCHANGE PATTERN		
Dairy . . . . . —	Fruit . . . . . —	
Bread . . . . . ½	Meat . . . . . —	
Fat 1	Veg. . . . . . . —	
NUTRITIONAL INFORMATION		
Carbohydrate 10		g
Protein 2		g
Total fat 4		g
Saturated fat 1		g
Cholesterol 0		mg
Sodium 42		mg
Potassium 39		mg
Fiber 0.1		g
Calcium 10		mg
Iron 0.4		mg

Mixed Berry Meringues; recipe page 159

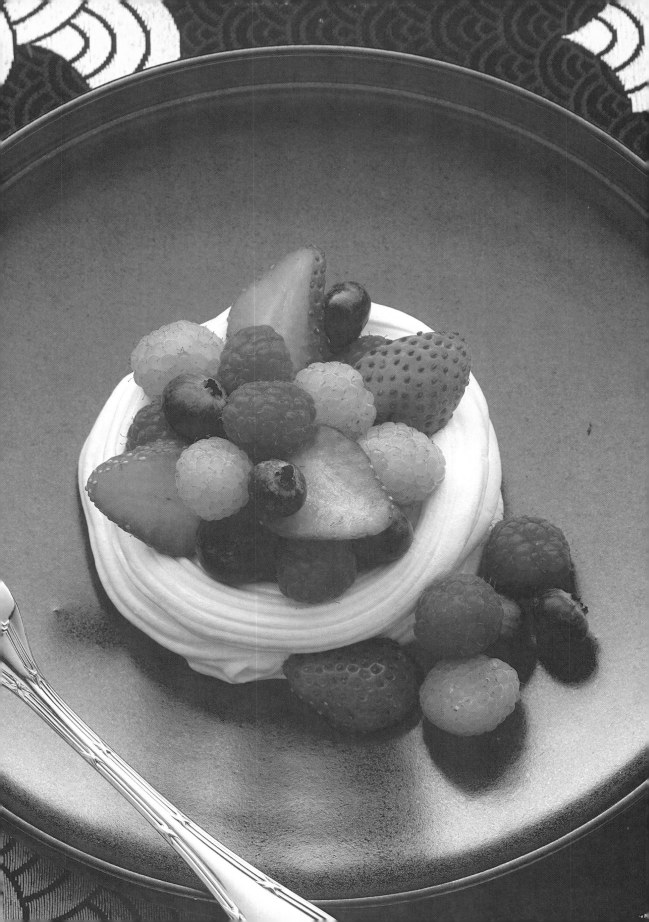

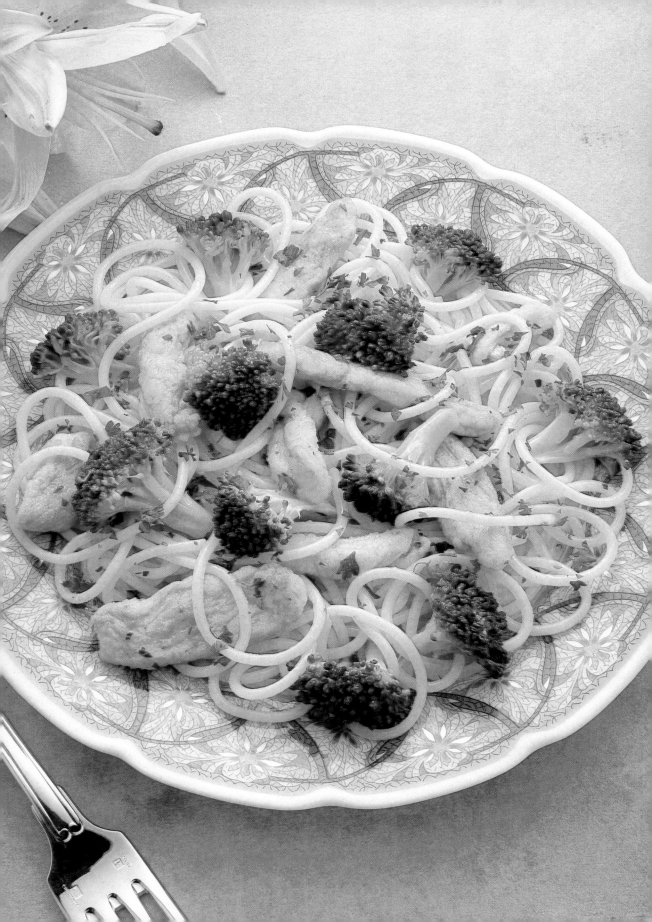

CHICKEN ENTREES

4

Carrot and Caraway Soup

St. Tropez Chicken Salad

Chinese Sesame Apples

Serves 4

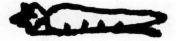

PER SERVING: 710 CALORIES			
MENU EXCHANGE PATTERN			
Dairy	—	Fruit	6
Bread	1½	Meat	1
Fat	4	Veg.	4
NUTRITIONAL INFORMATION			
Carbohydrate	118		g
Protein	15		g
Total fat	23		g
Saturated fat	3.9		g
Cholesterol	29		mg
Sodium	84		mg
Potassium	1128		mg
Fiber	3.6		g
Calcium	88		mg
Iron	3.4		mg

Pasta with Chicken and Broccoli; recipe page 161

Carrot and Caraway Soup

2 cups shredded carrots
2 tablespoons margarine
1/2 cup finely chopped onion
1 teaspoon caraway seed
1/2 teaspoon dried thyme

1/2 teaspoon freshly ground
    black pepper
2 tablespoons all-purpose flour
1 1/2 quarts hot Homemade
    Chicken Stock (page 36)

- Sauté carrots in margarine over medium-high heat until limp, about 5 minutes. Add onion, caraway, thyme, and pepper, then sauté until onion starts to change color to a light brown, about 3 to 4 minutes. Add flour, stirring constantly to form a roux, and cook about 5 minutes over medium heat. Gradually add stock, mixing constantly, then simmer 20 minutes, or until flavors are blended.

PER SERVING: 95 CALORIES		
MENU EXCHANGE PATTERN		
Dairy .... —	Fruit ..... —	
Bread .... —	Meat ..... —	
Fat 1	Veg. 2	
NUTRITIONAL INFORMATION		
Carbohydrate 10	g	
Protein 2	g	
Total fat 6	g	
Saturated fat 1.1	g	
Cholesterol 0	mg	
Sodium 28	mg	
Potassium 221	mg	
Fiber 1	g	
Calcium 34	mg	
Iron 0.7	mg	

St. Tropez Chicken Salad

8 leaves red-leaf lettuce
2 cups Boston or iceberg
    lettuce, torn into bite-size
    pieces
8 ounces skinned cooked
    chicken, shredded
1/2 avocado, peeled, pitted, and
    sliced

1 tomato, cut in wedges
1/2 cup alfalfa sprouts
2 bananas, peeled and sliced
12 cucumber slices
4 tablespoons Mustard
    Vinaigrette (recipe follows)

- Line sides of individual salad bowls with red lettuce leaves; set torn lettuce leaves in bottom of bowls. Arrange chicken, avocado, tomato wedges, alfalfa sprouts, bananas, and cucumber slices over lettuce bed. Serve with vinaigrette.

PER SERVING: 196 CALORIES		
MENU EXCHANGE PATTERN		
Dairy .... —	Fruit 1	
Bread .... —	Meat 1	
Fat 1	Veg. 2	
NUTRITIONAL INFORMATION		
Carbohydrate 20	g	
Protein 12	g	
Total fat 9	g	
Saturated fat 1.9	g	
Cholesterol 29	mg	
Sodium 38	mg	
Potassium 738	mg	
Fiber 1.4	g	
Calcium 38	mg	
Iron 2.3	mg	

Mustard Vinaigrette

1/3 cup white wine vinegar
1 tablespoon Dijon-style
    mustard

1 teaspoon dried oregano
1/3 cup safflower oil
Black pepper

- Combine vinegar, mustard, oregano, and pepper in a small bowl and whisk in oil until well blended. Makes about 2/3 cup; 1 serving = 1 tablespoon.

PER SERVING: 54 CALORIES		
MENU EXCHANGE PATTERN		
Dairy .... —	Fruit ..... —	
Bread .... —	Meat ..... —	
Fat 1	Veg. .... —	
NUTRITIONAL INFORMATION		
Carbohydrate 0	g	
Protein 0	g	
Total fat 6	g	
Saturated fat 0.5	g	
Cholesterol 0	mg	
Sodium 15	mg	
Potassium 8	mg	
Fiber 0	g	
Calcium 1	mg	
Iron 0.1	mg	

Chinese Sesame Apples

1¹/₃ cups sugar
4 apples, cored and cut in
  ¹/₂-inch slices
2 tablespoons toasted sesame
  seed
4 apple birds (garnish)

PER SERVING: 364 CALORIES		
MENU EXCHANGE PATTERN		
Dairy . . . . . —	Fruit 5	
Bread 1½	Meat . . . . . —	
Fat 1	Veg. . . . . . . —	
NUTRITIONAL INFORMATION		
Carbohydrate 88	g	
Protein 1	g	
Total fat 3	g	
Saturated fat 0.4	g	
Cholesterol 0	mg	
Sodium 2	mg	
Potassium 161	mg	
Fiber 1.2	g	
Calcium 15	mg	
Iron 0.4	mg	

- Melt sugar in a skillet over low heat until it begins to caramelize. Remove from heat immediately. Dip apple slices into sugar, coating evenly on both sides. Dip one side into toasted sesame seed; immediately dip into ice water. Serve on dessert plates garnished with apple birds; prepare apple birds as shown in Figure 7-1.

Note: Thin pear or pineapple slices may be substituted for apples.

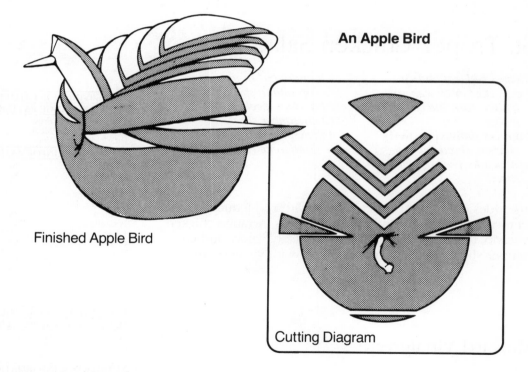

An Apple Bird

Finished Apple Bird

Cutting Diagram

Figure 7.1. Apple Bird Garnish

CHICKEN ENTREES

5

Cheese-Stuffed Tortillas

Caldo Xochitl

Pico de Gallo (page 90)

Papaya with Vanilla Yogurt

Serves 4

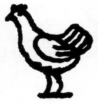

PER SERVING: 713 CALORIES		
MENU EXCHANGE PATTERN		
Dairy 1	Fruit 1	
Bread 2½	Meat 5	
Fat 2	Veg. 1½	
NUTRITIONAL INFORMATION		
Carbohydrate 69	g	
Protein 48	g	
Total fat 27	g	
Saturated fat 5.6	g	
Cholesterol. 99	mg	
Sodium 730	mg	
Potassium 1605	mg	
Fiber 4.5	g	
Calcium 334	mg	
Iron 3	mg	

Cheese-Stuffed Tortillas

4 teaspoons margarine
4 teaspoons dry sherry
1/2 cup chopped onion
1 1/3 cups chopped green
    bell pepper

1 cup chopped mushrooms
2 1/2 ounces (2/3 cup) grated low-
    fat, Monterey Jack-style
    cheese
4 corn tortillas

PER SERVING: 195 CALORIES		
MENU EXCHANGE PATTERN		
Dairy 1/2	Fruit	—
Bread 1	Meat	—
Fat 1	Veg.	1
NUTRITIONAL INFORMATION		
Carbohydrate 23		g
Protein 9		g
Total fat 7		g
Saturated fat 0.7		g
Cholesterol. 9		mg
Sodium 412		mg
Potassium 226		mg
Fiber 0.6		g
Calcium 179		mg
Iron . . . . 1.6 mg		

- Melt margarine in a nonstick skillet over medium heat. Add sherry, onion, bell pepper, and mushrooms and sauté until tender, about 10 minutes. Transfer vegetables to a small broilerproof dish and sprinkle with grated cheese. Place under broiler until cheese has melted. Warm tortillas. Divide cheese/vegetable mixture among tortillas and fold in the sides as for a crepe. Serve warm.

Caldo Xochitl

4 cups Caldo de Pollo (recipe
    follows)
4 chicken breasts, 4 ounces
    each, skinned and boned

2/3 avocado, peeled and pitted
4 tablespoons Pico de Gallo
    (page 90)
1 cup cooked rice

PER SERVING: 388 CALORIES		
MENU EXCHANGE PATTERN		
Dairy . . . . . —	Fruit	—
Bread 1	Meat	5
Fat 1	Veg.	—
NUTRITIONAL INFORMATION		
Carbohydrate 17		g
Protein 36		g
Total fat 19		g
Saturated fat 4		g
Cholesterol 88		mg
Sodium 282		mg
Potassium 773		mg
Fiber 0.9		g
Calcium 33		mg
Iron . . . . 2.4 mg		

- Pour Caldo de Pollo into a large saucepan. Add chicken breasts and poach just until firm and opaque, about 20 to 25 minutes. Shred meat and serve in individual soup bowls with 1/4 cup cooked rice, 1/6 avocado section, and 1 tablespoon Pico de Gallo per serving.

Caldo de Pollo (Chicken Broth)

1 gallon (16 cups) water
3 green bell peppers, cored,
    seeded, and quartered
2 medium tomatoes, cut into
    12 chunks

3 onions, cut into 18 chunks
1 stalk celery, coarsely chopped
3 cloves garlic, crushed
1 chicken, about 1 1/2 pounds

- Combine water, vegetables, and garlic in a large stockpot and boil over medium-high heat until vegetables are soft, about 10 minutes. Remove skin and as much fat as possible from chicken. When vegetables are cooked, add chicken to stockpot, cover and simmer for 20 to 30 minutes. Remove chicken and vegetables. Cool broth, refrigerate overnight, and skim fat from the top.

- Use chicken in recipes calling for cooked chicken, in chicken sandwiches, or in chicken salad.

PER SERVING: 67 CALORIES

MENU EXCHANGE PATTERN

Dairy	—	Fruit	—
Bread	1	Meat	—
Fat	—	Veg.	—

NUTRITIONAL INFORMATION

Carbohydrate	15	g
Protein	3	g
Total fat	0	g
Saturated fat	0	g
Cholesterol	0	mg
Sodium	130	mg
Potassium	756	mg
Fiber	1.6	g
Calcium	60	mg
Iron	1.2	mg

Papaya with Vanilla Yogurt

2 ripe papayas, peeled, halved,
*   and seeded*
1 cup low-fat vanilla yogurt
Mint sprigs (garnish)

- Set a papaya half on each dessert plate. Top with ¼ cup yogurt and garnish with a sprig of mint.

PER SERVING: 114 CALORIES

MENU EXCHANGE PATTERN

Dairy	½	Fruit	1
Bread	½	Meat	—
Fat	—	Veg.	—

NUTRITIONAL INFORMATION

Carbohydrate	25	g
Protein	3	g
Total fat	1	g
Saturated fat	0.5	g
Cholesterol	2	mg
Sodium	34	mg
Potassium	490	mg
Fiber	1.2	g
Calcium	114	mg
Iron	0.2	mg

MEAT ENTREES

1

Marinated Beef Salad

Warm Potato Salad

Melon-Fruit Compote

Serves 4

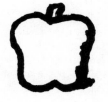

PER SERVING: 683 CALORIES			
MENU EXCHANGE PATTERN			
Dairy	—	Fruit	4
Bread	2	Meat	2
Fat	5½	Veg.	2
NUTRITIONAL INFORMATION			
Carbohydrate	80	g	
Protein	22	g	
Total fat	33	g	
Saturated fat	10.4	g	
Cholesterol	53	mg	
Sodium	287	mg	
Potassium	1834	mg	
Fiber	3.3	g	
Calcium	79	mg	
Iron	4.6	mg	

Marinated Beef Salad

2/3 pound beef sirloin, grilled,
    preferably over mesquite,
    and sliced into julienne
1 small green bell pepper,
    cored, seeded, and sliced
    into julienne
1 small red bell pepper, cored,
    seeded, and sliced into
    julienne
1/4 onion, sliced into julienne
2 green onions, sliced into
    julienne

1/4 cup Sherry Horseradish
    Dressing (recipe follows)
Black pepper
4 leaves Boston or Bibb lettuce
4 leaves radicchio
1 1/3 cups enoki mushrooms
1 grapefruit, peeled and
    sectioned
4 cherry tomatoes

- Toss beef with peppers, onion, green onions, and dressing.
  Season with pepper. Arrange lettuce and radicchio leaves on
  individual plates. Place marinated beef in center of lettuce.
  Add mushrooms, grapefruit sections, and tomatoes to each
  plate.

Note: To reduce fat intake, substitute a commercial low-calorie Italian dressing for the Sherry Horseradish Dressing. Adjusted analysis for dressing: calories = 16; exchange = 1/2 Fat.

PER SERVING: 262 CALORIES			
MENU EXCHANGE PATTERN			
Dairy ..... —	Fruit ..... —		
Bread .... —	Meat 2		
Fat 2	Veg. 2		
NUTRITIONAL INFORMATION			
Carbohydrate 10	g		
Protein 14	g		
Total fat 19	g		
Saturated fat 8.9	g		
Cholesterol 45	mg		
Sodium 60	mg		
Potassium 622	mg		
Fiber 1.1	g		
Calcium 1	mg		
Iron 2.8	mg		

Sherry Horseradish Dressing

2 cloves garlic, minced
1 1/2 teaspoons minced shallot
2 cups safflower oil
1 cup sherry
1/4 cup sugar
3/4 cup cider vinegar
1 tablespoon prepared
    horseradish

1 tablespoon Creole or Dijon-
    style mustard
2 1/4 teaspoons black pepper
2 1/4 teaspoons Worcestershire
    sauce
2 1/4 teaspoons each dried thyme,
    rosemary, chives, oregano,
    and basil

- In a medium skillet, sauté garlic and shallot in 1 tablespoon
  of the oil over medium heat for 3 minutes. Add sherry and
  simmer until reduced by half. Add sugar and vinegar and
  simmer 5 minutes. Combine all remaining ingredients in
  blender or food processor. Add sherry mixture and blend
  until dressing is emulsified. Chill before serving. Makes
  about 3 cups; 1 serving = 2 tablespoons.

PER SERVING: 69 CALORIES			
MENU EXCHANGE PATTERN			
Dairy ..... —	Fruit ..... —		
Bread .... —	Meat ..... —		
Fat 1 1/2	Veg. .... —		
NUTRITIONAL INFORMATION			
Carbohydrate 1	g		
Protein 0	g		
Total fat 7	g		
Saturated fat 0.6	g		
Cholesterol 0	mg		
Sodium 8	mg		
Potassium 10	mg		
Fiber 0	g		
Calcium 2	mg		
Iron 0	mg		

Warm Potato Salad

1 pound russet potatoes
*2 ounces lean ham, finely
  diced*
4 teaspoons safflower oil
⅔ onion, finely chopped
½ teaspoon minced garlic
1 teaspoon minced shallot
2 teaspoons honey
½ apple, cored and diced

*Pinch each of dried rosemary
  and thyme*
½ teaspoon Dijon-style mustard
*3 tablespoons unsweetened
  apple juice or cider*
1 tablespoon cider vinegar
*3 tablespoons Homemade
  Chicken Stock (page 36)*

PER SERVING: 192 CALORIES			
MENU EXCHANGE PATTERN			
Dairy	—	Fruit	—
Bread	2	Meat	—
Fat	2	Veg.	—

NUTRITIONAL INFORMATION		
Carbohydrate	30	g
Protein	6	g
Total fat	6	g
Saturated fat	0.9	g
Cholesterol	8	mg
Sodium	204	mg
Potassium	601	mg
Fiber	0.9	g
Calcium	20	mg
Iron	1.1	mg

- Boil potatoes until easily pierced with a skewer, about 10 to 15 minutes. Drain. When cool enough to handle, peel and slice. Sauté ham in oil in a nonstick skillet for about 5 minutes. Add onion, garlic, and shallot and sauté until tender, another 5 minutes. Add remaining ingredients except potatoes. Bring to a boil, pour over potatoes and toss lightly.

Melon-Fruit Compote

⅔ cup diced pineapple
⅔ cup honeydew melon balls
⅔ cup cantaloupe balls
⅔ cup watermelon balls
1½ grapefruits, sectioned

⅓ cup blueberries
*⅓ cup green, purple, or red
  grapes*
8 strawberries
1 orange, sectioned

Sauce

2 tablespoons honey
2 tablespoons yogurt
2 tablespoons orange juice

PER SERVING: 160 CALORIES			
MENU EXCHANGE PATTERN			
Dairy	—	Fruit	4
Bread	—	Meat	—
Fat	—	Veg.	—

NUTRITIONAL INFORMATION		
Carbohydrate	39	g
Protein	3	g
Total fat	1	g
Saturated fat	0.1	g
Cholesterol	0	mg
Sodium	15	mg
Potassium	601	mg
Fiber	1.3	g
Calcium	56	mg
Iron	0.7	mg

- Mix sauce ingredients and set aside.

- Arrange fruit on a dessert plate, and pour sauce over.

MEAT ENTREES

2

Vegetable Ravioli with Tomato Sauce

Summer Salad with Marinated Pepper Steak

Strawberry Yogurt Crepes with Orange Sauce

Serves 6

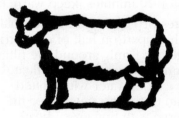

PER SERVING: 675 CALORIES		
MENU EXCHANGE PATTERN		
Dairy . . . . . . ½	Fruit . . . . . . ½	
Bread 3	Meat 3½	
Fat 2½	Veg. 4	
NUTRITIONAL INFORMATION		
Carbohydrate 78	g	
Protein 41	g	
Total fat 22	g	
Saturated fat 4.9	g	
Cholesterol 83	mg	
Sodium 256	mg	
Potassium 1623	mg	
Fiber 2.6	g	
Calcium 283	mg	
Iron 7.7	mg	

Vegetable Ravioli with Tomato Sauce

1/4 cup chopped oyster
   mushrooms, in 1/4-inch dice
1/4 cup diced carrots
2 tablespoons chopped shallot
1/4 cup tiny green beans
1/4 cup chopped zucchini
1 tablespoon safflower oil
1 quart Homemade Chicken
   Stock (page 36)

2 tablespoons instant tapioca
1 tablespoon chopped fresh
   basil
Black pepper
4 strips of fresh eggless pasta,
   12 × 4 inches each
2 egg substitutes, or 4 egg
   whites
1 cup cooked tiny green beans

Tomato Sauce

2 large tomatoes, peeled and
   seeded
1 tablespoon chopped shallot
1 tablespoon safflower oil
1/2 cup low-sodium tomato juice
1 tablespoon chopped fresh
   tarragon

1 tablespoon chopped fresh
   parsley
1 tablespoon chopped fresh
   chives

- In a large nonstick skillet, sauté vegetables in oil over medium heat until soft, 5 minutes. Add chicken stock and boil until reduced by half. Add tapioca and cook for 2 minutes. Season with basil and pepper. Let cool.

- For sauce, puree tomatoes in a blender. In a medium nonstick skillet, sauté shallot in oil over medium heat until translucent, about 3 minutes. Add tomato puree, tomato juice, and herbs and simmer for 20 minutes, keep warm.

- Brush pasta with egg substitutes or egg whites. Place small mounds of filling about 2 inches apart on half of each strip. Fold pasta over and press together firmly around the filling. Cut into squares and poach in hot water until they float, about 5 to 10 minutes. Remove from water with slotted spoon and transfer to saucepan of tomato sauce over medium heat to heat through. Serve with tiny green beans.

PER SERVING: 203 CALORIES		
MENU EXCHANGE PATTERN		
Dairy . . . . . —	Fruit . . . . . —	
Bread 1	Meat . . . . . —	
Fat 1	Veg. 3	
NUTRITIONAL INFORMATION		
Carbohydrate 33	g	
Protein 8	g	
Total fat 5	g	
Saturated fat 0.4	g	
Cholesterol 0	mg	
Sodium 82	mg	
Potassium 488	mg	
Fiber 1	g	
Calcium 57	mg	
Iron 2	mg	

Summer Salad with Marinated Pepper Steak

1 1/2 pounds flank steak, in one
   piece
1/2 cup sugar
1/2 cup Korean chili sauce
1/2 cup Oriental garlic paste
1/4 cup safflower oil

3 cups romaine lettuce torn
   into bite-size pieces
1 1/2 cups watercress
18 radicchio leaves
12 Belgian endive

PER SERVING: 348 CALORIES

MENU EXCHANGE PATTERN

Dairy	—	Fruit	—
Bread	1	Meat	3½
Fat	1	Veg.	1

NUTRITIONAL INFORMATION

Carbohydrate	25	g
Protein	27	g
Total fat	15	g
Saturated fat	4	g
Cholesterol	79	mg
Sodium	101	mg
Potassium	691	mg
Fiber	1	g
Calcium	60	mg
Iron	5	mg

- Sprinkle the steak with sugar and refrigerate for 24 hours. The following day spread chili, garlic paste, and oil on both sides; refrigerate for another 24 hours. Grill over mesquite to desired doneness, about 10 minutes for medium, and slice very thin. Arrange salad greens on plates and place beef in center.

Note: Korean chili sauce and Oriental garlic paste are sold in gourmet shops and groceries specializing in Asian and Southeast Asian foods.

Strawberry Yogurt Crepes with Orange Sauce

1 egg substitute, or 3 egg whites
2 tablespoons bread flour
½ teaspoon safflower oil

¼ cup skim milk
½ teaspoon grated orange rind
½ teaspoon grated lemon rind

Strawberry Filling

1 cup overripe strawberries
1½ cups plain low-fat yogurt
12 strawberries, hulled and chopped

Orange Sauce

4 oranges
2 teaspoons cornstarch

- Beat egg substitute (or egg whites) until frothy and gradually whisk in flour. Whisk in oil, then milk. Add orange and lemon rinds and let stand for 40 minutes. Strain batter. Spray a small omelet pan with nonstick spray to coat the bottom. Place over medium-high heat. When pan is hot, add 2 tablespoons batter and quickly tilt the pan to coat the bottom. Cook until bottom of crepe is browned, then turn and cook other side. Repeat with the remaining batter, stacking crepes between squares of waxed paper. Keep warm.

- For filling, puree the overripe strawberries in a blender and pass through a fine sieve. Stir puree into yogurt. Stir in the chopped strawberries. Set aside.

- Juice the oranges for the sauce and boil the juice in a non-aluminum saucepan until it is reduced by half. Add the cornstarch and whisk vigorously for 2 minutes. Spoon onto plates.

- Spoon a little strawberry filling onto each crepe. Fold over and serve on a pool of sauce.

PER SERVING: 124 CALORIES

MENU EXCHANGE PATTERN

Dairy	½	Fruit	1
Bread	½	Meat	—
Fat	½	Veg.	—

NUTRITIONAL INFORMATION

Carbohydrate	20	g
Protein	7	g
Total fat	2	g
Saturated fat	0.7	g
Cholesterol	4	mg
Sodium	73	mg
Potassium	444	mg
Fiber	0.6	g
Calcium	166	mg
Iron	0.7	mg

MEAT ENTREES

3

Caesar Salad

Veal Piccata

Fettuccine Florentine

Italian Sesame Cookies

Serves 4

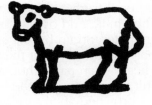

PER SERVING: 747 CALORIES		
MENU EXCHANGE PATTERN		
Dairy . . . . . —	Fruit . . . . . —	
Bread 3½	Meat 3½	
Fat 5½	Veg. 3	
NUTRITIONAL INFORMATION		
Carbohydrate 57	g	
Protein 38	g	
Total fat 41	g	
Saturated fat 11.4	g	
Cholesterol 178	mg	
Sodium 258	mg	
Potassium 834	mg	
Fiber 0.8	g	
Calcium 206	mg	
Iron 7.3	mg	

Caesar Salad

1 clove garlic	2 teaspoons drained capers
3 anchovies	4 cups torn leaf lettuce
2 teaspoons Dijon-style mustard	3 tablespoons red wine vinegar
3 tablespoons safflower oil	1/4 cup croutons
1 egg, warmed in warm water	2 tablespoons grated Parmesan
Juice of 1 lemon	cheese

- Using a fork, crush garlic in a bowl, spreading it around the bottom. Add the anchovies and mash them with the fork. Add mustard and 2 teaspoons oil. Separate egg; add yolk to the bowl. Gradually beat in oil; continue beating until mixture reaches a thick consistency. Beat in lemon juice; stir in capers. Add lettuce and pour vinegar over the leaves. Add croutons and toss. Sprinkle Parmesan over the top of the salad and serve.

Note: To further reduce fat, eliminate mustard, oil, egg, lemon, vinegar, and Parmesan. After crushing garlic and mixing anchovies into a paste, add lettuce and capers. Toss with croutons and 1/4 cup low-calorie Italian dressing. Adjusted analysis: calories = 47; exchange = 2 Vegetables.

PER SERVING: 161 CALORIES			
MENU EXCHANGE PATTERN			
Dairy	—	Fruit	—
Bread	—	Meat	—
Fat	2½	Veg.	2
NUTRITIONAL INFORMATION			
Carbohydrate		7	g
Protein		5	g
Total fat		13	g
Saturated fat		1.9	g
Cholesterol		71	mg
Sodium		133	mg
Potassium		209	mg
Fiber		0.4	g
Calcium		78	mg
Iron		1.7	mg

Veal Piccata

8 veal scallops (5 ounces each), cut 1/4 inch thick	3 tablespoons margarine
Black pepper	Juice of 1½ lemons
5 tablespoons all-purpose flour	2 tablespoons chopped fresh parsley

- Pound the veal between sheets of wax paper or plastic wrap to make them as thin as possible without tearing them. Season with pepper and dust with flour. Heat 2 tablespoons of the margarine in a large nonstick skillet over medium-high heat until golden. Add the veal a few pieces at a time and brown for about 2 minutes on each side. Transfer veal to a hot serving platter and keep warm. Add the lemon juice and parsley to the skillet. Remove from heat, slowly swirl in the remaining margarine and pour over the veal.

Note: Thinly pounded skinned chicken breasts may be substituted.

PER SERVING: 329 CALORIES			
MENU EXCHANGE PATTERN			
Dairy	—	Fruit	—
Bread	1	Meat	3
Fat	2	Veg.	—
NUTRITIONAL INFORMATION			
Carbohydrate		9	g
Protein		24	g
Total fat		21	g
Saturated fat		7.8	g
Cholesterol		100	mg
Sodium		81	mg
Potassium		416	mg
Fiber		0.2	g
Calcium		25	mg
Iron		3.7	mg

Fettuccine Florentine

6 ounces fettuccine
2/3 cup fresh spinach leaves
4 teaspoons chopped fresh
    parsley
2 teaspoons chopped fresh basil

1/3 cup skim-milk ricotta
3 tablespoons plain low-fat
    yogurt
Black pepper

- Cook fettuccine in 2 quarts boiling water until *al dente*, about 5 minutes. Drain in colander.

- Combine spinach, parsley, basil, ricotta, yogurt, and pepper to taste in a blender or processor and blend well. Toss with fettuccine and serve.

PER SERVING: 195 CALORIES		
MENU EXCHANGE PATTERN		
Dairy . . . . . —	Fruit . . . . . —
Bread 2	Meat . . . . . . ½
Fat . . . . —	Veg. 1

NUTRITIONAL INFORMATION		
Carbohydrate 34	g
Protein 9	g
Total fat 2	g
Saturated fat 1.1	g
Cholesterol 7	mg
Sodium 41	mg
Potassium 186	mg
Fiber 0	g
Calcium 97	mg
Iron 1.7	mg

Italian Sesame Cookies

3 cups all-purpose flour
1 cup sugar
2 teaspoons baking powder
1 cup margarine

3 egg substitutes, beaten
1/4 cup skim milk
1 cup sesame seed

- Preheat oven to 375°F. Mix flour, sugar, and baking powder. Cut in margarine until mixture resembles coarse meal. Add egg substitutes and milk and mix well. Divide dough in fourths and roll into ½-inch ropes. Cut into 1½-inch lengths and roll in sesame seeds. Place about ½ inch apart on cookie sheets coated with nonstick spray. Flatten each cookie slightly with a spatula. Bake until lightly browned, about 20 minutes. Makes 6 dozen; 1 serving = 1 cookie.

PER SERVING: 63 CALORIES		
MENU EXCHANGE PATTERN		
Dairy . . . . . —	Fruit . . . . . —
Bread . . . . . ½	Meat . . . . . —
Fat . . . . ½	Veg. . . . . . . —

NUTRITIONAL INFORMATION		
Carbohydrate 7	g
Protein 1	g
Total fat 4	g
Saturated fat 0.6	g
Cholesterol 0	mg
Sodium 3	mg
Potassium 23	mg
Fiber 0.2	g
Calcium 6	mg
Iron 0.2	mg

MEAT ENTREES

4

Marinated Pork Roast

Carrot "Pennies"

Cornbread

Fresh Fruit with Orange-Mint Sauce

Serves 8

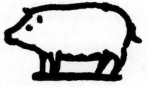

PER SERVING: 629 CALORIES			
MENU EXCHANGE PATTERN			
Dairy	—	Fruit	1
Bread	3	Meat	2½
Fat	4½	Veg.	2
NUTRITIONAL INFORMATION			
Carbohydrate	61	g	
Protein	24	g	
Total fat	34	g	
Saturated fat	9.6	g	
Cholesterol	75	mg	
Sodium	342	mg	
Potassium	1156	mg	
Fiber	2.6	g	
Calcium	174	mg	
Iron	3.0	mg	

Marinated Pork Roast

2 pounds boneless pork roast
1 teaspoon fennel seed
3 tablespoons all-purpose flour
1 teaspoon black pepper
1 tablespoon chopped fresh
   oregano, or 1 teaspoon
   dried

1 tablespoon chopped fresh
   thyme, or 1 teaspoon dried
2 cloves garlic
4 teaspoons safflower oil
1 1/2 onions, thinly sliced

- Trim meat of all visible fat. Grind fennel with mortar and pestle. Combine with flour, pepper, and herbs in a small bowl. Crush garlic with oil and rub onto meat. Place meat on a large piece of wax paper and rub the flour mixture over the entire surface. Arrange the onion slices over the meat. Wrap meat in the wax paper and then in a plastic bag or foil. Refrigerate at least overnight, preferably for 2 days.

- Preheat oven to 350°F. Remove wrappings from meat and place meat on rack in a roasting pan. Roast for 30 minutes to the pound, to an internal temperature of 165° to 170°F.

PER SERVING: 321 CALORIES		
MENU EXCHANGE PATTERN		
Dairy . . . . . —	Fruit . . . . . —	
Bread . . . . —	Meat 2½	
Fat 3½	Veg. 1	
NUTRITIONAL INFORMATION		
Carbohydrate 5	g	
Protein 17	g	
Total fat 26	g	
Saturated fat 8.6	g	
Cholesterol 73	mg	
Sodium 63	mg	
Potassium 362	mg	
Fiber 0.3	g	
Calcium 15	mg	
Iron . . . . 1.3 mg		

Carrot "Pennies"

2/3 cup cider vinegar
1 1/3 cups sugar
4 teaspoons mixed pickling
   spice
1 3-inch cinnamon stick,
   broken

1 1/2 teaspoons whole cloves
1 1/2 teaspoons whole allspice
1 1/3 pounds carrots, peeled and
   cut into 1/8-inch slices
1 1/3 cups water

- Combine vinegar, sugar, and spices in a medium nonaluminum saucepan (if desired, tie spices in a muslin bag). Simmer gently for 10 minutes. Strain syrup or remove spice bag. Let cool slightly.

- Cook carrots in water until just barely tender, about 5 to 10 minutes. Drain well.

- Pour spiced syrup over well-drained carrots. Refrigerate until ready to use.

PER SERVING: 84 CALORIES		
MENU EXCHANGE PATTERN		
Dairy . . . . . —	Fruit . . . . . —	
Bread 1	Meat . . . . . —	
Fat . . . . —	Veg. 1	
NUTRITIONAL INFORMATION		
Carbohydrate 21	g	
Protein 1	g	
Total fat 0	g	
Saturated fat 0	g	
Cholesterol 0	mg	
Sodium 56	mg	
Potassium 430	mg	
Fiber 1.3	g	
Calcium 46	mg	
Iron . . . . 0.9 mg		

Cornbread

1 cup yellow cornmeal
1 cup all-purpose or whole
    wheat flour
3 tablespoons sugar
1 tablespoon baking powder
1/3 cup nonfat dry milk powder

1/4 teaspoon salt
1 cup water
3 tablespoons safflower oil
2 egg whites, lightly beaten, or
    1 egg substitute

PER SERVING: 142 CALORIES		
MENU EXCHANGE PATTERN		
Dairy ..... —	Fruit ..... —	
Bread 1½	Meat ..... —	
Fat 1	Veg. ...... —	
NUTRITIONAL INFORMATION		
Carbohydrate 20		g
Protein 4		g
Total fat 5		g
Saturated fat 0.5		g
Cholesterol 0		mg
Sodium 201		mg
Potassium 119		mg
Fiber 0.4		g
Calcium 42		mg
Iron 0.6		mg

- Preheat oven to 425°F. Combine the cornmeal, flour, sugar, baking powder, milk powder, and salt in a medium bowl.

- Mix the water, oil, and egg whites. Add to the dry ingredients and mix just until blended. Bake in a greased 9-inch square pan until tester inserted in center comes out clean, about 20 to 25 minutes. Serve hot.

Fresh Fruit with Orange-Mint Sauce

1 cup plain low-fat yogurt
1 tablespoon honey
2 tablespoons unsweetened
    apple juice
2 drops green or red food
    coloring

1 orange
1/2 cup pineapple cubes
1 papaya, cut into cubes
1/2 cup grapes
1/2 cup strawberries
1/2 cup blueberries

Orange-Mint Oil

2 firmly packed cups orange
    mint leaves and tender stems
    (see note)
1/2 cup safflower oil

PER SERVING: 82 CALORIES		
MENU EXCHANGE PATTERN		
Dairy ..... —	Fruit 1	
Bread ..... ½	Meat ..... —	
Fat .... —	Veg. ...... —	
NUTRITIONAL INFORMATION		
Carbohydrate 14		g
Protein 2		g
Total fat 2		g
Saturated fat 0.5		g
Cholesterol 2		mg
Sodium 22		mg
Potassium 245		mg
Fiber 0.6		g
Calcium 71		mg
Iron 0.3	mg

- Combine mint and oil in blender and puree until smooth, turning blender off and on and pushing down leaves. Set aside 1 tablespoon for the sauce and refrigerate or freeze remainder in small containers.

- Combine 1 tablespoon mint oil, yogurt, honey, juice, and food coloring in a blender and mix well. Taste and adjust mint flavor and sweetness. Pour sauce over the fruit. Serve in individual dessert dishes or in a large, clear compote.

Note: Spearmint, apple mint, or peppermint may be substituted for orange mint.

MEAT ENTREES

5

Endive and Watercress Salad

Herbed Garlic Pork Chops

Wild and Patna Rice

Fresh Fruit Compote with Sauterne

Serves 2

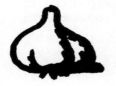

PER SERVING: 800 CALORIES		
MENU EXCHANGE PATTERN		
Dairy . . . . . —	Fruit 3	
Bread 4½	Meat 3½	
Fat 2½	Veg. 2	
NUTRITIONAL INFORMATION		
Carbohydrate 93	g	
Protein 34	g	
Total fat 27	g	
Saturated fat 8.6	g	
Cholesterol 90	mg	
Sodium 259	mg	
Potassium 1303	mg	
Fiber 3	g	
Calcium 123	mg	
Iron . . . . 4.6 mg		

Endive and Watercress Salad

1 medium Belgian endive
½ bunch watercress
2 Boston lettuce leaves

1 tomato, cut in 8 wedges
2 tablespoons commercial low-
   calorie Italian dressing

- Wash the endive, watercress, and lettuce thoroughly. Cut off the base of the endive and remove the outer leaves. Place the lettuce leaves on a plate and arrange the 5 endive leaves on it in a star pattern. Finely chop the heart of the endive and place it in the center of the star. Garnish with sprigs of watercress and tomato wedges. Drizzle dressing over salad.

Note: Recipe analysis includes dressing.

PER SERVING: 31 CALORIES		
MENU EXCHANGE PATTERN		
Dairy ..... —	Fruit ..... —	
Bread .... —	Meat ..... —	
Fat .... —	Veg. 1	
NUTRITIONAL INFORMATION		
Carbohydrate 6	g	
Protein 2	g	
Total fat 0	g	
Saturated fat 0	g	
Cholesterol 0	mg	
Sodium 16	mg	
Potassium 381	mg	
Fiber 0.9	g	
Calcium 68	mg	
Iron 1.4	mg	

Herbed Garlic Pork Chops

2 rib or loin pork chops,
   5 ounces each, well trimmed
1 clove garlic, mashed
1 teaspoon margarine
¼ cup dry white wine

½ teaspoon chopped fresh
   rosemary, or ¼ teaspoon
   dried
1 teaspoon fresh mint, or
   ¼ teaspoon dried

- Rub the chops with garlic. Melt the margarine in a large skillet over medium heat and brown the chops on both sides. The meat should be crusty outside and barely pink inside.

- Transfer the chops to serving plates and add wine and herbs to the pan drippings. Bring to a boil on top of the stove and simmer for 5 minutes, scraping loose all the browned particles. Spoon the pan juices over the chops and serve.

PER SERVING: 328 CALORIES		
MENU EXCHANGE PATTERN		
Dairy ..... —	Fruit ..... —	
Bread ..... ½	Meat 3½	
Fat 2	Veg. .... —	
NUTRITIONAL INFORMATION		
Carbohydrate 1	g	
Protein 26	g	
Total fat 22	g	
Saturated fat 8	g	
Cholesterol 90	mg	
Sodium 66	mg	
Potassium 357	mg	
Fiber 0	g	
Calcium 7	mg	
Iron 1	mg	

Wild and Patna Rice

1 teaspoon margarine
½ small onion, finely chopped
¼ cup Patna rice, washed and
   drained
¼ cup wild rice, washed and
   drained

½ teaspoon dried thyme
1 cup Homemade Chicken
   Stock (page 36)

- Melt the margarine in a large saucepan over medium heat, add the onion, and cook until soft, about 5 minutes. Add the rices and thyme, and cook for 2 minutes. Pour in the chicken stock and simmer until rice is tender, about 40 minutes. Fluff with a fork and serve.

PER SERVING: 213 CALORIES		
MENU EXCHANGE PATTERN		
Dairy ..... —	Fruit ..... —	
Bread 2½	Meat ..... —	
Fat .... —	Veg. 1	
NUTRITIONAL INFORMATION		
Carbohydrate 38	g	
Protein 5	g	
Total fat 2	g	
Saturated fat 0.4	g	
Cholesterol 0	mg	
Sodium 56	mg	
Potassium 134	mg	
Fiber 0.5	g	
Calcium 22	mg	
Iron 1.8	mg	

Fresh Fruit Compote
with Sauterne

1 small apple, cored and diced
1 peach, peeled, pitted, and
   sliced
⅓ cup diced fresh pineapple
⅓ cup Bing cherries, stemmed
   and pitted

½ lemon, thinly sliced
1 tablespoon sugar
¼ cup orange juice
¼ cup sauterne or other sweet
   white wine

- Combine the fruit in a large bowl.

- Heat the remaining ingredients in a saucepan until just boiling. Pour over the fruit. Stir, cover, and refrigerate until ready to serve.

PER SERVING: 213 CALORIES			
MENU EXCHANGE PATTERN			
Dairy	—	Fruit	3
Bread	1½	Meat	—
Fat	—	Veg.	—

NUTRITIONAL INFORMATION		
Carbohydrate	46	g
Protein	1	g
Total fat	1	g
Saturated fat	0.2	g
Cholesterol	0	mg
Sodium	3	mg
Potassium	429	mg
Fiber	1.6	g
Calcium	26	mg
Iron	0.6	mg

MEAT ENTREES

6

Beef Steamers

Steamed White Rice

Green and White Jade

Almond Cookies

Serves 6

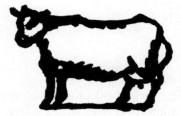

PER SERVING: 756 CALORIES			
MENU EXCHANGE PATTERN			
Dairy	—	Fruit	—
Bread 4½		Meat	4
Fat 2½		Veg.	4

NUTRITIONAL INFORMATION		
Carbohydrate 101	g
Protein 42	g
Total fat 21	g
Saturated fat 5	g
Cholesterol 91	mg
Sodium 530	mg
Potassium 1213	mg
Fiber 3.6	g
Calcium 157	mg
Iron 9.2	mg

Beef Steamers

$1\frac{1}{2}$ pounds beef flank steak
2 tablespoons soy sauce
6 tablespoons sweet bean paste
2 teaspoons Chinese hot sauce
3 tablespoons cornstarch
3 tablespoons dry white wine

2 tablespoons safflower oil
2 cups spicy rice powder
4 cups shredded green cabbage
2 tablespoons minced green
 onion

- Slice flank steak against the grain into 2 × 1 × ¼-inch pieces; pound pieces flat. Mix soy sauce, sweet bean paste, hot sauce, cornstarch, wine, and safflower oil in a large bowl. Add beef and marinate for 20 minutes, then dredge in rice powder.

- Line a steamer with half of the shredded cabbage and top with half of the beef. Steam over boiling water until cooked through, about 5 minutes. Repeat with remaining cabbage and beef. Transfer cabbage and beef to a warm serving platter, sprinkle with green onion, and serve with rice.

Note: Sweet bean paste, Chinese hot sauce, and spicy rice powder are available in Chinese groceries and the oriental section of some supermarkets.

PER SERVING: 371 CALORIES		
MENU EXCHANGE PATTERN		
Dairy . . . . . —	Fruit . . . . . —	
Bread 1½	Meat 4	
Fat . . . . —	Veg. 2	
NUTRITIONAL INFORMATION		
Carbohydrate 42	g	
Protein 34	g	
Total fat 8	g	
Saturated fat 3.2	g	
Cholesterol 80	mg	
Sodium 445	mg	
Potassium 829	mg	
Fiber 1.8	g	
Calcium 72	mg	
Iron 6.5	mg	

Steamed White Rice

$1\frac{1}{2}$ cups white rice
3 cups water

- Wash rice thoroughly. Bring water to a boil in a large saucepan set over medium-high heat and add rice. Bring water back to a boil, then cover, reduce heat to low, and simmer for about 20 minutes, or until water is absorbed. Fluff with a fork and serve.

PER SERVING: 177 CALORIES		
MENU EXCHANGE PATTERN		
Dairy . . . . . —	Fruit . . . . . —	
Bread 2½	Meat . . . . . —	
Fat . . . . —	Veg. . . . . . . —	
NUTRITIONAL INFORMATION		
Carbohydrate 39	g	
Protein 3	g	
Total fat 0	g	
Saturated fat 0	g	
Cholesterol 0	mg	
Sodium 3	mg	
Potassium 45	mg	
Fiber 0.1	g	
Calcium 12	mg	
Iron 1.4	mg	

Green and White Jade

2 cups cauliflower florets
6 medium broccoli stalks
   (about 2 cups)
1 cup diagonally sliced carrot
1 cup sliced mushrooms
2 tablespoons cornstarch
1/4 cup water

2 tablespoons safflower oil
2 teaspoons minced garlic
1 1/2 cups Homemade Chicken
   Stock (page 36)
1/4 teaspoon white pepper
1 teaspoon Oriental sesame oil

- Drop cauliflower into a large saucepan of boiling water and blanch for 1 minute. Remove cauliflower, then blanch broccoli, carrot, and mushrooms for 30 seconds. Drain well.

- Mix the cornstarch and water in a cup. Heat oil in a wok or large skillet over high heat. Add garlic and fry just until fragrant. Add the vegetables and stock and bring to a boil. Add white pepper, sesame oil, and cornstarch mixture and cook until vegetables are crisp-tender, about 3 to 4 minutes. Serve immediately.

PER SERVING: 98 CALORIES

MENU EXCHANGE PATTERN

Dairy	—	Fruit	—
Bread	—	Meat	—
Fat	1	Veg.	2

NUTRITIONAL INFORMATION

Carbohydrate	9	g
Protein	3	g
Total fat	6	g
Saturated fat	0.6	g
Cholesterol	0	mg
Sodium	20	mg
Potassium	335	mg
Fiber	1.5	g
Calcium	63	mg
Iron	0.9	mg

Almond Cookies

3/4 cup margarine
2/3 cup sugar
1 egg, lightly beaten
1 teaspoon almond extract
1 1/3 cups all-purpose flour
1/4 teaspoon baking soda

1/2 teaspoon baking powder
24 blanched whole almonds
   (about 1/3 cup)
1 egg white, mixed with 2
   tablespoons water

- Cream margarine, sugar, egg, and almond extract together with an electric beater. Sift flour, soda, and baking powder together and gradually blend into creamed mixture. Knead briefly and chill for at least 20 minutes.

- Preheat oven to 350°F. Roll chilled dough into 1-inch balls and arrange on a cookie sheet coated with nonstick spray. Flatten dough with the palm of your hand and top each cookie with an almond. Brush with egg white mixture. Bake until lightly browned, about 15 minutes. Transfer to racks to cool. Makes 2 dozen; 1 serving = 1 cookie.

PER SERVING: 110 CALORIES

MENU EXCHANGE PATTERN

Dairy	—	Fruit	—
Bread	1/2	Meat	—
Fat	1 1/2	Veg.	—

NUTRITIONAL INFORMATION

Carbohydrate	11	g
Protein	2	g
Total fat	7	g
Saturated fat	1.2	g
Cholesterol	11	mg
Sodium	19	mg
Potassium	46	mg
Fiber	0.2	g
Calcium	10	mg
Iron	0.4	mg

CHAPTER 8

COMPLETE DINNERS

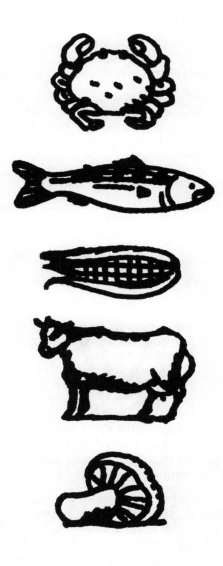

SHELLFISH

1

Fettuccine Primavera

Seafood Brochettes with Lemon Chive Sauce

Pecan Rice

Bananas Foster

Serves 4

PER SERVING: 1097 CALORIES		
MENU EXCHANGE PATTERN		
Dairy . . . . . . ½	Fruit 4	
Bread 5½	Meat 4½	
Fat 5	Veg. 3	
NUTRITIONAL INFORMATION		
Carbohydrate 128	g	
Protein 50	g	
Total fat 33	g	
Saturated fat 8	g	
Cholesterol 170	mg	
Sodium 797	mg	
Potassium 2072	mg	
Fiber 3.7	g	
Calcium 474	mg	
Iron 8.4	mg	

Fettuccine Primavera

2 carrots, sliced
1 cup broccoli florets
1 cup cauliflower florets
1 cup sliced zucchini
1/3 cup snow peas, ends
   trimmed
4 teaspoons margarine

1 teaspoon dried basil
Black pepper
1/4 cup Homemade Chicken
   Stock (page 36)
1/2 cup grated Parmesan cheese
1/3 pound fettuccine

- Blanch carrots, broccoli, and cauliflower by immersing in boiling water for about 1 minute. Remove and plunge into ice water. Drain and reserve. In a nonstick skillet over medium heat, sauté zucchini and snow peas in margarine until crisp-tender, about 3 to 4 minutes. Add carrots, broccoli, cauliflower, basil, and pepper to taste. Stir in chicken stock and Parmesan.

- Meanwhile, cook fettuccine until *al dente* and drain. Divide among serving plates and top with vegetable-cheese mixture. Serve immediately.

Photo opposite page 226.

PER SERVING: 276 CALORIES
MENU EXCHANGE PATTERN

Dairy	—	Fruit	—
Bread	2	Meat	1
Fat	1	Veg.	2

NUTRITIONAL INFORMATION

Carbohydrate	40	g
Protein	13	g
Total fat	8	g
Saturated fat	3	g
Cholesterol	8	mg
Sodium	216	mg
Potassium	615	mg
Fiber	2	g
Calcium	242	mg
Iron	2.7	mg

Seafood Brochettes

3/4 pound sea scallops, rinsed
   and drained
3/4 pound shrimp, shelled and
   deveined
1 small onion, chopped
2/3 cup whole mushrooms
8 cherry tomatoes

1 red bell pepper, small, cored,
   seeded, and cut into 1-inch
   squares
Pinch of black pepper
Lemon Chive Sauce (recipe
   follows)

- Alternate scallops, shrimp, and vegetables on 4 metal or wooden skewers. Sprinkle with pepper and grill over charcoal until seafood is just opaque and vegetables are crisp-tender. Serve immediately.

PER SERVING: 172 CALORIES
MENU EXCHANGE PATTERN

Dairy	—	Fruit	—
Bread	—	Meat	3½
Fat	—	Veg.	1

NUTRITIONAL INFORMATION

Carbohydrate	10	g
Protein	30	g
Total fat	1	g
Saturated fat	0	g
Cholesterol	153	mg
Sodium	344	mg
Potassium	733	mg
Fiber	0.8	g
Calcium	90	mg
Iron	3.4	mg

Lemon Chive Sauce

2/3 cup margarine
1 shallot, minced
Juice of 2 lemons
1/4 cup dry white wine

4 teaspoons evaporated skim
   milk
1/3 cup chopped fresh chives
White pepper to taste

Fish Stock

2/3 pound fish bones, rinsed
2/3 cup dry white wine
1 bay leaf

A few peppercorns
1 leek, coarsely chopped
1 stalk celery, coarsely chopped

- Place fish bones in large saucepan or stockpot. Pour in wine and enough water to cover. Add bay leaf, peppercorns, leek, and celery and bring to simmer. Simmer 45 minutes, then strain. Return liquid to pan and simmer until reduced by ½. Reserve ⅓ cup and save remainder for another use.

- Melt margarine in a nonstick saucepan over medium heat and sauté shallot until tender, about 3 minutes. Add ⅓ cup reduced stock, lemon juice, and wine and simmer until reduced by ½. Add milk and bring to a boil. Remove from heat. Stir in chives and pepper. Serve over Seafood Brochettes.

Note: If desired, substitute ⅓ cup Homemade Chicken Stock (page 36) for the reduced fish stock.

PER SERVING: 96 CALORIES		
MENU EXCHANGE PATTERN		
Dairy . . . . . —	Fruit . . . . . —	
Bread . . . . . ½	Meat . . . . . —	
Fat 1	Veg. . . . . . —	
NUTRITIONAL INFORMATION		
Carbohydrate 4	g	
Protein 1	g	
Total fat 8	g	
Saturated fat 1.5	g	
Cholesterol 14	mg	
Sodium 164	mg	
Potassium 102	mg	
Fiber 0.2	g	
Calcium 17	mg	
Iron 0.3	mg	

Pecan Rice

2 teaspoons margarine
½ small onion, chopped
⅔ cup rice
1⅓ cups Homemade Chicken
   Stock (page 36)
1 bay leaf

1 tablespoon Worcestershire
   sauce
White pepper
2 tablespoons chopped toasted
   pecans
⅓ cup chopped green onion

- Preheat oven to 350°F. Melt margarine in a nonstick, ovenproof saucepan and sauté onion over medium heat until translucent, about 5 minutes. Stir in rice and sauté 3 to 5 minutes. Add stock, bay leaf, and Worcestershire sauce. Cover and bake until rice is tender, about 20 minutes. Stir in pepper, pecans, and green onion; discard bay leaf and serve.

PER SERVING: 172 CALORIES		
MENU EXCHANGE PATTERN		
Dairy . . . . . —	Fruit . . . . . —	
Bread 2	Meat . . . . . —	
Fat 1	Veg. . . . . . —	
NUTRITIONAL INFORMATION		
Carbohydrate 29	g	
Protein 3	g	
Total fat 5	g	
Saturated fat 0.4	g	
Cholesterol 0	mg	
Sodium 16	mg	
Potassium 112	mg	
Fiber 0.4	g	
Calcium 21	mg	
Iron 1.3	mg	

Bananas Foster

3 bananas
3 tablespoons margarine
3 tablespoons firmly packed
   brown sugar
½ teaspoon ground cinnamon

3 tablespoons banana liqueur
½ cup light or dark rum
2 cups low-fat frozen vanilla
   yogurt

- Peel bananas; slice lengthwise twice and then in half crosswise. Melt margarine in a flat chafing dish or nonstick skillet. Add brown sugar and stir until sugar is melted. Add bananas and sauté until tender, about 3 minutes on each side, over medium-high heat. Sprinkle with cinnamon. Pour liqueur and rum over bananas, swirl pan to distribute, and ignite, shaking pan gently and basting the bananas with the sauce until the flames subside. Serve in individual dessert dishes over ½ cup frozen yogurt.

PER SERVING: 381 CALORIES		
MENU EXCHANGE PATTERN		
Dairy . . . . . . ½	Fruit 4	
Bread 1	Meat . . . . . —	
Fat 2	Veg. . . . . . —	
NUTRITIONAL INFORMATION		
Carbohydrate 45	g	
Protein 4	g	
Total fat 12	g	
Saturated fat 3.5	g	
Cholesterol 9	mg	
Sodium 57	mg	
Potassium 510	mg	
Fiber 0.4	g	
Calcium 104	mg	
Iron 0.7	mg	

SHELLFISH

2

Scallop Ceviche

Consommé Florentine with Orange

Lobster with Tomato-Tarragon Fettuccine

Sautéed Zucchini and Onions

Strawberry Shortcake

Serves 6

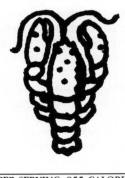

PER SERVING: 955 CALORIES		
MENU EXCHANGE PATTERN		
Dairy . . . . . —	Fruit 1½	
Bread 5	Meat 5	
Fat 3½	Veg. 4	
NUTRITIONAL INFORMATION		
Carbohydrate 117	g	
Protein 53	g	
Total fat 30	g	
Saturated fat 3.8	g	
Cholesterol 220	mg	
Sodium 1299	mg	
Potassium 2018	mg	
Fiber 2.3	g	
Calcium 317	mg	
Iron 7.9	mg	

Scallop Ceviche

3/4 pound bay scallops
1/2 cup lime juice
1/2 white onion, sliced into rings
  and blanched 2 minutes
1 large tomato, peeled and
  diced
1/4 cup fresh coriander
  (cilantro) or parsley leaves

2 tablespoons safflower oil
1 1/2 jalapeño chilies, seeded and
  chopped
6 leaves lettuce
Lime slices (garnish)

PER SERVING: 102 CALORIES			
MENU EXCHANGE PATTERN			
Dairy	—	Fruit	—
Bread	—	Meat	1
Fat	1	Veg.	—
NUTRITIONAL INFORMATION			
Carbohydrate 6			g
Protein 9			g
Total fat 5			g
Saturated fat 0			g
Cholesterol 23			mg
Sodium 147			mg
Potassium 358			mg
Fiber 0.3			g
Calcium 28			mg
Iron .... 1.3 mg			

- Place scallops in a glass or ceramic dish, add lime juice and stir. Cover and refrigerate at least 4 hours, stirring once. Add onion, tomato, cilantro, oil, and chilies and stir gently. Cover and refrigerate 4 hours. To serve, arrange on lettuce leaves and garnish with lime slices.

Consommé Florentine with Orange

2 cups orange juice
4 cups Homemade Chicken
  Stock (page 36)
1/4 teaspoon white pepper

1 tablespoon safflower oil
1/4 cup low-sodium soy sauce
1 pound spinach, stemmed and
  torn into bite-size pieces

PER SERVING: 99 CALORIES			
MENU EXCHANGE PATTERN			
Dairy	—	Fruit	1/2
Bread	1/2	Meat	—
Fat	1/2	Veg.	1
NUTRITIONAL INFORMATION			
Carbohydrate 12			g
Protein 6			g
Total fat 4			g
Saturated fat 0.5			g
Cholesterol 1			mg
Sodium 611			mg
Potassium 522			mg
Fiber 0.3			g
Calcium 49			mg
Iron 2			mg

- Combine juice, stock, pepper, and oil in a saucepan and bring to simmer. Place a handful of raw spinach into each bowl, cover with hot broth, and serve.

Lobster with Tomato-Tarragon Fettuccine

2 live lobsters, 1½ pounds each
   (about 1½ pounds total
   meat)
¼ cup olive oil
½ cup chopped onion
1 clove garlic
4 ripe tomatoes, chopped and
   seeded (4 cups)
2 tablespoons chopped fresh
   parsley

1 teaspoon dried thyme
1 tablespoon chopped fresh
   tarragon, or 1 teaspoon
   dried
Cayenne pepper to taste
½ cup dry white wine
3 tablespoons tomato paste
1 pound fettuccine

- Kill lobsters by severing spinal column at point where body and tail adjoin. Cut bodies lengthwise and clean, removing all green material (tomalley) and coral. Cut each body and tail into 4 crosswise pieces. Crack claws.

- In a heavy skillet, heat 3 tablespoons olive oil over medium-high heat and add lobster pieces. Cook about 10 minutes until shell turns pink and meat is opaque. Transfer lobster to a plate and remove meat from shell. Set aside.

- Add onion and garlic to skillet and sauté in remaining olive oil until onion is translucent, about 5 minutes. Add tomatoes, seasonings, white wine, and tomato paste. Stir, lower heat to a simmer, cover, and cook sauce for about 30 minutes.

- Bring 2 quarts water to a boil in a large saucepan. Add fettuccine and cook until *al dente*, about 5 minutes. Drain well.

- Add lobster meat to sauce. Cook 5 minutes to heat thoroughly. Then transfer fettuccine to dinner plates and top with lobster and sauce.

PER SERVING: 518 CALORIES

MENU EXCHANGE PATTERN

Dairy	—	Fruit	—
Bread	3½	Meat	4
Fat	—	Veg.	2

NUTRITIONAL INFORMATION

Carbohydrate	67	g
Protein	31	g
Total fat	12	g
Saturated fat	1.2	g
Cholesterol	193	mg
Sodium	350	mg
Potassium	853	mg
Fiber	0.8	g
Calcium	78	mg
Iron	3.9	mg

Sautéed Zucchini and Onions

2 white onions, thinly sliced
2 tablespoons safflower oil
3 small zucchini, thinly sliced

¼ teaspoon black pepper
¼ teaspoon dried rosemary

- In a large nonstick skillet, sauté onions in oil over medium heat until lightly brown, about 5 minutes. Add zucchini and cook until slightly softened, 5 to 10 minutes. Season with pepper and rosemary and serve immediately.

PER SERVING: 67 CALORIES

MENU EXCHANGE PATTERN

Dairy	—	Fruit	—
Bread	—	Meat	—
Fat	1	Veg.	1

NUTRITIONAL INFORMATION

Carbohydrate	6	g
Protein	1	g
Total fat	5	g
Saturated fat	0	g
Cholesterol	0	mg
Sodium	3	mg
Potassium	219	mg
Fiber	0.6	g
Calcium	31	mg
Iron	0.5	mg

Strawberry Shortcake

1 cup whole wheat pastry flour
1 teaspoon baking powder
1/4 teaspoon salt
1/4 teaspoon baking soda
2 tablespoons margarine,
   chilled

1/3 cup buttermilk
1 1/2 cups plain low-fat yogurt
2 tablespoons honey
1 teaspoon vanilla extract
2 cups sliced strawberries

- Preheat oven to 425°F. Combine all dry ingredients in a large bowl and toss with a fork. Cut in margarine with a pastry blender until mixture is the consistency of coarse crumbs. Pour in buttermilk all at once and stir just until dough holds together; mix as briefly as possible.

- Pat and roll dough quickly and lightly to 3/4-inch thickness. Cut with a floured 2½-inch biscuit cutter by pressing down firmly without twisting. Arrange biscuits on an ungreased cookie sheet and bake until golden, about 15 minutes.

- Combine yogurt, honey, and vanilla and mix well. Split biscuits in half, allowing one per person. Fill with yogurt mixture and strawberries and serve immediately.

Note: Whole wheat pastry flour is available in natural foods stores.

PER SERVING: 169 CALORIES			
MENU EXCHANGE PATTERN			
Dairy	—	Fruit	1
Bread	1	Meat	—
Fat	1	Veg.	—
NUTRITIONAL INFORMATION			
Carbohydrate	27		g
Protein	5		g
Total fat	5		g
Saturated fat	1		g
Cholesterol	4		mg
Sodium	188		mg
Potassium	256		mg
Fiber	0.3		g
Calcium	131		mg
Iron	0.4		mg

SHELLFISH

3

Shrimp Cocktail

Crawfish Étouffée with Rice

Southern-Style Spinach

Dilled Garlic Bread

Blueberry Cheesecake

Serves 6

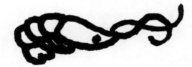

PER SERVING: 987 CALORIES
MENU EXCHANGE PATTERN

Dairy	1	Fruit	—
Bread	5½	Meat	5½
Fat	3½	Veg.	3

NUTRITIONAL INFORMATION

Carbohydrate	119	g
Protein	62	g
Total fat	29	g
Saturated fat	5.8	g
Cholesterol	254	mg
Sodium	1818	mg
Potassium	1129	mg
Fiber	1.5	g
Calcium	342	mg
Iron	7.3	mg

Shrimp Cocktail

24 large shrimp (1¼ pounds),
  shelled and deveined
Cocktail Sauce (recipe follows)
3 lemons, cut in wedges

- Cook shrimp in a large quantity of boiling water until pink, about 5 minutes. Drain and immediately drop into ice water until thoroughly cooled. Drain well. Serve on ice with Cocktail Sauce and lemon wedges.

PER SERVING: 86 CALORIES		
MENU EXCHANGE PATTERN		
Dairy .... —	Fruit .... —	
Bread .... —	Meat 2	
Fat .... —	Veg. ..... —	
NUTRITIONAL INFORMATION		
Carbohydrate 1		g
Protein 17		g
Total fat 1		g
Saturated fat 0		g
Cholesterol 132		mg
Sodium 132		mg
Potassium 207		mg
Fiber 0		g
Calcium 60		mg
Iron .... 1.5 mg		

Cocktail Sauce

¾ cup catsup
1 tablespoon lemon juice
Tabasco sauce
1 tablespoon prepared
  horseradish

1 tablespoon minced fresh
  parsley

- Combine all ingredients and chill thoroughly.

Note: Low-sodium catsup may be substituted for regular.

PER SERVING: 32 CALORIES		
MENU EXCHANGE PATTERN		
Dairy .... —	Fruit .... —	
Bread .... —	Meat ...... —	
Fat .... —	Veg. 1	
NUTRITIONAL INFORMATION		
Carbohydrate 7		g
Protein 1		g
Total fat 0		g
Saturated fat 0		g
Cholesterol 0		mg
Sodium 297		mg
Potassium 117		mg
Fiber 0.1		g
Calcium 9		mg
Iron .... 0.2 mg		

Crawfish Étouffée with Rice

1½ pounds cleaned crawfish
  tails
¼ teaspoon cayenne pepper
¼ cup margarine
1 onion, finely chopped
1 green bell pepper, cored,
  seeded, and finely chopped
2 teaspoons all-purpose flour
¾ cup water

1 lemon, thinly sliced
2 tablespoons tomato paste
1 clove garlic, minced
1 tablespoon chopped green
  onion
1 tablespoon chopped fresh
  parsley
6 cups cooked rice

- Season crawfish tails with cayenne. Melt margarine in a medium saucepan over medium heat. Add onion and green pepper and cook until tender, about 10 minutes. Blend in flour. Add water, lemon, tomato paste, and garlic and simmer for 20 minutes.

- Add crawfish tails, cover, and cook for 8 minutes. Taste and adjust seasoning. Stir in green onion and parsley and serve over rice.

PER SERVING: 413 CALORIES		
MENU EXCHANGE PATTERN		
Dairy .... —	Fruit .... —	
Bread 3	Meat 3	
Fat .... —	Veg. 1	
NUTRITIONAL INFORMATION		
Carbohydrate 54		g
Protein 25		g
Total fat 10		g
Saturated fat 1.5		g
Cholesterol 113		mg
Sodium 630		mg
Potassium 292		mg
Fiber 0.5		g
Calcium 85		mg
Iron .... 3.1 mg		

Southern-Style Spinach

1¹/₂ pounds fresh spinach
2 tablespoons margarine
1 small onion, grated
1 clove garlic, chopped

1¹/₂ tablespoons all-purpose
*   flour*
³/₄ cup skim milk

- Boil spinach in 1 quart water for 10 minutes; drain. Chop spinach. Melt margarine in a saucepan over medium heat. Add onion and garlic and sauté until translucent, about 5 minutes. Stir in flour. Add milk and cook, stirring, until thickened. Add spinach and cook 2 or 3 minutes. Serve immediately.

PER SERVING: 66 CALORIES			
MENU EXCHANGE PATTERN			
Dairy	—	Fruit	—
Bread	—	Meat	—
Fat	1	Veg.	1
NUTRITIONAL INFORMATION			
Carbohydrate	6	g	
Protein	3	g	
Total fat	4	g	
Saturated fat	0.8	g	
Cholesterol	0	mg	
Sodium	48	mg	
Potassium	275	mg	
Fiber	0.3	g	
Calcium	82	mg	
Iron	1.4	mg	

Dilled Garlic Bread

¹/₄ cup margarine
2 cloves garlic, mashed
¹/₄ cup grated Parmesan cheese

Dried dillweed
1 loaf French bread

- Whip margarine with garlic. Cover and let stand at room temperature for at least 30 minutes for flavor to develop.

- Preheat oven to 325°F. Cut French bread into 12 diagonal slices. Spread margarine mixture between slices and on top of bread. Sprinkle with cheese and dillweed. Wrap in aluminum foil and bake for 15 minutes. Serve hot. Makes 12 slices; 1 serving = 1 slice.

PER SERVING: 115 CALORIES			
MENU EXCHANGE PATTERN			
Dairy	—	Fruit	—
Bread	1	Meat	—
Fat	1	Veg.	—
NUTRITIONAL INFORMATION			
Carbohydrate	14	g	
Protein	3	g	
Total fat	5	g	
Saturated fat	1.2	g	
Cholesterol	1	mg	
Sodium	176	mg	
Potassium	28	mg	
Fiber	0.1	g	
Calcium	35	mg	
Iron	0.6	mg	

Blueberry Cheesecake

1 cup graham cracker crumbs
2 tablespoons margarine,
    melted
1 tablespoon safflower oil
1 package (3 ounces) lemon
    gelatin

1 cup boiling water
1½ pounds low-fat cottage
    cheese
¼ cup sugar

Blueberry Topping

1 cup fresh or frozen
    blueberries
½ cup water

2 tablespoons sugar
1½ teaspoons cornstarch
2 teaspoons lemon juice

- Combine crumbs, margarine, and oil and press into the bottom of an 8-inch springform pan. Set crust aside.

- Add gelatin to boiling water, stirring to dissolve. Cool to room temperature.

- Thoroughly mix cottage cheese and sugar in a blender or food processor. With machine running, slowly add gelatin. Pour into the prepared crust and chill thoroughly.

- Combine blueberries and water in a saucepan and bring to simmer. Blend sugar with cornstarch. Add to blueberries and cook, stirring constantly, until smooth. Stir in lemon juice. Let cool completely. When cheesecake is firm, pour cooled topping over. Refrigerate until serving time. Makes 8 servings; 1 serving = one 1-inch slice.

PER SERVING: 275 CALORIES			
MENU EXCHANGE PATTERN			
Dairy	1	Fruit	—
Bread	1½	Meat	½
Fat	1½	Veg.	—
NUTRITIONAL INFORMATION			
Carbohydrate		36	g
Protein		14	g
Total fat		9	g
Saturated fat		2.3	g
Cholesterol		7	mg
Sodium		535	mg
Potassium		210	mg
Fiber		0.5	g
Calcium		72	mg
Iron		0.5	mg

SHELLFISH

4

Raw Vegetables with Basil Dip

Skillet Scallops Italienne

Ratatouille

Hilltop Whole Wheat Bread

Spring Fruit Compote

Serves 4

PER SERVING: 896 CALORIES			
MENU EXCHANGE PATTERN			
Dairy	½	Fruit	5
Bread	2½	Meat	2½
Fat	4	Veg.	6
NUTRITIONAL INFORMATION			
Carbohydrate	113	g	
Protein	41	g	
Total fat	29	g	
Saturated fat	3.5	g	
Cholesterol	50	mg	
Sodium	665	mg	
Potassium	2845	mg	
Fiber	7.5	g	
Calcium	366	mg	
Iron	8.6	mg	

Raw Vegetables with Basil Dip

⅔ cup broccoli florets
2 carrots, peeled and cut into
    sticks
½ cup mushrooms

1 cucumber, peeled and cut
    into strips
1 tomato, cut into wedges

Basil Dip

2 teaspoons lemon juice
2 tablespoons fresh basil
½ clove garlic
1 tablespoon chopped fresh
    parsley

½ cup low-fat cottage cheese
2 tablespoons plain low-fat
    yogurt

PER SERVING: 76 CALORIES		
MENU EXCHANGE PATTERN		
Dairy . . . . . ½	Fruit . . . . . —	
Bread . . . . —	Meat . . . . . —	
Fat . . . . —	Veg. 1	
NUTRITIONAL INFORMATION		
Carbohydrate 11		g
Protein 7		g
Total fat 1		g
Saturated fat 0.4		g
Cholesterol 3		mg
Sodium 147		mg
Potassium 519		mg
Fiber 1.5		g
Calcium 102		mg
Iron . . . . 1.4 mg		

- Prepare dip. Combine lemon juice, basil, garlic, and parsley in a blender and mix until smooth. Add cottage cheese and yogurt and again blend until smooth.

- Arrange vegetables on salad plates and serve with dip.

Skillet Scallops Italienne

1 pound scallops
¼ cup all-purpose flour
3 tablespoons safflower oil
1 clove garlic, minced
¾ cup water or Homemade
    Chicken Stock (page 36)
1 teaspoon dried savory

4 teaspoons chopped pimiento
4 teaspoons lemon juice
1 tablespoon chopped fresh
    parsley
¾ pound green beans, ends
    trimmed

PER SERVING: 237 CALORIES		
MENU EXCHANGE PATTERN		
Dairy . . . . . —	Fruit . . . . . —	
Bread . . . . . ½	Meat 2½	
Fat 1	Veg. 1	
NUTRITIONAL INFORMATION		
Carbohydrate 16		g
Protein 20		g
Total fat 11		g
Saturated fat 0.9		g
Cholesterol 45		mg
Sodium 296		mg
Potassium 701		mg
Fiber 1.1		g
Calcium 83		mg
Iron . . . . 3.1 mg		

- Dust scallops with flour. Heat oil in a large nonstick skillet over medium-high heat. Add garlic and scallops and brown scallops lightly on all sides, about 5 minutes. Set aside.

- Meanwhile, bring water or stock to a boil with savory, pimiento, lemon juice, and parsley. Add green beans and cook until tender. Drain well.

- Toss beans with scallops and serve.

Ratatouille

³/₄ cup coarsely chopped onion
2 cloves garlic, chopped
3 tablespoons safflower oil
³/₄ cup coarsely chopped green
*   bell pepper*
1¹/₂ cups diced eggplant

1¹/₂ cups zucchini, sliced ¹/₂ inch
*   thick*
6 large tomatoes, diced
2 teaspoons dried basil, or
*   2 tablespoons fresh*
¹/₄ teaspoon dried thyme

- In a large nonstick saucepan, sauté onion and garlic in oil over medium heat until soft, about 10 minutes. Add green pepper and eggplant, cover, and cook over medium-low heat for 30 minutes. Add zucchini, tomatoes, basil, and thyme and continue cooking, covered, for 15 minutes; if necessary, uncover for last 10 minutes of cooking to reduce liquid. Serve hot or cold.

PER SERVING: 196 CALORIES			
MENU EXCHANGE PATTERN			
Dairy	—	Fruit	1
Bread	—	Meat	—
Fat	2	Veg.	3

NUTRITIONAL INFORMATION		
Carbohydrate	23	g
Protein	5	g
Total fat	11	g
Saturated fat	0.9	g
Cholesterol	0	mg
Sodium	15	mg
Potassium	1015	mg
Fiber	2.9	g
Calcium	69	mg
Iron	2.3	mg

Hilltop Whole Wheat Bread

1 cup skim milk
¹/₂ cup margarine
1 cup cold water
¹/₂ cup firmly packed brown
*   sugar*
1¹/₂ teaspoons salt
2 envelopes active dry yeast
1¹/₂ tablespoons wheat germ
2 tablespoons soy flour

1 tablespoon Hilltop Herb Farm
*   Good 'n Nuff Seasoning (see*
*   note)*
3 cups whole wheat flour
2 egg substitutes
3 cups unbleached all-purpose
*   flour*
Margarine, melted

- Scald milk and add ¹/₂ cup margarine. Stir to melt margarine and remove from heat. Add cold water and let cool to luke-warm.

- In large bowl of electric mixer, combine brown sugar, salt, yeast, wheat germ, soy flour, seasoning, and 2 cups of the whole wheat flour. Add cooled milk mixture and beat 1 minute at medium speed. Add egg substitutes and beat at high speed for 2 minutes. By hand stir in remaining 1 cup whole wheat flour and the unbleached flour. Place dough in a greased large bowl, cover and refrigerate for 2 hours.

- Shape dough into 2 loaves and place in greased 9 × 5-inch loaf pans. Cover with a towel, place in a warm area and let rise until doubled in volume, about 1 hour.

- Preheat oven to 350°F. Bake loaves until they sound hollow when tapped, about 40 to 45 minutes. Remove from pans and brush tops lightly with melted margarine while hot. Let loaves cool on racks before slicing. Each loaf makes 10 slices; 1 serving = 1 slice.

Note: One teaspoon each of ground coriander, cumin, and fennel may be substituted.

PER SERVING: 196 CALORIES			
MENU EXCHANGE PATTERN			
Dairy	—	Fruit	—
Bread	2	Meat	—
Fat	1	Veg.	—

NUTRITIONAL INFORMATION		
Carbohydrate	33	g
Protein	6	g
Total fat	5	g
Saturated fat	1	g
Cholesterol	0	mg
Sodium	177	mg
Potassium	154	mg
Fiber	0.5	g
Calcium	36	mg
Iron	1.1	mg

Spring Fruit Compote

3/4 cup raspberries
1 1/2 peaches
3/4 cup cantaloupe

3/4 cup blueberries
1/2 cup plain low-fat yogurt

Marinade

1 1/2 cups dry white wine
3 tablespoons sugar
2-inch piece of vanilla bean, cut into small pieces
2 teaspoons cassia buds

1/3 cup fresh basil, or 2 1/2 tablespoons dried
1/3 cup rose geranium leaves
Rind of 1/2 lemon, cut into strips

- Prepare marinade. Combine all ingredients in a heavy saucepan, bring to a boil and cook 1 minute. Remove from heat and let steep 15 to 20 minutes, stirring occasionally. Cool to room temperature. Strain syrup.

- Cut fruit into bite-size pieces and combine with yogurt in a large bowl. Pour marinade over fruit and refrigerate for several hours before serving.

Note: Cassia buds and rose geranium leaves are available in specialty food stores and gourmet shops.

PER SERVING: 191 CALORIES			
MENU EXCHANGE PATTERN			
Dairy	—	Fruit	4
Bread	—	Meat	—
Fat	—	Veg.	1

NUTRITIONAL INFORMATION		
Carbohydrate	30	g
Protein	3	g
Total fat	1	g
Saturated fat	0.3	g
Cholesterol	2	mg
Sodium	30	mg
Potassium	456	mg
Fiber	1.5	g
Calcium	76	mg
Iron	0.7	mg

SHELLFISH

5

Spicy Squid

Four-Season Tossed Green Salad

Crab Leg Do-Fu

Steamed White Rice (page 185)

Almond Gelatin with Fruit

Serves 2

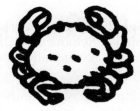

PER SERVING: 799 CALORIES		
MENU EXCHANGE PATTERN		
Dairy . . . . . —	Fruit 2½	
Bread 2½	Meat 5½	
Fat 3½	Veg. 3	
NUTRITIONAL INFORMATION		
Carbohydrate 83	g	
Protein 46	g	
Total fat 32	g	
Saturated fat 3.1	g	
Cholesterol 57	mg	
Sodium 1040	mg	
Potassium 757	mg	
Fiber 2.1	g	
Calcium 282	mg	
Iron 7.6	mg	

Spicy Squid

6 ounces baby squid
1 tablespoon safflower oil
1 teaspoon minced garlic
1 teaspoon minced chili pepper
1 teaspoon low-sodium soy
   sauce

1 tablespoon chopped green
   onion
1 teaspoon dry white wine
1/2 teaspoon Oriental sesame oil

- Place squid flat on a cutting board. Hold the body of the squid with one hand and pull out the tentacles and clear inner "quill" with the other hand. Peel off spotted skin. Cut cleaned squid into 1/2-inch pieces, wash thoroughly, and drain.

- Heat 2 teaspoons safflower oil in a wok or large saucepan over high heat. Add squid and stir-fry until it begins to turn white, about 1 to 2 minutes. Remove squid and drain.

- Reheat wok or saucepan with remaining 1 teaspoon safflower oil. Stir in garlic, chili, and soy sauce and heat until fragrant. Add squid and onion and stir-fry for another minute. Sprinkle with wine and seasame oil and serve immediately.

PER SERVING: 170 CALORIES

MENU EXCHANGE PATTERN

Dairy	. . . . —	Fruit	. . . . . —
Bread	. . . . —	Meat	. . . 2½
Fat	. . . . ½	Veg.	. . . . . . —

NUTRITIONAL INFORMATION

Carbohydrate	 2	g
Protein	 17	g
Total fat	 10	g
Saturated fat	. . . . 0.9	g
Cholesterol	 0	mg
Sodium	 172	mg
Potassium	 21	mg
Fiber	 0	g
Calcium	 13	mg
Iron	. . . . 0.5	mg

Four-Season Tossed Green Salad

2 cups shredded lettuce
2/3 cup bean sprouts
1/3 cup shredded carrot
Four-Season Salad Dressing
   (recipe follows)

- Arrange shredded lettuce on individual salad plates. Cover with a layer of bean sprouts and a second layer of shredded carrot. Pour dressing over salad and serve.

Note: To reduce fat intake, substitute a commercial low-calorie Italian dressing. Adjusted analysis for dressing: calories = 16; exchange = 1/2 Fat.

PER SERVING: 45 CALORIES

MENU EXCHANGE PATTERN

Dairy	. . . . —	Fruit	. . . . . —
Bread	. . . . —	Meat	. . . . . —
Fat	. . . . —	Veg.	 2

NUTRITIONAL INFORMATION

Carbohydrate	 7	g
Protein	 3	g
Total fat	 0	g
Saturated fat	 0	g
Cholesterol	 0	mg
Sodium	 22	mg
Potassium	 268	mg
Fiber	. . . . 0.8	g
Calcium	 51	mg
Iron	. . . . 1.7	mg

Four-Season Salad Dressing

4 teaspoons safflower oil
2 teaspoons black peppercorns
1/2 teaspoon minced garlic

2 teaspoons sugar
1/3 cup rice or cider vinegar

- Prepare peppercorn oil by heating safflower oil in a small saucepan to 400°F. Add peppercorns and heat, stirring, until aromatic, about 2 to 3 minutes. Strain oil to remove peppercorns. Let oil cool.

- Mix garlic, sugar, vinegar, and pepper oil and pour over salad.

PER SERVING: 103 CALORIES		
MENU EXCHANGE PATTERN		
Dairy . . . . . —	Fruit 1/2	
Bread . . . . . —	Meat . . . . . . —	
Fat 2	Veg. . . . . —	
NUTRITIONAL INFORMATION		
Carbohydrate 7		g
Protein 0		g
Total fat 9		g
Saturated fat 0.8		g
Cholesterol 0		mg
Sodium 1		mg
Potassium 48		mg
Fiber 0		g
Calcium 3		mg
Iron 0.3		mg

Crab Leg Do-Fu

1/2 pound firm bean curd
1 tablespoon safflower oil
1 teaspoon shredded ginger
1 teaspoon minced garlic
1/4 cup Homemade Chicken
    Stock (page 36)

1/4 pound crab legs
1/2 cup snow peas
1 tablespoon oyster sauce

- Cut bean curd into 1/2-inch cubes. Heat oil in a wok or large skillet over high heat. Add ginger and garlic and stir-fry for 10 seconds. Add bean curd and stock and simmer for 2 to 3 minutes, stirring frequently.

- Add crab legs and snow peas and simmer until peas are cooked but still crisp, about 2 to 3 minutes. Stir in oyster sauce and serve with steamed rice.

PER SERVING: 232 CALORIES		
MENU EXCHANGE PATTERN		
Dairy . . . . . —	Fruit . . . . . —	
Bread . . . . . —	Meat 3	
Fat 1	Veg. 1	
NUTRITIONAL INFORMATION		
Carbohydrate 9		g
Protein 22		g
Total fat 13		g
Saturated fat 1.4		g
Cholesterol 57		mg
Sodium 835		mg
Potassium 264		mg
Fiber 0.9		g
Calcium 182		mg
Iron 3.6		mg

Almond Gelatin with Fruit

1/8 ounce agar-agar, or
    1 envelope unflavored
    gelatin
1 1/2 cups water
2 tablespoons skim milk

1/2 teaspoon almond extract
2 tablespoons sugar
1 peach, peeled, pitted, and
    diced; or 1 cup seedless
    grapes, halved

- Mince agar-agar, add water, and soak for 3 minutes. Transfer to a saucepan and place over low heat until agar-agar dissolves. (If using gelatin, sprinkle over the water and soak for 5 minutes, then heat until gelatin dissolves.)

- Blend milk, almond extract, and sugar and stir into the dissolved agar-agar. Pour into an 8-inch square pan and chill until set, about 30 minutes. Cut gelatin into bite-size cubes. Toss cubes gently with fruit, transfer to dessert glasses and serve.

PER SERVING: 72 CALORIES		
MENU EXCHANGE PATTERN		
Dairy . . . . . —	Fruit 2	
Bread . . . . . —	Meat . . . . . . —	
Fat . . . . —	Veg. . . . . —	
NUTRITIONAL INFORMATION		
Carbohydrate 18		g
Protein 1		g
Total fat 0		g
Saturated fat 0		g
Cholesterol 0		mg
Sodium 8		mg
Potassium 111		mg
Fiber 0.3		g
Calcium 21		mg
Iron 0.1		mg

FIN FISH

1

Sautéed Mushrooms

Trout Amandine

Rice Pilaf

Braised Carrots with Onions

Fresh Peach Crumble

Serves 4

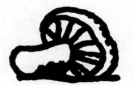

PER SERVING: 894 CALORIES		
MENU EXCHANGE PATTERN		
Dairy . . . . . —	Fruit 3	
Bread 2½	Meat 5	
Fat 5	Veg. 3	
NUTRITIONAL INFORMATION		
Carbohydrate 85	g	
Protein 40	g	
Total fat 43	g	
Saturated fat 4.5	g	
Cholesterol 78	mg	
Sodium 111	mg	
Potassium 1542	mg	
Fiber 2.6	g	
Calcium 161	mg	
Iron 5.6	mg	

Sautéed Mushrooms

2 teaspoons margarine
2 teaspoons dry sherry
1/2 teaspoon black pepper
1 1/3 cups sliced mushrooms

- Melt margarine in a large skillet over medium heat. Add sherry and pepper, then mushrooms. Sauté until most of liquid has evaporated, 10 to 15 minutes, and serve immediately.

PER SERVING: 27 CALORIES			
MENU EXCHANGE PATTERN			
Dairy . . . . . —	Fruit . . . . . —		
Bread . . . . . —	Meat . . . . . —		
Fat . . . . —	Veg. 1		
NUTRITIONAL INFORMATION			
Carbohydrate 1	g		
Protein 0	g		
Total fat 2	g		
Saturated fat 0	g		
Cholesterol 0	mg		
Sodium 4	mg		
Potassium 101	mg		
Fiber 0	g		
Calcium 3	mg		
Iron 0	mg		

Trout Amandine

1/2 teaspoon paprika
1/3 cup all-purpose flour
4 skinless trout fillets, 5 ounces each
4 teaspoons safflower oil
4 teaspoons margarine, melted

1/4 cup dry sherry
Juice of 1 lemon
1/3 cup blanched sliced almonds, lightly toasted
1/4 cup finely chopped fresh parsley

- Combine paprika and flour. Dredge trout in flour mixture to coat lightly. Heat oil in a large nonstick skillet over medium-high heat, add trout, and sauté until tender and flaky, about 10 minutes, turning at least once during cooking. Melt margarine in a small saucepan. Add sherry and lemon juice and heat thoroughly. Pour sherry sauce over trout and let stand for 3 to 4 minutes. Remove trout from sauce. Transfer to a warm platter, sprinkle with almonds and parsley, and serve.

PER SERVING: 447 CALORIES			
MENU EXCHANGE PATTERN			
Dairy . . . . . —	Fruit . . . . . —		
Bread . . . . . —	Meat 5		
Fat 3	Veg. 1		
NUTRITIONAL INFORMATION			
Carbohydrate 5	g		
Protein 33	g		
Total fat 31	g		
Saturated fat 3	g		
Cholesterol 78	mg		
Sodium 58	mg		
Potassium 817	mg		
Fiber 0.4	g		
Calcium 68	mg		
Iron 2.3	mg		

Rice Pilaf

4 teaspoons margarine
1/3 cup chopped onion
1 clove garlic, minced

2/3 cup rice
1 1/3 cups water or Homemade Chicken Stock (page 36)

- Melt margarine in a nonstick skillet over medium heat. Add onion and garlic and sauté until golden, about 8 to 10 minutes. Add rice and sauté 5 minutes. Add stock, cover, and cook over low heat until liquid is absorbed, about 20 minutes.

Note: To further reduce fat, simmer onion and garlic in about 1/2 cup of water or chicken stock until softened. Add remaining water or stock and rice and cook according to directions above. Adjusted analysis: calories = 112; exchange = 1 1/2 Bread.

PER SERVING: 157 CALORIES			
MENU EXCHANGE PATTERN			
Dairy . . . . . —	Fruit . . . . . —		
Bread 1 1/2	Meat . . . . . —		
Fat 1	Veg. . . . . . —		
NUTRITIONAL INFORMATION			
Carbohydrate 27	g		
Protein 2	g		
Total fat 4	g		
Saturated fat 0	g		
Cholesterol 0	mg		
Sodium 3	mg		
Potassium 56	mg		
Fiber 0	g		
Calcium 13	mg		
Iron 1	mg		

Braised Carrots with Onions

4 carrots, peeled and sliced
   into julienne
8 small white onions, peeled
1 teaspoon safflower oil

2 teaspoons margarine
2 teaspoons sugar
1/2 cup water

PER SERVING: 72 CALORIES		
MENU EXCHANGE PATTERN		
Dairy . . . . . —	Fruit	1
Bread . . . . . —	Meat	—
Fat . . . . —	Veg.	1
NUTRITIONAL INFORMATION		
Carbohydrate 15		g
Protein 2		g
Total fat 1		g
Saturated fat 0.1		g
Cholesterol 0		mg
Sodium 40		mg
Potassium 346		mg
Fiber 1.2		g
Calcium 44		mg
Iron . . . . 0.8 mg		

- Combine carrots and onions in a saucepan and cover with water. Bring to a boil and simmer for 5 minutes. Drain.

- Heat safflower oil in a large nonstick skillet over medium heat. Add carrots and onions and sauté until onions start to brown. Add margarine and sprinkle vegetables with sugar. Add water and cook, stirring often, until vegetables are tender but not overcooked, about 10 minutes. Serve immediately.

Fresh Peach Crumble

2 cups sliced peeled peaches
2 teaspoons lemon juice
1/2 teaspoon almond extract
2 tablespoons sugar
1/3 cup whole wheat flour
1/3 cup firmly packed brown
   sugar

2 teaspoons safflower oil
1/2 teaspoon ground cinnamon
2 tablespoons chopped
   blanched almonds

PER SERVING: 191 CALORIES		
MENU EXCHANGE PATTERN		
Dairy . . . . . —	Fruit	2
Bread 1	Meat	—
Fat 1	Veg.	—
NUTRITIONAL INFORMATION		
Carbohydrate 37		g
Protein 3		g
Total fat 5		g
Saturated fat 0.4		g
Cholesterol 0		mg
Sodium 6		mg
Potassium 222		mg
Fiber 0.6		g
Calcium 33		mg
Iron . . . . 1.2 mg		

- Preheat oven to 375°F. Mix peaches, lemon juice, almond extract, and sugar in a large bowl. Transfer to a 9 × 5-inch loaf pan lightly coated with nonstick spray. Bake 30 minutes.

- Blend flour, brown sugar, oil, cinnamon, and almonds. Sprinkle over fruit and continue baking until topping is lightly browned, 15 to 20 minutes. Serve warm.

Note: To further reduce fat, eliminate chopped almonds. Adjusted analysis: calories = 191; exchanges = 1 Bread, 3 Fruit, 1/2 Fat.

FIN FISH

2

Prosciutto with Melon

Trout Bollita

Thin Spaghetti with Fresh Basil

Zucchini Oregano

Gelato with Whiskey and Espresso

Serves 4

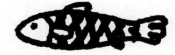

PER SERVING: 730 CALORIES		
MENU EXCHANGE PATTERN		
Dairy . . . . . . ½	Fruit 1	
Bread 3	Meat 5½	
Fat 2½	Veg. 1	
NUTRITIONAL INFORMATION		
Carbohydrate 67	g	
Protein 48	g	
Total fat 30	g	
Saturated fat 3.6	g	
Cholesterol 102	mg	
Sodium 221	mg	
Potassium 1828	mg	
Fiber 1.5	g	
Calcium 229	mg	
Iron 3.9	mg	

Prosciutto with Melon

1 cantaloupe
4 lettuce leaves
4 paper-thin slices prosciutto
1 lemon, thinly sliced

- Quarter the cantaloupe and remove rind and seeds. Place each quarter on a lettuce leaf and cover with 1 slice of prosciutto. Garnish with a twisted lemon slice.

PER SERVING: 58 CALORIES		
MENU EXCHANGE PATTERN		
Dairy . . . . . —	Fruit 1	
Bread . . . . . —	Meat . . . . . . ½	
Fat . . . . —	Veg. . . . . . . —	
NUTRITIONAL INFORMATION		
Carbohydrate 12	g	
Protein 2	g	
Total fat 0	g	
Saturated fat 0.1	g	
Cholesterol 3	mg	
Sodium 74	mg	
Potassium 441	mg	
Fiber 0.5	g	
Calcium 17	mg	
Iron . . . . 0.4 mg		

Trout Bollita

1½ pounds trout fillets
1 lemon, cut in wedges
4 sprigs Italian parsley

Poaching Broth

2 quarts water
½ cup dry white wine
½ teaspoon dried thyme
1 bay leaf

1 sprig Italian parsley
1 stalk celery, cut in large pieces
1 carrot, cut in large pieces

- Prepare poaching broth. Combine all ingredients in a large saucepan, cover, and bring to a simmer. Let broth simmer very slowly for 30 minutes, then strain.

- Place fish in poacher and cover with hot (but not boiling) poaching broth. Cover and simmer very slowly until fish is firm and opaque, about 15 minutes, then let stand, covered, for 5 minutes. Lift fish out of broth and transfer to a platter. Surround with the lemon wedges and parsley sprigs.

PER SERVING: 331 CALORIES		
MENU EXCHANGE PATTERN		
Dairy . . . . . —	Fruit . . . . . —	
Bread 1	Meat 5	
Fat 1	Veg. . . . . . . —	
NUTRITIONAL INFORMATION		
Carbohydrate 0	g	
Protein 37	g	
Total fat 19	g	
Saturated fat 1.6	g	
Cholesterol 93	mg	
Sodium 66	mg	
Potassium 799	mg	
Fiber 0	g	
Calcium 32	mg	
Iron . . . . 1.7 mg		

Thin Spaghetti with Fresh Basil

1 large bunch fresh basil, preferably small-leaf
2 tablespoons safflower oil
3 large cloves garlic, peeled and finely chopped or thinly sliced

1⅓ cups fresh plum tomatoes, seeded, drained, and coarsely chopped
Black pepper
⅓ pound angel hair spaghetti

- Pull off all the basil leaves from the stalks, rinse them briefly in cold water, and chop coarsely. There should be 1 to 1½ cups leaves.

- Heat oil in a large saucepan, add garlic and cook until lightly colored but not brown, about 5 minutes. Add the basil, tomatoes, and about 6 grinds of pepper and cook uncovered over medium-high heat for 15 minutes.

- Drop the spaghetti into 3 quarts boiling water and cook just until *al dente.* Drain well and transfer quickly to a heated large bowl. Add the sauce and toss to coat the pasta. Serve immediately.

PER SERVING: 214 CALORIES			
MENU EXCHANGE PATTERN			
Dairy	—	Fruit	—
Bread	2	Meat	—
Fat	1½	Veg.	½
NUTRITIONAL INFORMATION			
Carbohydrate	32		g
Protein	6		g
Total fat	7		g
Saturated fat	0.6		g
Cholesterol	0		mg
Sodium	3		mg
Potassium	233		mg
Fiber	0.4		g
Calcium	19		mg
Iron	1.4		mg

Zucchini Oregano

1 pound zucchini, sliced
4 teaspoons minced shallot
⅓ cup water
2 teaspoons lemon juice
1 teaspoon chopped fresh
*   oregano*

2 teaspoons chopped fresh
*   parsley*
Black pepper

PER SERVING: 16 CALORIES			
MENU EXCHANGE PATTERN			
Dairy	—	Fruit	—
Bread	—	Meat	—
Fat	—	Veg.	½
NUTRITIONAL INFORMATION			
Carbohydrate	4		g
Protein	1		g
Total fat	0		g
Saturated fat	0		g
Cholesterol	0		mg
Sodium	1		mg
Potassium	150		mg
Fiber	0.4		g
Calcium	21		mg
Iron	0.3		mg

- Combine zucchini, shallot, and water in a large saucepan, cover, and bring to a boil. Lower heat and simmer just until zucchini is tender, about 5 minutes; do not overcook. Drain zucchini and stir in lemon juice, oregano, parsley, and pepper to taste. Serve immediately.

Gelato with Whiskey and Espresso

2 cups low-fat frozen vanilla
*   yogurt*
¼ cup bourbon
1 teaspoon ground espresso
*   coffee beans*

PER SERVING: 111 CALORIES			
MENU EXCHANGE PATTERN			
Dairy	½	Fruit	—
Bread	1	Meat	—
Fat	—	Veg.	—
NUTRITIONAL INFORMATION			
Carbohydrate	19		g
Protein	4		g
Total fat	2		g
Saturated fat	1.3		g
Cholesterol	6		mg
Sodium	77		mg
Potassium	205		mg
Fiber	0.2		g
Calcium	140		mg
Iron	0.1		mg

- Place ½ cup frozen yogurt in each dessert dish. Pour ½ ounce (1 tablespoon) bourbon over yogurt and sprinkle ¼ teaspoon espresso on top of each serving.

FIN FISH

3

Lobster Bisque

Bibb Lettuce Dijonnaise

Trout Zielinski

Scalloped Potatoes

Steamed Broccoli with Lemon

Cherries Jubilee

Serves 6

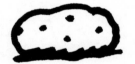

PER SERVING: 1126 CALORIES			
MENU EXCHANGE PATTERN			
Dairy	—	Fruit	4
Bread	4½	Meat	6
Fat	5	Veg.	4
NUTRITIONAL INFORMATION			
Carbohydrate	113	g	
Protein	57	g	
Total fat	43	g	
Saturated fat	6.2	g	
Cholesterol	184	mg	
Sodium	420	mg	
Potassium	2622	mg	
Fiber	4.5	g	
Calcium	474	mg	
Iron	7.6	mg	

Lobster Bisque

1 small live lobster, about
    ³/₄ pound
1 tablespoon olive oil
6 tablespoons brandy
1 small stalk celery, chopped
1 small onion, chopped
1 small carrot, diced
1 clove garlic, chopped

¹/₄ teaspoon paprika
¹/₃ cup all-purpose flour
1 tablespoon tomato puree
¹/₂ cup dry white wine
3 cups fish stock or Homemade
    Chicken Stock (page 36)
¹/₂ cup skim milk

• Kill and clean lobster (see page 193). In a large skillet, sauté in hot olive oil over medium-high heat until the shell turns light red, about 5 to 10 minutes. Pour in brandy and ignite, shaking pan gently until flames subside. Add vegetables and sauté over low heat for 5 minutes. Add paprika, flour, tomato puree, wine, and stock and simmer for 10 minutes. Remove the lobster and cut the tail and claw meat into small chunks; reserve. Pound or chop the lobster shell into pieces and return to the soup. Add the milk and simmer for 30 minutes, adding water if the soup becomes too thick. Strain soup and stir in the chunks of lobster. Serve immediately.

PER SERVING: 169 CALORIES		
MENU EXCHANGE PATTERN		
Dairy . . . . . —	Fruit . . . . . —	
Bread . . . . . ½	Meat 1½	
Fat . . . . ½	Veg. 1	
NUTRITIONAL INFORMATION		
Carbohydrate 10	g	
Protein 11	g	
Total fat 6	g	
Saturated fat 0.4	g	
Cholesterol 97	mg	
Sodium 227	mg	
Potassium 305	mg	
Fiber 0.3	g	
Calcium 54	mg	
Iron 0.8	mg	

Bibb Lettuce Dijonnaise

2 heads Boston or Bibb lettuce,
    about 6 cups
6 tablespoons Dijonnaise
    Dressing (recipe follows)
Black pepper

• Tear lettuce into bite-size pieces and place in a salad bowl. Add dressing and toss to coat lettuce. Season with pepper and serve on individual salad plates. (Analysis does not include dressing.)

Note: To reduce fat intake, substitute a commercial low-calorie Italian dressing for the Dijonnaise Dressing. Adjusted analysis for dressing: calories = 16; exchange = ¹/₂ Fat.

PER SERVING: 8 CALORIES		
MENU EXCHANGE PATTERN		
Dairy . . . . . —	Fruit . . . . . —	
Bread . . . . —	Meat . . . . . —	
Fat . . . . —	Veg. . . . . ½	
NUTRITIONAL INFORMATION		
Carbohydrate 1	g	
Protein 1	g	
Total fat 0	g	
Saturated fat 0	g	
Cholesterol 0	mg	
Sodium 5	mg	
Potassium 144	mg	
Fiber 0.3	g	
Calcium 19	mg	
Iron 1.1	mg	

Dijonnaise Dressing

1/4 cup wine vinegar
1 teaspoon grated onion
1/2 teaspoon black pepper

1 teaspoon sugar
2 teaspoons Dijon-style mustard
1/2 cup safflower or olive oil

- Combine vinegar, onion, pepper, sugar, and mustard in a jar and shake well. Add oil and shake to mix thoroughly. Makes 3/4 cup; 1 serving = 1 tablespoon.

PER SERVING: 83 CALORIES		
MENU EXCHANGE PATTERN		
Dairy ..... —	Fruit ..... —	
Bread .... —	Meat ..... —	
Fat 2	Veg. ...... —	
NUTRITIONAL INFORMATION		
Carbohydrate 0		g
Protein 0		g
Total fat 9		g
Saturated fat 0.8		g
Cholesterol 0		mg
Sodium 11		mg
Potassium 6		mg
Fiber 0.1		g
Calcium 1		mg
Iron 0		mg

Trout Zielinski

6 trout fillets, 5 ounces each
Black pepper
1/2 cup lemon juice
1/3 cup all-purpose flour
1 tablespoon safflower oil
1 tablespoon margarine
2 cucumbers, peeled, seeded,
  and thinly sliced

1 tablespoon diced pimiento
1 tablespoon chopped green
  onion
2 tablespoons chopped fresh
  parsley
4 lemons, cut in wedges
Parsley sprigs (garnish)

- Season the fillets with pepper and marinate in lemon juice for 5 minutes. Drain the fillets and pat dry; reserve lemon juice. Dip fillets in flour to coat lightly. Heat oil in a large nonstick skillet over medium-high heat. Add fillets and cook until golden brown, about 10 minutes. Remove from skillet and keep warm.

- Melt 1 tablespoon margarine in another skillet and sauté the cucumber and pimientos over medium heat until cucumbers are softened, about 5 minutes. Add green onion and parsley; season with pepper and reserved lemon juice to taste. Top fillets with cucumber mixture. Garnish with lemon wedges and parsley.

PER SERVING: 357 CALORIES		
MENU EXCHANGE PATTERN		
Dairy ..... —	Fruit 1	
Bread .... —	Meat 4½	
Fat 1	Veg. .... ½	
NUTRITIONAL INFORMATION		
Carbohydrate 11		g
Protein 32		g
Total fat 20		g
Saturated fat 2.6		g
Cholesterol 78		mg
Sodium 59		mg
Potassium 838		mg
Fiber 0.6		g
Calcium 54		mg
Iron 2.4		mg

Scalloped Potatoes

3 cups peeled and thinly sliced
    Idaho potatoes
1/2 cup minced onion
2 tablespoons all-purpose flour

White pepper
1 1/2 cups skim milk
2 tablespoons margarine

- Preheat oven to 350°F. Lightly coat a 1-quart casserole dish with nonstick spray. Layer half of the sliced potatoes on bottom of dish. Sprinkle half of the onion, flour, and pepper over the potatoes. Repeat the layers. Pour milk over the potatoes and dot with margarine. Cover and bake for 30 minutes, then uncover and continue to bake until potatoes are tender, 30 to 40 minutes longer.

PER SERVING: 126 CALORIES

MENU EXCHANGE PATTERN

Dairy .... —	Fruit .... —
Bread 1½	Meat ..... —
Fat ....½	Veg. .... —

NUTRITIONAL INFORMATION

Carbohydrate 19	g
Protein 4	g
Total fat 4	g
Saturated fat 0.8	g
Cholesterol 1	mg
Sodium 36	mg
Potassium 440	mg
Fiber 1	g
Calcium 87	mg
Iron 0.6	mg

Steamed Broccoli with Lemon

3 cups broccoli florets
Juice of 1 lemon
Black pepper

- Steam broccoli until crisp-tender, about 5 to 10 minutes. Toss with lemon juice and pepper and serve.

PER SERVING: 41 CALORIES

MENU EXCHANGE PATTERN

Dairy .... —	Fruit .... —
Bread .... —	Meat ..... —
Fat .... —	Veg. 2

NUTRITIONAL INFORMATION

Carbohydrate 8	g
Protein 4	g
Total fat 0	g
Saturated fat 0	g
Cholesterol 0	mg
Sodium 18	mg
Potassium 470	mg
Fiber 1.8	g
Calcium 126	mg
Iron 1.4	mg

Cherries Jubilee

1 can (30 ounces) pitted Bing
    cherries, drained
1/2 cup firmly packed brown
    sugar

6 tablespoons cherry brandy
1/4 cup Kirsch
3 cups frozen low-fat vanilla
    yogurt

- Heat the cherries and sugar in a skillet. Add cherry brandy and Kirsch and ignite, shaking pan gently until flames subside. Simmer for 3 to 5 minutes. Pour over frozen yogurt and serve immediately.

PER SERVING: 342 CALORIES

MENU EXCHANGE PATTERN

Dairy .... —	Fruit 3
Bread 2½	Meat ..... —
Fat 1	Veg. .... —

NUTRITIONAL INFORMATION

Carbohydrate 64	g
Protein 4	g
Total fat 2	g
Saturated fat 1.6	g
Cholesterol 8	mg
Sodium 64	mg
Potassium 419	mg
Fiber 0.5	g
Calcium 133	mg
Iron 1.2	mg

FIN FISH

4

Crawfish Bisque

Trout with Lemon Sauce

Baked Potatoes

Grilled Tomato Slices

Bread Pudding

Serves 8

PER SERVING: 961 CALORIES
MENU EXCHANGE PATTERN
Dairy . . . . . . ½ Fruit . . . . . . ½
Bread . . . . . 4 Meat 6
Fat . . . . 3½ Veg. 5
NUTRITIONAL INFORMATION
Carbohydrate 92   g
Protein 57   g
Total fat 41   g
Saturated fat . . . . 4.2   g
Cholesterol 110   mg
Sodium 603   mg
Potassium 2437   mg
Fiber . . . . 2.6   g
Calcium 318   mg
Iron . . . . 5.9 mg

Crawfish Bisque

¼ cup safflower oil
¼ cup all-purpose flour
1 large onion, chopped
2 cloves garlic, mashed
2 stalks celery, chopped
1½ cups chopped fresh tomato
8 cups water
1 bay leaf
Black and cayenne pepper

1 tablespoon margarine
2 tablespoons chopped green
    onion
2 tablespoons chopped fresh
    parsley
4 ounces crawfish tails
8 teaspoons filé powder
2 cups cooked rice

- Heat oil in a large saucepan over medium heat. Add flour and cook, stirring constantly, until deep golden brown, about 10 to 15 minutes. Add onion, garlic, and celery and cook, stirring, until soft. Add tomato and cook 5 minutes. Add water, bay leaf, and peppers and bring to a boil. Reduce heat to simmer, cover tightly, and cook 1 hour.

- Melt margarine in a large skillet over medium heat. Add green onion, parsley, and crawfish tails and cook 2 to 3 minutes, then add to gumbo. Serve in soup plates with ¼ cup hot cooked rice per serving. Sprinkle each serving with 1 teaspoon filé powder.

PER SERVING: 174 CALORIES		
MENU EXCHANGE PATTERN		
Dairy . . . . . —	Fruit . . . . . —	
Bread . . . . . ½	Meat . . . . . . ½	
Fat 1	Veg. 3	
NUTRITIONAL INFORMATION		
Carbohydrate 20	g	
Protein 5	g	
Total fat 9	g	
Saturated fat 0.9	g	
Cholesterol 14	mg	
Sodium 293	mg	
Potassium 226	mg	
Fiber 0.6	g	
Calcium 32	mg	
Iron 1.1	mg	

Trout with Lemon Sauce

8 trout fillets, skinned
    (6 ounces each)
White pepper

⅓ cup sliced almonds
Parsley sprigs (garnish)
2 lemons, cut into wedges

Lemon Sauce

3 tablespoons margarine,
    melted
¼ cup lemon juice
1 teaspoon Worcestershire
    sauce

- Combine all ingredients for sauce. Set aside.

- Preheat broiler. Sprinkle fillets with white pepper. Arrange on a broiler pan and pour lemon sauce over. Broil just until fish is firm and opaque, about 10 minutes, turning once. Sprinkle with almonds and return to broiler for 2 to 3 minutes to brown. Garnish with parsley and serve with lemon wedges.

PER SERVING: 420 CALORIES		
MENU EXCHANGE PATTERN		
Dairy . . . . . —	Fruit . . . . . . ½	
Bread . . . . . —	Meat 5½	
Fat 2	Veg. . . . . . . —	
NUTRITIONAL INFORMATION		
Carbohydrate 4	g	
Protein 38	g	
Total fat 28	g	
Saturated fat 2.4	g	
Cholesterol 94	mg	
Sodium 75	mg	
Potassium 907	mg	
Fiber 0.3	g	
Calcium 59	mg	
Iron 2.3	mg	

Baked Potatoes

8 medium-size Idaho potatoes

- Preheat oven to 400°F. Scrub potatoes. Bake until tender when pierced with a fork, about 1 hour.

PER SERVING: 144 CALORIES			
MENU EXCHANGE PATTERN			
Dairy . . . . . —		Fruit . . . . . . —	
Bread 2		Meat . . . . . . —	
Fat . . . . —		Veg. . . . . . . —	
NUTRITIONAL INFORMATION			
Carbohydrate 32			g
Protein 4			g
Total fat 0			g
Saturated fat 0			g
Cholesterol 0			mg
Sodium 6			mg
Potassium 781			mg
Fiber 1.2			g
Calcium 14			mg
Iron 1			mg

Grilled Tomato Slices

4 tomatoes, cut in ¹/₂-inch slices
Black pepper
2 teaspoons sugar
2 tablespoons margarine,
  melted

¹/₂ cup fine dry breadcrumbs
Paprika

- Preheat broiler. Season tomato slices with pepper and sugar. Dip in melted margarine, and then in breadcrumbs. Dust with paprika. Arrange on a cookie sheet coated with non-stick spray. Broil about 4 inches from the heat source for 5 minutes, then turn, and cook 5 minutes longer. Serve hot.

PER SERVING: 74 CALORIES			
MENU EXCHANGE PATTERN			
Dairy . . . . . —		Fruit . . . . . —	
Bread . . . . —		Meat . . . . . —	
Fat . . . . ½		Veg. 2	
NUTRITIONAL INFORMATION			
Carbohydrate 10			g
Protein 2			g
Total fat 3			g
Saturated fat 0.6			g
Cholesterol 0			mg
Sodium 49			mg
Potassium 232			mg
Fiber 0.5			g
Calcium 20			mg
Iron 0.7			mg

Bread Pudding

4 slices stale white bread
1¹/₃ cups skim milk
1¹/₃ cups evaporated skim milk
2 egg substitutes, well beaten
8 tablespoons sugar

1 teaspoon vanilla extract
3 egg whites
1 teaspoon lemon juice
Pinch of nutmeg

- Soak the bread in skim and evaporated milk for at least 1 hour. Preheat oven to 400°F. Beat egg substitutes and 5 tablespoons sugar until creamy. Add bread (with milk) and vanilla. Pour into a lightly oiled 1-quart baking dish and bake until a toothpick inserted in center comes out clean, 20 to 30 minutes. Beat egg whites until soft peaks form. Gradually add 3 tablespoons sugar and lemon juice and beat until stiff. Sprinkle pudding with nutmeg and place meringue in 3 or 4 mounds on top. Return to the oven and bake 2 to 3 minutes. Serve hot or cold.

PER SERVING: 149 CALORIES			
MENU EXCHANGE PATTERN			
Dairy . . . . . . ½		Fruit . . . . . —	
Bread 1½		Meat . . . . . —	
Fat . . . . —		Veg. . . . . . . —	
NUTRITIONAL INFORMATION			
Carbohydrate 26			g
Protein 9			g
Total fat 1			g
Saturated fat 0.3			g
Cholesterol 2			mg
Sodium 180			mg
Potassium 291			mg
Fiber 0			g
Calcium 193			mg
Iron 0.8			mg

FIN FISH

5

Watercress, Apple, and Pecan Salad

Grilled Salmon with Julienne of Vegetables

Champagne Ice

Serves 2

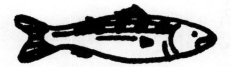

PER SERVING: 630 CALORIES			
MENU EXCHANGE PATTERN			
Dairy	—	Fruit	4
Bread	½	Meat	3½
Fat	3	Veg.	4
NUTRITIONAL INFORMATION			
Carbohydrate	65	g	
Protein	32	g	
Total fat	26	g	
Saturated fat	6.1	g	
Cholesterol	41	mg	
Sodium	164	mg	
Potassium	1772	mg	
Fiber	2.5	g	
Calcium	219	mg	
Iron	3.3	mg	

Watercress, Apple, and Pecan Salad

1 cup watercress leaves
1 apple, peeled, seeded, and
   sliced into julienne
2 teaspoons lemon juice
1 teaspoon minced shallot

Apple Salad Dressing (recipe
   follows)
1/4 cup toasted croutons
2 tablespoons toasted pecans
   (see note)

- Toss together watercress, apple, lemon juice, and shallot. Add dressing and toss lightly. Arrange on salad plates and garnish with croutons and pecans.

Note: To further reduce fat, eliminate pecans from recipe. Adjusted analysis: calories = 80; exchanges = 1/2 Bread, 1/2 Fruit.

PER SERVING: 142 CALORIES		
MENU EXCHANGE PATTERN		
Dairy . . . . . —	Fruit 1/2	
Bread 1/2	Meat . . . . . —	
Fat 1 1/2	Veg. . . . . . . —	
NUTRITIONAL INFORMATION		
Carbohydrate 19		g
Protein 2		g
Total fat 7		g
Saturated fat 0.6		g
Cholesterol 0		mg
Sodium 73		mg
Potassium 208		mg
Fiber 0.9		g
Calcium 49		mg
Iron 0.9		mg

Apple Salad Dressing

1 teaspoon lemon juice
2 teaspoons minced shallot
1/2 cup plain low-fat yogurt

1/4 cup unsweetened apple juice
1/4 teaspoon black pepper

- Stir all ingredients together. Refrigerate any unused dressing. Makes about 3/4 cup; 1 serving = 1 tablespoon.

PER SERVING: 19 CALORIES		
MENU EXCHANGE PATTERN		
Dairy . . . . . —	Fruit 1/2	
Bread . . . . . —	Meat . . . . . —	
Fat . . . . —	Veg. . . . . . . —	
NUTRITIONAL INFORMATION		
Carbohydrate 3		g
Protein 1		g
Total fat 0		g
Saturated fat 0.2		g
Cholesterol 1		mg
Sodium 14		mg
Potassium 68		mg
Fiber 0		g
Calcium 36		mg
Iron 0.1		mg

Grilled Salmon with Julienne of Vegetables

2 salmon fillets (4 ounces
   each), cut about 1 inch thick
Black pepper
1 carrot, sliced into julienne
1/2 zucchini, sliced into julienne
1/2 red bell pepper, sliced into
   julienne

1/3 cup snow peas, ends
   trimmed
1/2 teaspoon margarine
1 lemon, cut in wedges

Marinade

1 teaspoon chopped shallot
1 teaspoon margarine
2 teaspoons port
1/2 teaspoon green peppercorns
2 teaspoons dry white wine

4 teaspoons Homemade
   Chicken Stock (page 36)
1 teaspoon brandy
Pinch of dried rosemary

- Prepare marinade. Sauté shallot in margarine in a nonstick saucepan. Add port and peppercorns and remove from heat. In a separate pan, combine white wine and chicken stock and boil until reduced by half, then add brandy. Reduce again by half and stir in shallot mixture and rosemary.

- Brush salmon fillets with marinade and sprinkle with pepper. Grill over mesquite fire until firm and opaque, about 10 minutes, turning once during cooking. (Cooking time will depend on thickness of fish.) Meanwhile, in a nonstick skillet sauté vegetables in margarine for about 5 minutes. Arrange around salmon. Serve with lemon wedges.

Photo opposite page 227.

PER SERVING: 344 CALORIES

MENU EXCHANGE PATTERN

Dairy . . . . . —	Fruit . . . . . —
Bread . . . . . —	Meat 3½
Fat 1½	Veg. 3

NUTRITIONAL INFORMATION

Carbohydrate 13	g
Protein 28	g
Total fat 18	g
Saturated fat 5.3	g
Cholesterol 40	mg
Sodium 76	mg
Potassium 805	mg
Fiber 1.5	g
Calcium 130	mg
Iron . . . . 2.2 mg

Champagne Ice

1½ cups water
¾ cup sugar
¼ cup lemon juice
¼ cup pineapple juice

¼ cup champagne
2 plums, preferably Santa Rosa, peeled and pureed (¼ cup puree)

- Bring water and sugar to a boil. Boil until sugar is dissolved, about 3 minutes. Let cool. Stir in the remaining ingredients and pour into a 1-quart container. Place in freezer and stir every 30 minutes until frozen, about 3 to 4 hours. Makes about 1 quart; 1 serving = ½ cup.

PER SERVING: 125 CALORIES

MENU EXCHANGE PATTERN

Dairy . . . . . —	Fruit 3
Bread . . . . . —	Meat . . . . . —
Fat . . . . —	Veg. . . . . . . —

NUTRITIONAL INFORMATION

Carbohydrate 30	g
Protein 0	g
Total fat 0	g
Saturated fat 0	g
Cholesterol 0	mg
Sodium 1	mg
Potassium 74	mg
Fiber 0.1	g
Calcium 4	mg
Iron . . . . 0.1 mg

FIN FISH

6

Frogs Legs Soup

Watercress Salad with Yogurt Dressing

Grilled Salmon with Pesto

Sautéed New Potatoes with Parsley

Blueberry-Filled Meringue Shells

Serves 4

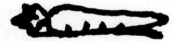

PER SERVING: 883 CALORIES		
MENU EXCHANGE PATTERN		
Dairy . . . . . —	Fruit 2	
Bread 2½	Meat 7	
Fat 4½	Veg. 2½	
NUTRITIONAL INFORMATION		
Carbohydrate 55	g	
Protein 58	g	
Total fat 42	g	
Saturated fat 9.6	g	
Cholesterol. 117	mg	
Sodium 542	mg	
Potassium 1404	mg	
Fiber 2.1	g	
Calcium 296	mg	
Iron 5	mg	

Frogs Legs Soup

16 frogs legs
4 tablespoons margarine
⅓ cup chopped onion
⅓ cup chopped carrot
⅓ cup chopped celery
4 teaspoons all-purpose flour
2½ cups fish stock or
   Homemade Chicken Stock
   (page 36), heated

1 bay leaf
2 teaspoons dried tarragon
1 teaspoon white pepper
1 tablespoon dry sherry
1 tablespoon brandy
⅔ cup plain low-fat yogurt

- Cut frogs legs in half at joint and brown in a large skillet in 2 tablespoons margarine. Cool. Pick all meat off bones and reserve. Melt 2 tablespoons margarine in a heavy nonstick skillet over medium-high heat. Add onion, carrot, and celery and sauté until onion is translucent, about 5 minutes. Sprinkle in flour and mix thoroughly. Whisk in hot stock. Reduce heat, cover, and simmer for 15 minutes, stirring occasionally. Add bay leaf, tarragon, white pepper, sherry, and brandy and simmer for 30 minutes. Remove from heat and let cool slightly.

- Place yogurt in a mixing bowl. Gradually add 1 to 2 cups hot soup, stirring constantly. Add meat and remaining soup. Transfer to a heavy saucepan and reheat gently; do not boil or soup will curdle. Serve immediately.

Note: If desired, substitute 12 chicken wings for the 16 frogs legs.

PER SERVING: 231 CALORIES		
MENU EXCHANGE PATTERN		
Dairy . . . . . —	Fruit . . . . . —	
Bread . . . . . —	Meat 2½	
Fat 1	Veg. 2	
NUTRITIONAL INFORMATION		
Carbohydrate 7	g	
Protein 19	g	
Total fat 12	g	
Saturated fat 2.5	g	
Cholesterol 52	mg	
Sodium 42	mg	
Potassium 183	mg	
Fiber 0.2	g	
Calcium 100	mg	
Iron 1.7	mg	

Watercress Salad with Yogurt Dressing

Juice of ½ lemon
2 tablespoons water
2 Red Delicious apples, cored
   and diced

2 tablespoons chopped toasted
   pecans
2 cups watercress, stemmed

Dressing

Juice of 1 lemon
¼ cup plain low-fat yogurt
2 tablespoons buttermilk
¼ tablespoon white pepper

- For the dressing, combine the lemon juice, yogurt, buttermilk, and white pepper and blend well.

- For salad, mix lemon juice with water and sprinkle over apples. Add pecans and watercress. Pour dressing over salad and toss gently.

PER SERVING: 71 CALORIES		
MENU EXCHANGE PATTERN		
Dairy . . . . . —	Fruit 1	
Bread . . . . . —	Meat . . . . . —	
Fat . . . . ½	Veg. . . . . . . ½	
NUTRITIONAL INFORMATION		
Carbohydrate 13	g	
Protein 1	g	
Total fat 3	g	
Saturated fat 0.2	g	
Cholesterol 0	mg	
Sodium 10	mg	
Potassium 169	mg	
Fiber 0.8	g	
Calcium 38	mg	
Iron 0.6	mg	

Grilled Salmon with Pesto

Grated rind of 1 lemon
Black pepper
4 salmon fillets, 5 ounces each
2¹/₂ tablespoons Pesto Sauce
    (recipe follows)

• Blend lemon rind and pepper and sprinkle over salmon. Grill (or broil) salmon, skin side down, until just opaque, about 10 to 15 minutes. Remove skin with spatula. Serve 1 tablespoon pesto with each fillet.

PER SERVING: 307 CALORIES		
MENU EXCHANGE PATTERN		
Dairy . . . . . —	Fruit . . . . . . —	
Bread . . . . —	Meat 4½	
Fat 1	Veg. . . . . . . —	
NUTRITIONAL INFORMATION		
Carbohydrate 0	g	
Protein 32	g	
Total fat 19	g	
Saturated fat 6	g	
Cholesterol 60	mg	
Sodium 68	mg	
Potassium 554	mg	
Fiber 0	g	
Calcium 111	mg	
Iron 1.2	mg	

Pesto Sauce

2 cloves garlic
1 cup parsley leaves
1 cup basil leaves

2 tablespoons pine nuts
¹/₄ cup grated Parmesan cheese
3 tablespoons safflower oil

• Mince garlic in a food processor. Add parsley, basil, nuts, and cheese and process until coarsely chopped. Slowly blend in the oil. Store any unused portion tightly covered in refrigerator. Makes about ½ cup; 1 serving = 2 teaspoons.

PER SERVING: 43 CALORIES		
MENU EXCHANGE PATTERN		
Dairy . . . . . —	Fruit . . . . . —	
Bread . . . . —	Meat . . . . . —	
Fat 1	Veg. . . . . . —	
NUTRITIONAL INFORMATION		
Carbohydrate 1	g	
Protein 1	g	
Total fat 4	g	
Saturated fat 0.3	g	
Cholesterol. 5	mg	
Sodium 7	mg	
Potassium 76	mg	
Fiber 0	g	
Calcium 111	mg	
Iron 0.6	mg	

Sautéed New Potatoes with Parsley

1 pound new potatoes, peeled
    and shaped into ovals
¹/₂ teaspoon salt

4 teaspoons margarine
¹/₄ teaspoon white pepper
¹/₃ cup chopped fresh parsley

• Boil potatoes in salted water until tender; drain. Melt margarine in large saucepan, add potatoes and heat through. Add white pepper and parsley, stir to coat potatoes and serve.

Note: To reduce fat, eliminate margarine from recipe. Adjusted analysis: calories = 57; exchange = 1 Bread.

PER SERVING: 93 CALORIES		
MENU EXCHANGE PATTERN		
Dairy . . . . . —	Fruit . . . . . —	
Bread 1	Meat . . . . . —	
Fat 1	Veg. . . . . . —	
NUTRITIONAL INFORMATION		
Carbohydrate 13	g	
Protein 2	g	
Total fat 4	g	
Saturated fat 0.7	g	
Cholesterol 0	mg	
Sodium 360	mg	
Potassium 344	mg	
Fiber 0.5	g	
Calcium 19	mg	
Iron 0.8	mg	

Blueberry-Filled Meringue Shells

4 egg whites
1 teaspoon vanilla extract
Pinch of cream of tartar

5 tablespoons amaretto
1/2 cup confectioners sugar
1 cup blueberries

- Beat egg whites until foamy. Blend in vanilla, cream of tartar, and 1 tablespoon amaretto. Gradually add sugar, beating constantly until mixture forms stiff peaks. Preheat oven to 300°F. Spoon meringue into pastry bag and line a cookie sheet with parchment paper. Pipe out four flat 3-inch rounds on the cookie sheet to serve as bottoms of the shells. Then pipe eight 3-inch rings, which will eventually be used to build the sides of the shells. Bake for 25 minutes. Using a little extra raw meringue to cement the layers together, place 2 baked rings on top of each round, making 4 meringue shells. Continue to bake for another 30 minutes. Turn oven off and let meringues rest in oven for 5 minutes. Cool shells completely.

- Sprinkle blueberries with remaining 4 tablespoons amaretto. Spoon into shells and serve.

PER SERVING: 138 CALORIES

MENU EXCHANGE PATTERN

Dairy ..... —	Fruit 1
Bread 1½	Meat ..... —
Fat .... —	Veg. ...... —

NUTRITIONAL INFORMATION

Carbohydrate 20	g
Protein 4	g
Total fat 0	g
Saturated fat 0	g
Cholesterol 0	mg
Sodium 52	mg
Potassium 78	mg
Fiber 0.5	g
Calcium 6	mg
Iron 0.1	mg

FIN FISH

7

Dong Ting Bean Curd Soup

Steamed Baby Red Snapper

Spicy Noodles

Lord Han's Vegetable Delight

Bathing Royal Concubine

Serves 4

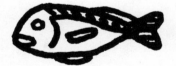

PER SERVING: 737 CALORIES			
MENU EXCHANGE PATTERN			
Dairy	—	Fruit	2
Bread	2½	Meat	4½
Fat	2½	Veg.	5½
NUTRITIONAL INFORMATION			
Carbohydrate		80	g
Protein		49	g
Total fat		22	g
Saturated fat		2.6	g
Cholesterol		101	mg
Sodium		857	mg
Potassium		1799	mg
Fiber		5	g
Calcium		218	mg
Iron		6.7	mg

Fettuccine Primavera;
recipe page 189

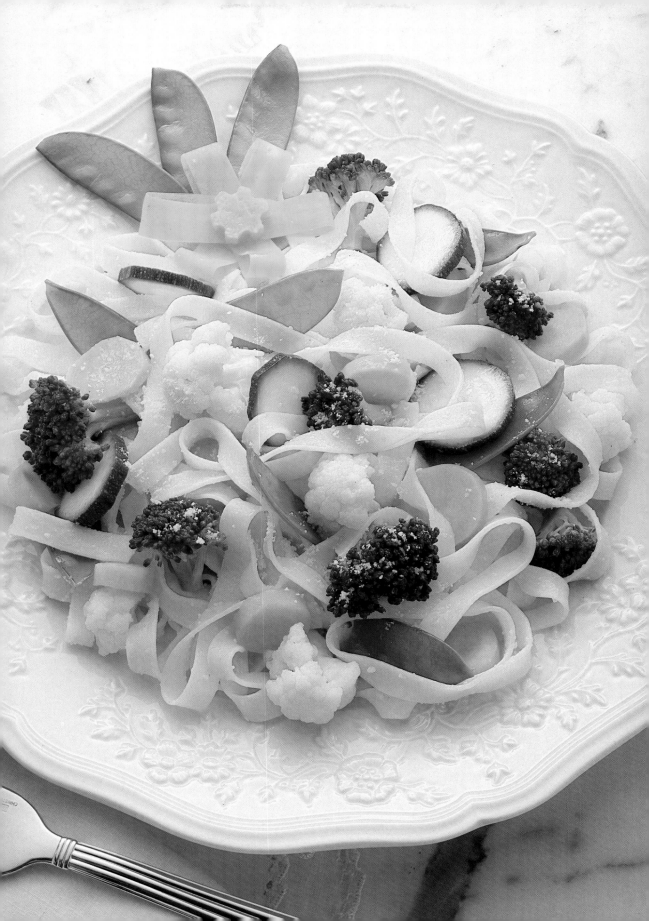

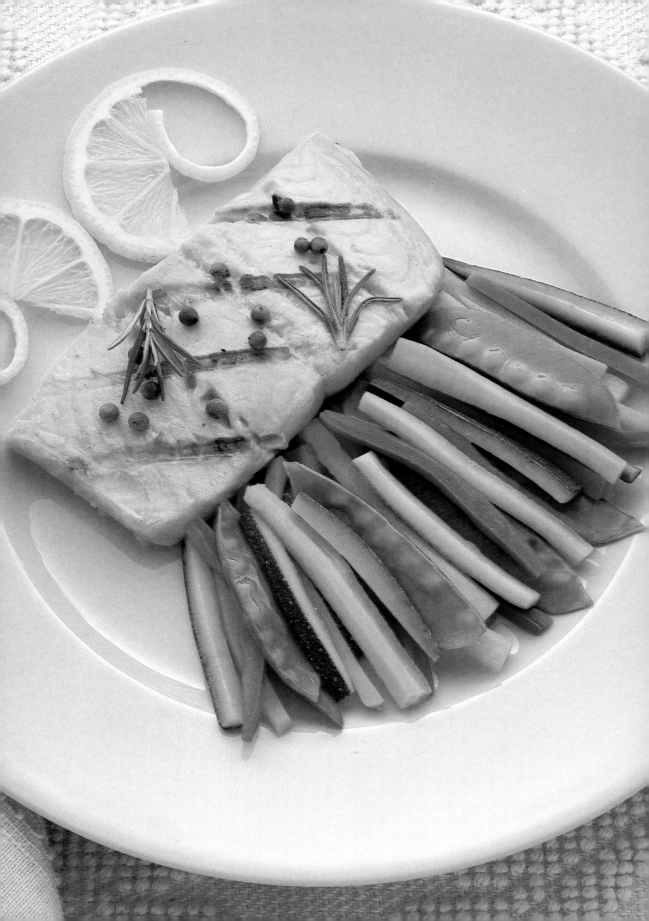

Dong Ting Bean Curd Soup

*1/2 ounce dried Chinese black
  mushrooms*
1/4 pound firm bean curd
*6 cups Homemade Chicken
  Stock (page 36)*

1/4 teaspoon white pepper
*2 teaspoons shredded cooked
  lean ham*

- Cover dried mushrooms with warm water and soak for 45 minutes. Shred caps, discarding hard stems. Cut bean curd into thin slices, then shred into julienne strips. Transfer to a large saucepan, add stock and white pepper and simmer over low heat for 10 minutes. Add ham and mushrooms and simmer for 5 more minutes. Serve immediately.

PER SERVING: 28 CALORIES		
MENU EXCHANGE PATTERN		
Dairy ..... —	Fruit ..... —	
Bread .... —	Meat 1/2	
Fat .... —	Veg. ...... —	
NUTRITIONAL INFORMATION		
Carbohydrate 1	g	
Protein 3	g	
Total fat 2	g	
Saturated fat 0.3	g	
Cholesterol 2	mg	
Sodium 49	mg	
Potassium 33	mg	
Fiber 0		
Calcium 37	mg	
Iron .... 0.6 mg		

Steamed Baby Red Snapper

*2 red snapper (12 ounces
  each), scaled and cleaned*
*1/4 cup Chinese fermented black
  beans*
*3 to 4 Serrano chilies, thinly
  sliced on the diagonal*

2 teaspoons minced ginger
*4 green onions, cut in 1-inch
  pieces*
2 tablespoons dry white wine
1 teaspoon white pepper

- Make three or four 1/4-inch deep diagonal cuts on each side of the fish. Scatter half of the fermented black beans, chili slices, ginger, and green onion on a platter large enough to hold both fish.

- Place fish on top of bean mixture and top with the remaining beans, chilies, ginger, and green onions. Sprinkle with wine and white pepper.

- Transfer platter to a steamer rack set over boiling water. Steam until fish flakes with a fork, about 15 to 20 minutes. Serve at once.

PER SERVING: 246 CALORIES		
MENU EXCHANGE PATTERN		
Dairy ..... —	Fruit ..... —	
Bread .... —	Meat 4	
Fat .... —	Veg. 1	
NUTRITIONAL INFORMATION		
Carbohydrate 11	g	
Protein 36	g	
Total fat 5	g	
Saturated fat 0.7	g	
Cholesterol.......... 99	mg	
Sodium 166	mg	
Potassium 810	mg	
Fiber 1	g	
Calcium 111	mg	
Iron .... 3.1 mg		

Spicy Noodles

*1/4 pound dried Chinese
  noodles, or 1/2 pound fresh*
2 tablespoons safflower oil
*1/2 teaspoon fresh finely ground
  black pepper*
*2 tablespoons low-sodium soy
  sauce*
*2 tablespoons sesame paste
  (tahini)*

1/2 teaspoon Chinese chili paste
1/2 teaspoon cayenne pepper
2 teaspoons minced garlic
1/2 cup shredded cucumber
1/2 cup shredded peeled carrot
1/2 cup alfalfa sprouts

*Grilled Salmon with
Julienne of Vegetables;
recipe page 220*

227

- Cook Chinese noodles in boiling water until soft, about 3 to 4 minutes; drain well. Chill noodles for about 20 minutes.

- Heat safflower oil in a very small skillet, and then add oil to pepper, soy sauce, sesame paste, chili paste, cayenne, and garlic and blend to make a sauce.

- Transfer chilled noodles to a serving dish and top with cucumber, carrot, and alfalfa sprouts. Pour sauce over vegetables and noodles and chill. Toss well before serving.

PER SERVING: 232 CALORIES

MENU EXCHANGE PATTERN

Dairy	—	Fruit	—
Bread	1½	Meat	—
Fat	2	Veg.	1½

NUTRITIONAL INFORMATION

Carbohydrate	26	g
Protein	7	g
Total fat	11	g
Saturated fat	1.3	g
Cholesterol	0	mg
Sodium	571	mg
Potassium	210	mg
Fiber	0.4	g
Calcium	24	mg
Iron	1.6	mg

Lord Han's Vegetable Delight

1 cup shredded celery
½ cup peeled and diagonally
   sliced carrot
½ cup sliced water chestnuts
½ cup sliced bamboo shoots
4 ears of baby corn
½ cup sliced mushrooms
½ cup snow peas

2 teaspoons safflower oil
½ teaspoon minced garlic
⅓ cup Homemade Chicken
   Stock (page 36)
1 teaspoon cornstarch
1 tablespoon water
½ teaspoon Oriental sesame oil

- Drop celery, carrot, water chestnuts, bamboo shoots, baby corn, mushrooms, and snow peas into a large pot of boiling water and blanch for 1 minute. Drain well.

- Heat safflower oil in a wok or skillet over high heat. Add garlic and vegetables and stir-fry for 2 minutes. Add stock and bring to a boil. Mix cornstarch with water, stir into the sauce, and return to boil. Stir in sesame oil and serve immediately.

PER SERVING: 94 CALORIES

MENU EXCHANGE PATTERN

Dairy	—	Fruit	—
Bread	—	Meat	—
Fat	½	Veg.	3

NUTRITIONAL INFORMATION

Carbohydrate	15	g
Protein	3	g
Total fat	3	g
Saturated fat	0.3	g
Cholesterol	0	mg
Sodium	54	mg
Potassium	515	mg
Fiber	1.3	g
Calcium	23	mg
Iron	1	mg

Bathing Royal Concubine

24 fresh litchi
½ cup chilled red Dubonnet
1 cup chilled club soda

- Shell and seed litchi. Refrigerate fruit for about 30 minutes. Add Dubonnet and soda, mix well, and transfer to individual dessert bowls. Serve immediately.

PER SERVING: 137 CALORIES

MENU EXCHANGE PATTERN

Dairy	—	Fruit	2
Bread	1	Meat	—
Fat	—	Veg.	—

NUTRITIONAL INFORMATION

Carbohydrate	27	g
Protein	1	g
Total fat	1	g
Saturated fat	0	g
Cholesterol	0	mg
Sodium	17	mg
Potassium	231	mg
Fiber	2.3	g
Calcium	23	mg
Iron	0.4	mg

FIN FISH

8

Onion and Apple Soup

Grilled Red Snapper Fillets with Basil Tomato Sauce

Wild Rice with Mushrooms

Green Beans with Dill

Lemon Chiffon

Serves 6

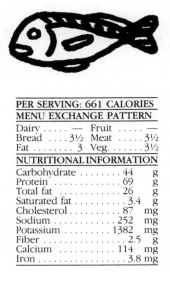

PER SERVING: 661 CALORIES		
MENU EXCHANGE PATTERN		
Dairy . . . . . —	Fruit . . . . . —	
Bread 3½	Meat 3½	
Fat 3	Veg. 3½	
NUTRITIONAL INFORMATION		
Carbohydrate 44	g	
Protein 69	g	
Total fat 26	g	
Saturated fat 3.4	g	
Cholesterol 87	mg	
Sodium 252	mg	
Potassium 1382	mg	
Fiber 2.5	g	
Calcium 114	mg	
Iron 3.8	mg	

Onion and Apple Soup

3 tablespoons margarine or
   safflower oil
3 onions, thinly sliced
2 cloves garlic, minced
2 apples, cored, peeled, and
   thinly sliced crosswise

1 1/2 quarts Homemade Chicken
   Stock (page 36)
1 teaspoon dried thyme
1/4 cup Calvados or applejack
Black pepper

PER SERVING: 175 CALORIES		
MENU EXCHANGE PATTERN		
Dairy . . . . . —	Fruit . . . . . —	
Bread 1	Meat . . . . . —	
Fat 2	Veg. 1	
NUTRITIONAL INFORMATION		
Carbohydrate 19	g	
Protein 4	g	
Total fat 11	g	
Saturated fat 1.1	g	
Cholesterol 0	mg	
Sodium 110	mg	
Potassium 201	mg	
Fiber 0.9	g	
Calcium 28	mg	
Iron . . . . 0.5 mg		

- Heat margarine or oil in a large nonstick skillet over medium heat. Add onion and garlic and sauté until tender but not brown, about 10 minutes, stirring frequently. Add apple, stock, and thyme and bring to a boil. Reduce heat to low and simmer for 40 minutes. Stir in Calvados, season with pepper to taste, and serve.

Grilled Red Snapper Fillets

6 red snapper fillets, 5 ounces
   each
Black pepper
Dried lemon rind
2 teaspoons dried thyme

2 teaspoons curry powder
3 tablespoons safflower oil
1 cup Basil Tomato Sauce
   (recipe follows)

PER SERVING: 201 CALORIES		
MENU EXCHANGE PATTERN		
Dairy . . . . . —	Fruit . . . . . —	
Bread . . . . . —	Meat 3½	
Fat . . . . —	Veg. . . . . —	
NUTRITIONAL INFORMATION		
Carbohydrate 0	g	
Protein 30	g	
Total fat 8	g	
Saturated fat 1.2	g	
Cholesterol 87	mg	
Sodium 77	mg	
Potassium 636	mg	
Fiber 0	g	
Calcium 18	mg	
Iron 1	mg	

- Sprinkle both sides of snapper fillets with pepper, lemon rind, thyme, and curry powder. Dip fish into safflower oil and drain off excess. Grill or broil until fish is lightly browned, about 4 to 5 minutes on each side. Serve with sauce.

Basil Tomato Sauce

2 tablespoons olive oil
1 clove garlic, finely chopped
1 tablespoon finely chopped
   shallots
1 onion, quartered
3 cups chopped fresh plum
   tomatoes, seeded

1/2 Idaho potato, peeled and
   quartered
1 cup water
10 fresh basil leaves

PER SERVING: 40 CALORIES		
MENU EXCHANGE PATTERN		
Dairy . . . . . —	Fruit . . . . . —	
Bread . . . . . —	Meat . . . . . —	
Fat . . . . ½	Veg. 1	
NUTRITIONAL INFORMATION		
Carbohydrate 5	g	
Protein 1	g	
Total fat 2	g	
Saturated fat 0.3	g	
Cholesterol 0	mg	
Sodium 3	mg	
Potassium 160	mg	
Fiber 0.4	g	
Calcium 10	mg	
Iron . . . . 0.3 mg		

- Heat olive oil in a saucepan over medium heat. Add garlic, shallots, and onion and sauté until translucent but not browned, about 5 minutes. Add tomato and simmer 30 minutes. Add potato, water, and basil and simmer 30 minutes longer. Transfer to a blender and puree. Makes about 2 cups; 1 serving = 3 tablespoons.

Wild Rice with Mushrooms

1 cup finely chopped onion
1 cup sliced mushrooms
1 tablespoon margarine
1 cup wild rice

2½ cups water
2 tablespoons chopped fresh
   parsley

PER SERVING: 132 CALORIES		
MENU EXCHANGE PATTERN		
Dairy . . . . . —	Fruit . . . . . —	
Bread 1½	Meat . . . . . —	
Fat . . . . —	Veg. 1	
NUTRITIONAL INFORMATION		
Carbohydrate 26	g
Protein 5	g
Total fat 2	g
Saturated fat 0.4	g
Cholesterol 0	mg
Sodium 7	mg
Potassium 165	mg
Fiber 0.6	g
Calcium 17	mg
Iron . . . . 1.5 mg	

- In a large nonstick saucepan, sauté onion and mushrooms in margarine over medium heat until onion is translucent, about 10 minutes. Stir in rice and water and bring to a boil. Cover, reduce heat to a simmer, and cook until liquid is absorbed, about 40 to 45 minutes. Stir in parsley and serve.

Green Beans with Dill

3 cups fresh green beans (ends
   trimmed), or 2 packages
   (7 ounces each) frozen
½ cup chopped onion

1 tablespoon margarine
½ teaspoon dried dillweed
Black pepper

PER SERVING: 40 CALORIES		
MENU EXCHANGE PATTERN		
Dairy . . . . . —	Fruit . . . . . —	
Bread . . . . —	Meat . . . . . —	
Fat . . . . ½	Veg. 1	
NUTRITIONAL INFORMATION		
Carbohydrate 5	g
Protein 1	g
Total fat 2	g
Saturated fat 0.4	g
Cholesterol 0	mg
Sodium 5	mg
Potassium 156	mg
Fiber 0.6	g
Calcium 35	mg
Iron . . . . 0.5 mg	

- Boil green beans in a small amount of water until crisp-tender, about 5 minutes. In a medium nonstick skillet, sauté onion in margarine over medium heat until translucent, about 5 minutes. Drain beans and combine with onion. Stir in dillweed and pepper to taste and heat through briefly. Serve immediately.

Lemon Chiffon

½ cup water
6 tablespoons lemon juice
6 tablespoons sugar
1 tablespoon cornstarch

1 tablespoon water
6 egg whites
Lemon peel twists (garnish)

PER SERVING: 73 CALORIES		
MENU EXCHANGE PATTERN		
Dairy . . . . . —	Fruit . . . . . —	
Bread 1	Meat . . . . . —	
Fat . . . . —	Veg. . . . . . . —	
NUTRITIONAL INFORMATION		
Carbohydrate 15	g
Protein 3	g
Total fat 0	g
Saturated fat 0	g
Cholesterol 0	mg
Sodium 50	mg
Potassium 64	mg
Fiber 0	g
Calcium 5	mg
Iron . . . . 0 mg	

- Combine water, lemon juice, and sugar in a nonaluminum saucepan and bring to boil. Dissolve cornstarch in 1 tablespoon water. Gradually stir several tablespoons of hot lemon mixture into cornstarch mixture, then stir back into saucepan and cook 5 more minutes, stirring constantly.

- Whip egg whites until stiff peaks form. Slowly beat in lemon mixture. Pour into dessert glasses and chill thoroughly. Garnish with lemon peel.

FIN FISH

9

Eggplant Caviar

Red Snapper Brazilian Style

Green Beans Vinaigrette

Bulgur Pilaf

Pineapple Chiffon

Serves 4

PER SERVING: 708 CALORIES		
MENU EXCHANGE PATTERN		
Dairy 1	Fruit 1	
Bread 1	Meat 4	
Fat 3	Veg. 6	
NUTRITIONAL INFORMATION		
Carbohydrate 73	g	
Protein 43	g	
Total fat 28	g	
Saturated fat 3.4	g	
Cholesterol 113	mg	
Sodium 399	mg	
Potassium 1687	mg	
Fiber 3.6	g	
Calcium 211	mg	
Iron 5.6	mg	

Eggplant Caviar

1 eggplant
1/4 cup chopped bell pepper
1/3 cup chopped onion
2 cloves garlic
1/3 cup chopped fresh or canned
   tomatoes

2 teaspoons lemon juice
Black pepper
1 1/2 teaspoons chopped fresh
   basil
Chopped fresh parsley (garnish)

- Preheat oven to 325°F. Bake whole eggplant until soft, about 30 to 40 minutes. Cool until eggplant can be handled, then cut in half. Scoop out meat and chop finely.

- In a nonstick skillet or a skillet coated with nonstick spray, sauté pepper, onion, and garlic over medium heat until soft but not brown, about 10 minutes. Add eggplant, tomatoes, lemon juice, pepper, and basil and cook over low heat until thick and nearly smooth, about 20 minutes. Garnish with chopped parsley and serve hot or cold.

PER SERVING: 38 CALORIES			
MENU EXCHANGE PATTERN			
Dairy	—	Fruit	—
Bread	—	Meat	—
Fat	—	Veg.	1 1/2
NUTRITIONAL INFORMATION			
Carbohydrate	8	g	
Protein	2	g	
Total fat	0	g	
Saturated fat	0	g	
Cholesterol	0	mg	
Sodium	5	mg	
Potassium	294	mg	
Fiber	1.2	g	
Calcium	19	mg	
Iron	0.9	mg	

Red Snapper Brazilian Style

3 tablespoons safflower oil
1/2 onion, halved and very
   thinly sliced
3 tablespoons chopped green
   bell pepper
1 clove garlic, chopped
1 tablespoon chopped mild
   green chilies
2 pounds fresh tomatoes,
   chopped
1/3 cup dry white wine

4 teaspoons lemon juice
2 teaspoons chopped fresh
   coriander (cilantro)
1 1/2 teaspoons Hilltop Herb
   Farm Good-'n-Nuff (see
   note)
1 pound snapper fillets, skinned
1/3 pound shrimp, shelled and
   deveined
1/3 cup chopped fresh parsley

- Heat oil in a large nonstick skillet over medium heat and sauté onion, pepper, and garlic until soft but not browned, about 10 minutes. Add chilies, tomatoes, wine, lemon juice, cilantro, and seasoning. Bring to a boil, reduce heat, and simmer 25 to 30 minutes.

- Preheat oven to 325°F. Arrange fish in a greased baking dish; arrange shrimp over and between fillets. Pour sauce over seafood and bake just until fish flakes with a fork, about 20 minutes. Garnish with parsley and serve.

Note: 1/2 teaspoon each of ground coriander, cumin, and fennel may be substituted.

PER SERVING: 274 CALORIES			
MENU EXCHANGE PATTERN			
Dairy	—	Fruit	—
Bread	—	Meat	4
Fat	—	Veg.	2
NUTRITIONAL INFORMATION			
Carbohydrate	11	g	
Protein	28	g	
Total fat	12	g	
Saturated fat	1.2	g	
Cholesterol	109	mg	
Sodium	150	mg	
Potassium	911	mg	
Fiber	1.0	g	
Calcium	74	mg	
Iron	2.7	mg	

Green Beans Vinaigrette

*¾ pound green beans, ends
    trimmed
1 small red onion, thinly sliced
1 tablespoon drained capers
3 tablespoons safflower oil
3 tablespoons red wine vinegar
2 teaspoons sugar*

*1 clove garlic, minced
Choice of fresh herb: marjoram,
    rosemary, savory, or lemon
    thyme
Black pepper
Red bell pepper slices (garnish)*

PER SERVING: 125 CALORIES		
MENU EXCHANGE PATTERN		
Dairy .... —	Fruit .... —	
Bread .... —	Meat .... —	
Fat 2	Veg. 1	
NUTRITIONAL INFORMATION		
Carbohydrate 8		g
Protein 1		g
Total fat 10		g
Saturated fat 0.9		g
Cholesterol 0		mg
Sodium 7		mg
Potassium 143		mg
Fiber 0.5		g
Calcium 25		mg
Iron 0.5		mg

- Steam green beans until crisp-tender, about 5 minutes. Drain and toss with onion and capers.

- Combine oil, vinegar, sugar, and garlic in a small bowl and whisk until thick. Pour dressing over the green beans and season with herbs and pepper. Chill, stirring occasionally. Garnish with red pepper slices.

Bulgur Pilaf

*4 teaspoons margarine
1 clove garlic, chopped
⅓ cup chopped celery
⅓ cup chopped onion
⅓ cup grated carrot*

*⅔ cup bulgur
1⅓ cups Homemade Chicken
    Stock (page 36)
¼ teaspoon dried oregano*

PER SERVING: 144 CALORIES		
MENU EXCHANGE PATTERN		
Dairy ..... —	Fruit ..... —	
Bread 1	Meat ..... —	
Fat 1	Veg. 1½	
NUTRITIONAL INFORMATION		
Carbohydrate 24		g
Protein 4		g
Total fat 4		g
Saturated fat 0.7		g
Cholesterol 0		mg
Sodium 17		mg
Potassium 145		mg
Fiber 0.7		g
Calcium 19		mg
Iron 1.2		mg

- Melt margarine in a large nonstick skillet over medium heat. Add garlic, celery, onion, and carrot and sauté until soft, about 10 minutes. Add bulgur and sauté 10 minutes. Add stock and oregano, cover, and cook until liquid is absorbed, about 15 minutes. Fluff with a fork and serve.

Pineapple Chiffon

1/4 cup sugar
1/2 cup pineapple juice (drained from canned pineapple)
1 cup skim milk
1 egg substitute
2 envelopes unflavored gelatin
2 cups low-fat cottage cheese
1 can unsweetened (1 pound 4 ounces) crushed pineapple, drained

2 tablespoons lemon juice
4 teaspoons sugar
1/2 teaspoon mace
2 tablespoons chopped mint
3 egg whites
2 tablespoons sugar
Cookie crumbs or nuts (garnish)
Mint sprigs (garnish)

- Combine 1/4 cup sugar, pineapple juice, milk, egg substitute, and gelatin in a small heavy saucepan and mix well with a fork. Let stand until gelatin is softened, about 5 minutes. Cook over medium heat, stirring constantly, until slightly thickened and gelatin is dissolved. Remove from heat and cool slightly.

- Transfer about 1/2 cup cooked mixture to blender. Add 1 cup cottage cheese and blend until smooth; add remaining cottage cheese and again blend until smooth. Stir into remaining cooked mixture. Add crushed pineapple, lemon juice, 4 teaspoons sugar, mace, and mint and chill until thickened but not set. (Mixture can also be set over a bowl of ice to chill; stir occasionally while cooling.)

- While base is cooling, beat egg whites until soft peaks form. Gradually add 2 tablespoons sugar and continue beating until stiff but not dry. Using a rubber spatula, gently fold egg whites into cooled base. Transfer to 2-quart soufflé dish or individual serving dishes. Garnish with cookie crumbs or nuts and sprigs of mint. Chill until serving time. Serves 10; 1 serving = 1 1/4 cups.

PER SERVING: 129 CALORIES

MENU EXCHANGE PATTERN

Dairy	1	Fruit	1
Bread	—	Meat	—
Fat	—	Veg.	—

NUTRITIONAL INFORMATION

Carbohydrate	21	g
Protein	9	g
Total fat	1	g
Saturated fat	0.6	g
Cholesterol	4	mg
Sodium	220	mg
Potassium	194	mg
Fiber	0.2	g
Calcium	74	mg
Iron	0.3	mg

FIN FISH

10

Ceviche Salad with Radicchio

Wild Mushroom and Barley Soup

Red Snapper Fillets with
Tomato-Ginger Vinaigrette

Lime-Marinated Figs with
Raspberry Yogurt Sauce

Serves 4

PER SERVING: 947 CALORIES		
MENU EXCHANGE PATTERN		
Dairy . . . . . —	Fruit 4½	
Bread 2½	Meat 7	
Fat 2	Veg. 4	
NUTRITIONAL INFORMATION		
Carbohydrate 103	g	
Protein 70	g	
Total fat 32	g	
Saturated fat 3.7	g	
Cholesterol 134	mg	
Sodium 689	mg	
Potassium 3058	mg	
Fiber 5.9	g	
Calcium 289	mg	
Iron 8.9	mg	

Ceviche Salad with Radicchio

1 pound bay scallops
2 lemons
3 limes
3 sprigs fresh oregano
2 1/2 tomatoes, peeled, seeded,
  and chopped

1/4 cup chopped onion
1/2 teaspoon white pepper
2 tablespoons chopped fresh
  coriander (cilantro) leaves
1/2 head radicchio
4 teaspoons safflower oil

- Rinse and drain scallops. Squeeze lemon and lime juice into a bowl and stir in oregano, tomato, onion, pepper, and cilantro. Add scallops, toss to coat in marinade, and refrigerate for 24 hours.

- Place 1 radicchio leaf on each plate. Remove scallops from marinade with slotted spoon and place on leaves.

- Measure 3 tablespoons remaining marinade and gradually whisk in safflower oil. Spoon over the scallops. Spoon remaining tomatoes and herbs onto scallops and serve.

PER SERVING: 186 CALORIES			
MENU EXCHANGE PATTERN			
Dairy	—	Fruit	1
Bread	—	Meat	2
Fat	—	Veg.	2
NUTRITIONAL INFORMATION			
Carbohydrate	18		g
Protein	20		g
Total fat	5		g
Saturated fat	0.4		g
Cholesterol	45		mg
Sodium	296		mg
Potassium	870		mg
Fiber	1.1		g
Calcium	76		mg
Iron	3.4		mg

Wild Mushroom and Barley Soup

5 cups Homemade Chicken
  Stock (page 36)
5 egg whites
1 cup chopped chicken meat
  (about 4 ounces)
3 whole carrots
1 white onion, peeled and
  quartered

1 bay leaf
2 tablespoons white
  peppercorns
10 ounces dried shiitake
  mushrooms
3 ounces oyster mushroom
1 1/2 cups cooked barley

- Simmer stock, egg whites, chicken, carrots, onion, bay leaf, and peppercorns until clarified, about 20 to 30 minutes, skimming foam as it accumulates. Simmer for 1 hour longer, then strain broth through cheesecloth. Discard vegetables and chicken.

- Soak dried mushrooms in warm water until soft, about 45 minutes. Add mushrooms and barley to consommé, heat through and serve.

PER SERVING: 226 CALORIES			
MENU EXCHANGE PATTERN			
Dairy	—	Fruit	—
Bread	2	Meat	1
Fat	—	Veg.	1
NUTRITIONAL INFORMATION			
Carbohydrate	34		g
Protein	17		g
Total fat	2		g
Saturated fat	0.5		g
Cholesterol	2		mg
Sodium	197		mg
Potassium	816		mg
Fiber	1.1		g
Calcium	32		mg
Iron	2.5		mg

Red Snapper Fillets

¼ cup safflower oil
4 teaspoons chopped fresh dill
4 red snapper fillets, 6 ounces
*   each*
Tomato-Ginger Vinaigrette
*   (recipe follows)*

- Combine oil and dill; marinate snapper in mixture for 30 minutes.

- Remove snapper from marinade and drain. Grill over mesquite or under broiler until fish flakes easily with a fork, about 10 to 15 minutes. Serve with vinaigrette.

PER SERVING: 254 CALORIES

MENU EXCHANGE PATTERN

Dairy	—	Fruit	—
Bread	—	Meat	4
Fat	½	Veg.	—

NUTRITIONAL INFORMATION

Carbohydrate	0	g
Protein	28	g
Total fat	15	g
Saturated fat	1.6	g
Cholesterol	85	mg
Sodium	133	mg
Potassium	581	mg
Fiber	0	g
Calcium	20	mg
Iron	1.3	mg

Tomato-Ginger Vinaigrette

2 teaspoons coarse-grained
*   mustard*
⅓ cup fruit vinegar
2½ tablespoons safflower oil
1 small shallot, chopped

2 tomatoes, peeled, seeded, and
*   chopped*
2 teaspoons finely grated fresh
*   ginger*
Black pepper

- Whisk together mustard and vinegar; gradually whisk in oil. Stir in shallot, tomato, ginger, and pepper. Makes about 2 cups; 1 serving = ½ cup.

PER SERVING: 95 CALORIES

MENU EXCHANGE PATTERN

Dairy	—	Fruit	—
Bread	—	Meat	—
Fat	1½	Veg.	1

NUTRITIONAL INFORMATION

Carbohydrate	5	g
Protein	1	g
Total fat	9	g
Saturated fat	0.7	g
Cholesterol	0	mg
Sodium	33	mg
Potassium	190	mg
Fiber	0.4	g
Calcium	12	mg
Iron	0.5	mg

Lime-Marinated Figs with Raspberry Yogurt Sauce

12 fresh figs
Juice of 1½ limes
1 cup very ripe raspberries
¾ cup plain low-fat yogurt

- Sprinkle the figs with lime juice and refrigerate for 1 hour, tossing occasionally. Force the raspberries through a fine sieve, then blend with the yogurt. Place figs in center of serving plate and surround with raspberry yogurt sauce.

PER SERVING: 186 CALORIES

MENU EXCHANGE PATTERN

Dairy	—	Fruit	3½
Bread	½	Meat	—
Fat	—	Veg.	—

NUTRITIONAL INFORMATION

Carbohydrate	45	g
Protein	4	g
Total fat	1	g
Saturated fat	0.5	g
Cholesterol	2	mg
Sodium	30	mg
Potassium	601	mg
Fiber	3.3	g
Calcium	149	mg
Iron	1	mg

FIN FISH

11

Marinated Fennel Salad

Snapper Charlotte

Herbed Rice

Green Peas and Pimientos

Amaretto Custard Romanoff

Serves 6

PER SERVING: 850 CALORIES		
MENU EXCHANGE PATTERN		
Dairy 1	Fruit 2½	
Bread 4	Meat 3	
Fat 3½	Veg. 2	
NUTRITIONAL INFORMATION		
Carbohydrate 108	g	
Protein 42	g	
Total fat 25	g	
Saturated fat 3.5	g	
Cholesterol 79	mg	
Sodium 257	mg	
Potassium 1276	mg	
Fiber 4.0	g	
Calcium 332	mg	
Iron 6.8	mg	

Marinated Fennel Salad

6 fennel bulbs, stalks removed
Onion Vinaigrette (page 133)
6 leaves romaine lettuce

2 tomatoes, cut in wedges
6 black olives
Parsley sprigs (garnish)

- Boil the fennel in water to cover until tender but still firm, about 10 minutes. Drain and cool, then slice fennel at an angle. Marinate slices in vinaigrette overnight in the refrigerator.

- Arrange lettuce leaves on individual plates; place fennel in center. Surround with tomato wedges and olives; garnish with parsley.

PER SERVING: 154 CALORIES			
MENU EXCHANGE PATTERN			
Dairy	—	Fruit	—
Bread	1	Meat	—
Fat	2	Veg.	—

NUTRITIONAL INFORMATION		
Carbohydrate	15	g
Protein	3	g
Total fat	10	g
Saturated fat	0.9	g
Cholesterol	0	mg
Sodium	69	mg
Potassium	45	mg
Fiber	1.7	g
Calcium	66	mg
Iron	1.5	mg

Snapper Charlotte

6 red snapper fillets, 6 ounces
   each
Black pepper
1/3 cup all-purpose flour
1 tablespoon safflower oil
1 tablespoon margarine
1 clove garlic, chopped
2 tablespoons chopped shallot
1 tablespoon chopped fresh
   parsley

1 tablespoon chopped fresh
   chives
Rind of 1 lemon, sliced into
   fine julienne
1/2 cup red Burgundy
Juice of 1 lemon
Cayenne pepper

Brown Sauce

1 tablespoon margarine
1 tablespoon all-purpose flour
1/2 cup skim milk or water

- Season fillets with pepper and dust with flour. Heat oil and margarine in a large nonstick skillet over medium heat. Add snapper and sauté on both sides about 10 to 15 minutes; just until fish flakes easily with a fork, do not overcook. Transfer to a heated platter and keep warm.

- Prepare sauce. Melt margarine in a small saucepan over medium heat. Add flour and cook, stirring constantly, until well browned, about 5 to 10 minutes. Whisk in liquid very slowly and simmer, whisking, until thickened. Set aside.

- Add garlic, shallot, parsley, chives, and lemon rind to skillet and sauté until shallot is translucent, about 5 minutes. Pour in wine and boil 1 to 2 minutes. Add sauce and boil until reduced to desired sauce consistency. Stir in lemon juice, black pepper, and cayenne to taste. Pour over fish and serve.

PER SERVING: 209 CALORIES			
MENU EXCHANGE PATTERN			
Dairy	—	Fruit	—
Bread	—	Meat	3
Fat	—	Veg.	1½

NUTRITIONAL INFORMATION		
Carbohydrate	4	g
Protein	24	g
Total fat	9	g
Saturated fat	1.6	g
Cholesterol	71	mg
Sodium	112	mg
Potassium	540	mg
Fiber	0.1	g
Calcium	28	mg
Iron	1.4	mg

Herbed Rice

2 teaspoons margarine
2 green onions, finely chopped
1½ cups white rice
½ cup chopped fresh parsley
¼ teaspoon dried thyme
White pepper

- Melt margarine in a large saucepan, add green onions, and sauté for 1 to 2 minutes. Add remaining ingredients, cover, and bring to a boil. Reduce heat and simmer until all water is absorbed, about 20 minutes. Fluff rice with a fork.

PER SERVING: 193 CALORIES			
MENU EXCHANGE PATTERN			
Dairy ..... —		Fruit ..... —	
Bread 2		Meat ..... —	
Fat .... ½		Veg. 1	
NUTRITIONAL INFORMATION			
Carbohydrate 40			g
Protein 4			g
Total fat 1			g
Saturated fat 0.3			g
Cholesterol 0			mg
Sodium 5			mg
Potassium 101			mg
Fiber 0.3			g
Calcium 26			mg
Iron 1.8			mg

Green Peas and Pimientos

3 cups green peas
⅓ cup water
2 teaspoons lemon juice
Black pepper
⅓ cup coarsely chopped
canned pimientos

- Combine all ingredients except pimientos in a saucepan, cover and bring to a boil. Reduce heat and simmer just until peas are tender, about 5 minutes. Drain. Stir in pimientos.

PER SERVING: 63 CALORIES			
MENU EXCHANGE PATTERN			
Dairy ..... —		Fruit ..... —	
Bread 1		Meat ..... —	
Fat .... —		Veg. .... —	
NUTRITIONAL INFORMATION			
Carbohydrate 11			g
Protein 5			g
Total fat 0			g
Saturated fat 0			g
Cholesterol 0			mg
Sodium 1			mg
Potassium 231			mg
Fiber 1.5			g
Calcium 20			mg
Iron 1.5			mg

Amaretto Custard Romanoff

2 cups skim milk
½ cup sugar
2 envelopes unflavored gelatin
¼ cup cold water
½ teaspoon almond extract
2 tablespoons amaretto
1 teaspoon vanilla extract
1 cup plain low-fat yogurt
¼ cup toasted slivered almonds
Mint leaves (garnish)

Romanoff Sauce
2 cups hulled strawberries or
raspberries
⅓ cup sugar
2 tablespoons lemon juice
2 tablespoons strawberry or
raspberry liqueur

- Combine milk and sugar in a heavy saucepan and bring to a boil, being careful not to scorch. Remove from heat. Sprinkle gelatin over water and let stand until softened, about 5 minutes. Add gelatin, almond extract, amaretto, and vanilla to milk and stir until gelatin is dissolved. Cool over ice. When mixture begins to set, fold in yogurt. Pour into individual molds and chill until firm. Dip into hot water for a few seconds to unmold.

- Prepare sauce. Combine berries and sugar in a saucepan and simmer over medium heat for 5 minutes. Remove from heat and cool. Add lemon juice and liqueur and puree in blender until smooth. Top with sauce and toasted almonds. Garnish with mint leaves.

PER SERVING: 230 CALORIES			
MENU EXCHANGE PATTERN			
Dairy 1		Fruit 2½	
Bread ..... —		Meat ..... —	
Fat 1		Veg. .... —	
NUTRITIONAL INFORMATION			
Carbohydrate 38			g
Protein 6			g
Total fat 4			g
Saturated fat 0.7			g
Cholesterol 4			mg
Sodium 70			mg
Potassium 359			mg
Fiber 0.4			g
Calcium 191			mg
Iron 0.6			mg

FIN FISH

12

Hickory-Smoked Shrimp

Beer-Batter Fried Redfish

Oven-Fried Potatoes

Green Beans with Tomatoes

Pecan Chocolate Sundae

Serves 2

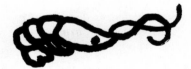

PER SERVING: 793 CALORIES		
MENU EXCHANGE PATTERN		
Dairy . . . . . —	Fruit . . . . . . ½	
Bread 4	Meat 5½	
Fat 2½	Veg. 1	

NUTRITIONAL INFORMATION		
Carbohydrate 78	g
Protein 52	g
Total fat 29	g
Saturated fat 5.9	g
Cholesterol 190	mg
Sodium 392	mg
Potassium 1706	mg
Fiber 1.7	g
Calcium 341	mg
Iron 5.2	mg

*Vegi-Nachos;
recipe page 269*

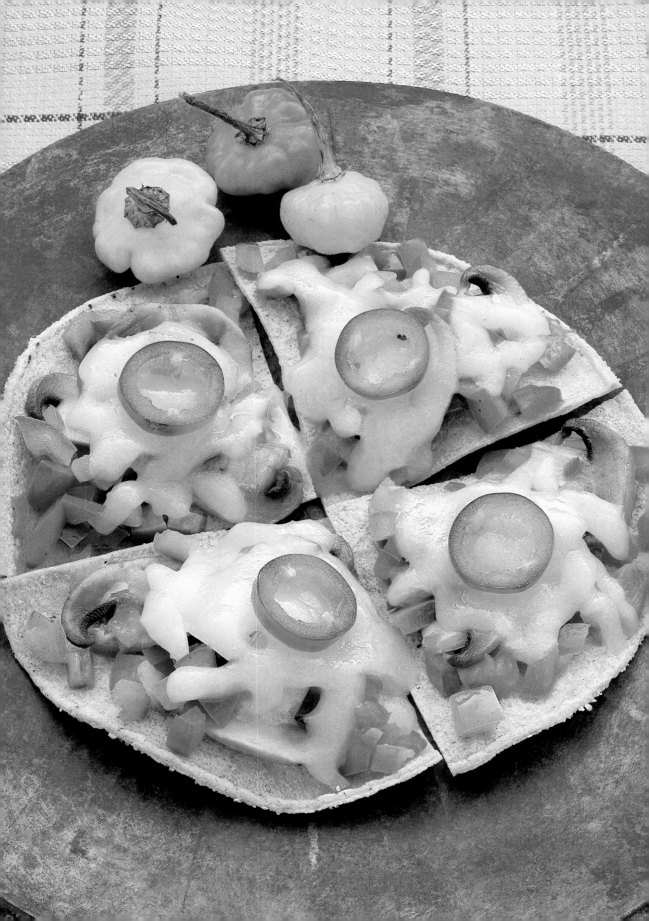

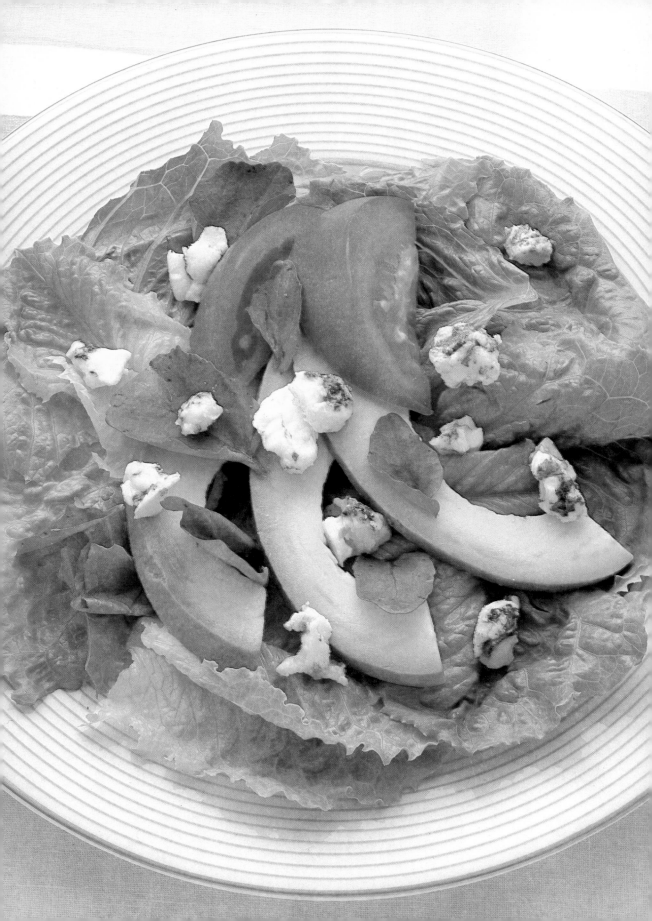

Hickory-Smoked Shrimp

1 tablespoon margarine, melted
2 teaspoons Worcestershire
   sauce
2 teaspoons lemon juice

10 shrimp, shelled and
   deveined, with tails left on
2 parsley sprigs and lemon
   wedges (garnish)

- Blend margarine, Worcestershire, and lemon juice. Brush mixture on shrimp and place on broiler pan. Broil until just pink and opaque about 6 to 8 minutes. Serve 5 shrimp on each plate; garnish each serving with a sprig of parsley and a lemon wedge.

PER SERVING: 126 CALORIES

MENU EXCHANGE PATTERN

Dairy	—	Fruit	—
Bread	—	Meat	1½
Fat	1	Veg.	—

NUTRITIONAL INFORMATION

Carbohydrate	3	g
Protein	14	g
Total fat	6	g
Saturated fat	1	g
Cholesterol	105	mg
Sodium	155	mg
Potassium	221	mg
Fiber	0	g
Calcium	56	mg
Iron	1.5	mg

Beer-Batter Fried Redfish

1 redfish, about 1 pound
¼ cup all-purpose flour
½ cup beer

Paprika
1 tablespoon margarine
Juice of 1 lemon

- Fillet, skin, and bone fish (final weight of fish will be about ⅔ pound). Preheat oven to 400°F. Combine flour and beer to form smooth batter. Coat with batter, then season with paprika. Melt margarine in a wide nonstick skillet. Add fish and sauté for 5 minutes, turning once. Transfer fish to baking dish and drizzle with lemon juice. Bake until fish is firm and opaque, about 15 to 20 minutes.

PER SERVING: 298 CALORIES

MENU EXCHANGE PATTERN

Dairy	—	Fruit	—
Bread	1	Meat	4
Fat	—	Veg.	—

NUTRITIONAL INFORMATION

Carbohydrate	16	g
Protein	30	g
Total fat	10	g
Saturated fat	1.7	g
Cholesterol	75	mg
Sodium	146	mg
Potassium	587	mg
Fiber	0.2	g
Calcium	83	mg
Iron	1.8	mg

Oven-Fried Potatoes

1 large Idaho potato, peeled
2 teaspoons safflower oil

- Preheat oven to 475°F. Cut potato into strips about ½ inch wide; pat dry with paper towels. Coat with oil by tossing in a bowl. Spread potato in a single layer on a baking sheet and bake for 35 minutes, turning periodically to brown all sides. For additional browning, place potatoes under broiler for 1 to 2 minutes.

PER SERVING: 89 CALORIES

MENU EXCHANGE PATTERN

Dairy	—	Fruit	—
Bread	1	Meat	—
Fat	½	Veg.	—

NUTRITIONAL INFORMATION

Carbohydrate	16	g
Protein	2	g
Total fat	2	g
Saturated fat	0	g
Cholesterol	0	mg
Sodium	3	mg
Potassium	370	mg
Fiber	0	g
Calcium	7	mg
Iron	0.5	mg

Wilhelmina Salad;
recipe page 280

Green Beans with Tomatoes

1 cup green beans, ends
   trimmed
1 teaspoon margarine
¼ cup chopped onion

1 small tomato, peeled, seeded
   and chopped
¼ teaspoon paprika
Black pepper

PER SERVING: 56 CALORIES			
MENU EXCHANGE PATTERN			
Dairy	—	Fruit	—
Bread	—	Meat	—
Fat	½	Veg.	1

NUTRITIONAL INFORMATION		
Carbohydrate	9	g
Protein	2	g
Total fat	2	g
Saturated fat	0.4	g
Cholesterol	0	mg
Sodium	8	mg
Potassium	314	mg
Fiber	1	g
Calcium	45	mg
Iron	0.9	mg

- Blanch green beans in boiling water for 5 minutes. Drain and run cold water over beans to cool.

- Melt margarine in a saucepan over medium heat. Add onion and sauté until translucent, about 5 minutes. Stir in beans, tomato, and seasonings and simmer until beans and tomato are cooked, about 5 minutes.

Pecan Chocolate Sundae

2 teaspoons margarine
2 teaspoons unsweetened cocoa
   powder
2 teaspoons white corn syrup
2 tablespoons sugar

2½ tablespoons evaporated
   skim milk
1 teaspoon vanilla extract
1 cup ice milk
2 teaspoons chopped pecans

PER SERVING: 224 CALORIES			
MENU EXCHANGE PATTERN			
Dairy	—	Fruit	½
Bread	2	Meat	—
Fat	1½	Veg.	—

NUTRITIONAL INFORMATION		
Carbohydrate	35	g
Protein	4	g
Total fat	8	g
Saturated fat	2.6	g
Cholesterol	10	mg
Sodium	80	mg
Potassium	214	mg
Fiber	0	g
Calcium	151	mg
Iron	0.5	mg

- Melt the margarine in a saucepan and blend in the cocoa, syrup, and sugar. Add the milk, bring to a boil, and stir until smooth. Remove from heat and stir in the vanilla.

- Serve 1 teaspoon sauce warm or cold over each ½ cup scoop of ice milk. Top with 1 teaspoon chopped pecans.

FIN FISH

13

Marinated Mushrooms

Baked Stuffed Fish

Savory Rice

Seasoned Broccoli and Carrots

Fruit Sorbet

Serves 4

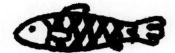

PER SERVING: 984 CALORIES		
MENU EXCHANGE PATTERN		
Dairy ..... —	Fruit 2½	
Bread 4	Meat 6½	
Fat 2	Veg. 5½	
NUTRITIONAL INFORMATION		
Carbohydrate 111	g	
Protein 63	g	
Total fat 30	g	
Saturated fat 4.3	g	
Cholesterol 21	mg	
Sodium 596	mg	
Potassium 2353	mg	
Fiber 4.5	g	
Calcium 357	mg	
Iron 8.6	mg	

Marinated Mushrooms

2 cups mushroom caps
4 teaspoons lemon juice
1/2 teaspoon sugar
4 teaspoons chopped shallot
4 teaspoons safflower oil
1/4 teaspoon dried basil
1 clove garlic, minced

3 tablespoons white wine
    vinegar
1/8 teaspoon black pepper
1/2 red bell pepper, cored,
    seeded, and chopped
4 leaves lettuce

PER SERVING: 85 CALORIES		
MENU EXCHANGE PATTERN		
Dairy .... —	Fruit .... —	
Bread .... —	Meat .... —	
Fat 1	Veg. 1½	
NUTRITIONAL INFORMATION		
Carbohydrate 7	g
Protein 3	g
Total fat 5	g
Saturated fat 0.4	g
Cholesterol 0	mg
Sodium 9	mg
Potassium 288	mg
Fiber 0.8	g
Calcium 24	mg
Iron 1	mg

- Drop mushrooms into a large saucepan of boiling water and blanch for 2 minutes; drain. Combine lemon juice, sugar, shallot, oil, basil, garlic, vinegar, and pepper. Pour over mushrooms, adding red pepper. Marinate at least 8 hours in refrigerator. Serve on lettuce leaves.

Baked Stuffed Fish

1 whole dressed bass, sea trout
    or red snapper, about
    2 pounds
Black pepper
4 tablespoons margarine
4 green onions, sliced
6 mushrooms, sliced
1 clove garlic, minced
1/3 cup chopped celery
1/3 cup chopped fresh parsley

1 tablespoon chopped fresh dill,
    or 1 teaspoon dried
1 cup fresh breadcrumbs
1 egg white
1/2 cup fish stock or Homemade
    Chicken Stock (page 36)
2/3 cup flaked fresh crabmeat
    (about 3 ounces)
Juice of 1 lemon

- Preheat oven to 425°F. Wash the fish and pat dry. Enlarge the pocket of the body cavity with a sharp knife. Sprinkle inside with pepper.

- Melt 2 tablespoons margarine in a heavy large skillet over medium heat. Add the green onion, mushrooms, garlic, celery, and parsley and sauté until golden, about 5 minutes. Let cool. Combine the sautéed vegetables with dill, breadcrumbs, egg white, stock, and crabmeat in a large bowl.

- Stuff the fish with the breadcrumb mixture and close the opening with skewers and thread. Melt remaining 2 tablespoons of margarine and mix with the lemon juice. Brush one side of fish with lemon mixture and lay greased side down in a foil-lined shallow baking pan. Brush the top of the fish with the remaining lemon mixture. Bake on the middle oven rack for 25 to 30 minutes before you test the flesh nearest the backbone with a fork. If it is opaque and separates easily from the bone, the fish is cooked.

- Lift the fish gently by the foil and transfer to a platter. Remove the skewers and thread and trim away excess foil.

PER SERVING: 491 CALORIES		
MENU EXCHANGE PATTERN		
Dairy ..... —	Fruit ..... —	
Bread 1	Meat 6½	
Fat .... —	Veg. 2	
NUTRITIONAL INFORMATION		
Carbohydrate 24	g
Protein 52	g
Total fat 20	g
Saturated fat 3.3	g
Cholesterol 21	mg
Sodium 545	mg
Potassium 1078	mg
Fiber 0.7	g
Calcium 179	mg
Iron 4.2	mg

Savory Rice

2 teaspoons safflower oil
1 small onion, finely chopped
1 clove garlic, chopped
2 whole cloves
1 teaspoon ground turmeric

$^1/_2$ teaspoon ground cumin
$^2/_3$ cup white rice, washed and
   drained
$1^1/_3$ cups boiling water

- Heat the oil in a skillet over medium heat. Add the onion, garlic, and cloves and sauté until onion is translucent, about 5 minutes. Add ground turmeric and cumin and sauté for 1 minute. Stir in the rice and sauté for 5 minutes. Pour in boiling water, cover and simmer until the rice is cooked and all liquid is absorbed, about 15 to 20 minutes, stirring occasionally to prevent sticking. Fluff rice with a fork.

PER SERVING: 154 CALORIES

MENU EXCHANGE PATTERN

Dairy . . . . . —	Fruit . . . . . —
Bread 2	Meat . . . . . —
Fat . . . . $^1/_2$	Veg. . . . . . . —

NUTRITIONAL INFORMATION

Carbohydrate 30	g
Protein 3	g
Total fat 2	g
Saturated fat 0.2	g
Cholesterol 0	mg
Sodium 6	mg
Potassium 100	mg
Fiber 0.4	g
Calcium 20	mg
Iron 1.2	mg

Seasoned Broccoli and Carrots

2 teaspoons margarine
$^2/_3$ cup diagonally sliced carrot
$^1/_2$ small onion, sliced
$^1/_2$ cup sliced broccoli
2 tablespoons water

1 teaspoon grated lemon rind
$^1/_4$ teaspoon dried thyme
1 tablespoon chopped fresh
   parsley

- Melt margarine in a medium saucepan over medium heat. Add carrot and onion and sauté for 5 minutes. Add broccoli, water, lemon rind, and thyme; cover and cook until vegetables are crisp-tender, about 5 minutes. Add parsley and toss.

PER SERVING: 69 CALORIES

MENU EXCHANGE PATTERN

Dairy . . . . . —	Fruit . . . . . —
Bread . . . . . —	Meat . . . . . —
Fat . . . . $^1/_2$	Veg. 2

NUTRITIONAL INFORMATION

Carbohydrate 11	g
Protein 4	g
Total fat 2	g
Saturated fat 0.4	g
Cholesterol 0	mg
Sodium 33	mg
Potassium 507	mg
Fiber 1.9	g
Calcium 114	mg
Iron 1.4	mg

Fruit Sorbet

3 cups coarsely chopped fruit,
   such as apricots, plums,
   pears, apples, peaches,
   strawberries, or melon

$^1/_2$ cup sugar or honey
$^2/_3$ cup dry white wine or
   Champagne
Mint sprigs (garnish)

- Puree the fruit in a blender, food processor, or food mill. Combine the sugar and wine in a nonaluminum saucepan and simmer until the sugar is dissolved. Stir in the fruit puree. Pour mixture into an 8-inch-square pan and place in the freezer. Stir every 15 minutes until creamy, then cover and freeze until hard.

- Scoop into serving dishes and garnish with mint sprigs. Makes about 1 quart; 1 serving = 1 cup.

Note: Though almost any fruit can be used in this recipe, apricots and pears are particularly good. The more you beat the partially frozen mixture, the finer its consistency will be; for the best results of all, churn the sorbet in an ice cream maker. Sorbet should be served slightly soft, so remove it from the freezer 10 minutes before serving.

PER SERVING: 185 CALORIES

MENU EXCHANGE PATTERN

Dairy . . . . . —	Fruit . . . . . $2^1/_2$
Bread 1	Meat . . . . . —
Fat . . . . —	Veg. . . . . . . —

NUTRITIONAL INFORMATION

Carbohydrate 39	g
Protein 2	g
Total fat 1	g
Saturated fat 0	g
Cholesterol 0	mg
Sodium 3	mg
Potassium 380	mg
Fiber 0.7	g
Calcium 20	mg
Iron 0.8	mg

FIN FISH

14

Hot and Sour Soup

Pine Nut Fish

Steamed White Rice (page 185)

Sautéed Snow Peas

Glazed Bananas

Serves 4

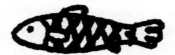

PER SERVING: 1035 CALORIES			
MENU EXCHANGE PATTERN			
Dairy	—	Fruit	4
Bread	4½	Meat	5½
Fat	3½	Veg.	4

NUTRITIONAL INFORMATION		
Carbohydrate	133	g
Protein	47	g
Total fat	36	g
Saturated fat	3.6	g
Cholesterol	69	mg
Sodium	491	mg
Potassium	1428	mg
Fiber	2.7	g
Calcium	122	mg
Iron	6.8	mg

Hot and Sour Soup

$1/_2$ *cup dried lily buds*
$1/_2$ *cup dried wood ear fungus*
2 ounces chicken, shredded
1 teaspoon cornstarch
6 cups Homemade Chicken
    Stock (page 36)
$1/_2$ *teaspoon white pepper*
2 tablespoons rice or cider
    vinegar

1 tablespoon low-sodium soy
    sauce
2 tablespoons cornstarch
$1/_4$ *cup water*
$1/_4$ *pound bean curd*
1 egg white lightly beaten
1 teaspoon Oriental sesame oil

- Soak lily buds and wood ears in warm water to cover for about 2 hours to soften. Rinse thoroughly and drain. Shred wood ears. Mix shredded chicken with cornstarch in a small bowl and set aside.

- Combine stock, white pepper, vinegar, and soy sauce in a nonaluminum saucepan and bring to a boil. Stir 2 table-spoons cornstarch into $1/_4$ cup water; gradually stir into soup.

- Add bean curd, shredded wood ears, and lily buds to the soup and cook over low heat for 8 minutes. Slowly stir in egg white. Remove from heat; immediately add sesame oil and serve.

PER SERVING: 80 CALORIES

MENU EXCHANGE PATTERN

Dairy . . . . . —	Fruit . . . . . —
Bread . . . . —	Meat 1
Fat . . . . —	Veg. 1

NUTRITIONAL INFORMATION

Carbohydrate 7	g
Protein 6	g
Total fat 3	g
Saturated fat 0.7	g
Cholesterol 7	mg
Sodium 281	mg
Potassium 144	mg
Fiber 0.2	g
Calcium 41	mg
Iron 1	mg

Pine Nut Fish

1 pound sea trout fillets
2 egg whites, lightly beaten
1 teaspoon white pepper
2 tablespoons cornstarch
2 tablespoons safflower oil
2 teaspoons minced ginger
2 teaspoons minced green
    onion
1 teaspoon Chinese hot sauce,
    or $1/_4$ *teaspoon Tabasco*

1 teaspoon minced jalapeño
    chili
$1/_4$ *cup lightly toasted pine nuts*
2 tablespoons dry white wine
1 teaspoon Oriental sesame oil
2 tablespoons minced fresh
    coriander (cilantro)

- Dice trout into $1/_4$-inch cubes. Combine egg whites with white pepper and cornstarch. Toss diced trout with mixture and marinate for 20 minutes. Heat 5 teaspoons safflower oil in a wok or large skillet over high heat. Add trout and stir-fry until cooked through, about 2 to 3 minutes. Remove and drain off excess oil.

- Reheat wok or skillet with remaining 1 teaspoon safflower oil. Add ginger, green onion, hot sauce, and jalapeño and stir-fry until fragrant, about 1 minute. Add trout and pine nuts and heat thoroughly. Stir in wine, sesame oil, and cilantro, remove from heat, and serve.

PER SERVING: 369 CALORIES

MENU EXCHANGE PATTERN

Dairy . . . . . —	Fruit . . . . . —
Bread . . . . —	Meat 4
Fat 2½	Veg. 1

NUTRITIONAL INFORMATION

Carbohydrate 6	g
Protein 27	g
Total fat 25	g
Saturated fat 1.9	g
Cholesterol 62	mg
Sodium 70	mg
Potassium 578	mg
Fiber 0.2	g
Calcium 30	mg
Iron 1.6	mg

Sautéed Snow Peas

1 tablespoon safflower oil
1 tablespoon sliced garlic
1/2 teaspoon minced ginger
2 cups snow peas, ends
    trimmed

1/4 teaspoon white pepper
2 tablespoons pumpkin seeds
1 teaspoon dry white wine

PER SERVING: 119 CALORIES		
MENU EXCHANGE PATTERN		
Dairy .... —	Fruit	.. —
Bread .... —	Meat	..... 1/2
Fat 1	Veg.	 2
NUTRITIONAL INFORMATION		
Carbohydrate 12		g
Protein 6		g
Total fat 6		g
Saturated fat 0.7		g
Cholesterol 0		mg
Sodium 2		mg
Potassium 242		mg
Fiber 1.6		g
Calcium 22		mg
Iron .... 1.9 mg		

- Heat oil in a wok or skillet over high heat. Add garlic and ginger and stir-fry until fragrant, about 1 to 2 minutes; do not brown garlic. Add snow peas and white pepper, reduce heat slightly, and stir-fry just until snow peas are crisp-tender. Stir in pumpkin seeds and wine and serve.

Glazed Bananas

2 firm bananas
1 egg substitute
1/4 cup cornstarch
1/4 cup all-purpose flour

1 teaspoon baking powder
3/4 cup sugar
1/4 cup water

- Preheat oven to 450°F. Peel bananas and cut into 1/2-inch-thick slices. Combine egg substitute, cornstarch, flour, and baking powder in a small mixing bowl and stir until well blended. Coat banana slices in batter and transfer to a cookie sheet coated with nonstick spray. Bake until batter has set (hardened) without browning, about 5 to 10 minutes. Remove banana slices from oven and set aside.

- Combine sugar and water in a small saucepan and bring to a boil, stirring constantly. Continue to cook, without stirring, until syrup reaches 300°F (hard crack stage) on a candy thermometer.

- Prepare a large bowl of ice water. Dip cooked banana slices individually into hot syrup, coating evenly. Immediately drop into ice water to harden. Remove banana slices from water and blot dry with a paper towel. Transfer to dessert plates and serve.

PER SERVING: 290 CALORIES		
MENU EXCHANGE PATTERN		
Dairy ..... —	Fruit	 4
Bread 2	Meat	..... —
Fat .... —	Veg.	...... —
NUTRITIONAL INFORMATION		
Carbohydrate 70		g
Protein 4		g
Total fat 1		g
Saturated fat 0.3		g
Cholesterol 0		mg
Sodium 136		mg
Potassium 419		mg
Fiber 0.6		g
Calcium 17		mg
Iron .... 0.9 mg		

FIN FISH

15

Oysters Landry

Stuffed Flounder Fillets

Creole Green Beans with Potatoes

Jalapeño Cornbread

Frozen Yogurt with Rum

Serves 6

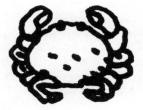

PER SERVING: 763 CALORIES		
MENU EXCHANGE PATTERN		
Dairy 1	Fruit . . . . . —	
Bread 2½	Meat 6	
Fat 3½	Veg. 1	
NUTRITIONAL INFORMATION		
Carbohydrate 57		g
Protein 61		g
Total fat 31		g
Saturated fat 5		g
Cholesterol 194		mg
Sodium 1361		mg
Potassium 1399		mg
Fiber 1.5		g
Calcium 418		mg
Iron 7.3		mg

Oysters Landry

1½ tablespoons margarine
¼ cup finely chopped onion or
   green onion
¼ cup finely chopped celery
2 teaspoons all-purpose flour
¾ cup milk
White and cayenne pepper
Pinch of nutmeg
⅓ cup grated low-fat American-
   style cheese

1 egg substitute
2 tablespoons lemon juice
½ pound crabmeat
30 raw oysters
Rock salt
1½ tablespoons fine dry
   breadcrumbs
Paprika

- Preheat oven to 375°F. Melt margarine in a saucepan over medium heat. Add onion and celery and cook until onion is soft and translucent but not brown, about 5 minutes. Sift in flour and briskly stir in milk. Add peppers, nutmeg, and grated cheese. Remove from heat and add egg substitute, lemon juice, and crabmeat.

- Clean and shuck oysters; replace each in its bottom shell. Arrange in a bed of rock salt. Top each oyster with 2 tablespoons crab mixture. Sprinkle with breadcrumbs and paprika. Bake until top is brown and crusty, 15 to 20 minutes. Serve immediately.

PER SERVING: 155 CALORIES		
MENU EXCHANGE PATTERN		
Dairy ...... ½	Fruit ..... —	
Bread .... —	Meat 2	
Fat .... —	Veg. ...... —	
NUTRITIONAL INFORMATION		
Carbohydrate 7	g	
Protein 17	g	
Total fat 6	g	
Saturated fat 0.7	g	
Cholesterol 76	mg	
Sodium 462	mg	
Potassium 91	mg	
Fiber 0.1	g	
Calcium 71	mg	
Iron .... 4.1 mg		

Stuffed Flounder Fillets

6 flounder fillets (2 pounds)
½ teaspoon cayenne pepper
2 tablespoons margarine
1 tablespoon all-purpose flour
½ cup evaporated skim milk
1 small onion, finely chopped

2 tablespoons chopped celery
Garlic powder
½ pound crabmeat
1 egg substitute, well beaten
1 lemon, cut into wedges

- Preheat oven to 350°F. Season fish with cayenne. Melt 1 tablespoon margarine in a small saucepan over medium heat. Add flour and stir constantly for 1 minute; do not brown. Stir in milk and cook until thickened. In another saucepan, sauté onion and celery in remaining 1 tablespoon margarine until tender, about 10 minutes. Add garlic powder to taste, crabmeat, and egg substitute. Place half of fillets dark side down on individual squares of greased aluminum foil. Spread with stuffing. Cover with the remaining fillets, skin side up. Fold foil over and seal.

- Preheat oven to 350°F. Place foil-wrapped fish on a cookie sheet and bake until fish flakes easily with a fork, is opaque, and crab stuffing is heated through, 30 to 35 minutes or longer. Serve with lemon wedges.

PER SERVING: 233 CALORIES		
MENU EXCHANGE PATTERN		
Dairy ..... —	Fruit ..... —	
Bread ..... ½	Meat 4	
Fat .... —	Veg. ...... —	
NUTRITIONAL INFORMATION		
Carbohydrate 8	g	
Protein 34	g	
Total fat 6	g	
Saturated fat 1.2	g	
Cholesterol 109	mg	
Sodium 402	mg	
Potassium 656	mg	
Fiber 0.1	g	
Calcium 110	mg	
Iron .... 1.9 mg		

Creole Green Beans with Potatoes

1 pound green beans
6 new potatoes, peeled and
 sliced
1 small onion, chopped

1 teaspoon sugar
1/4 teaspoon black pepper
1 1/2 cups water

- Combine all ingredients in a saucepan, bring to a boil, and cook over medium heat for 5 minutes. Reduce heat to low and cook until beans are crisp-tender, about 15 more minutes. Serve immediately.

PER SERVING: 52 CALORIES			
MENU EXCHANGE PATTERN			
Dairy ..... —	Fruit ..... —		
Bread 1/2	Meat ..... —		
Fat .... —	Veg. 1		
NUTRITIONAL INFORMATION			
Carbohydrate 12	g
Protein 2	g
Total fat 0	g
Saturated fat 0	g
Cholesterol 0	mg
Sodium 62	mg
Potassium 302	mg
Fiber 0.8	g
Calcium 37	mg
Iron 0.7	mg

Jalapeño Cornbread

1 small onion, finely chopped
1/4 cup safflower oil
1/2 cup yellow cornmeal
1/2 teaspoon salt
1 teaspoon baking powder
1 cup cooked fresh or frozen
 corn

1/3 cup grated low-fat cheddar-
 style cheese
2 jalapeño chilies, finely
 chopped
2/3 cup buttermilk
1/2 teaspoon baking soda
2 egg whites, lightly beaten

- Preheat oven to 400°F. In a small skillet, sauté onion in oil over medium heat until tender, about 5 minutes. Combine cornmeal, salt, and baking powder in a large bowl. Add corn, onion mixture, cheese, and jalapeños. Mix buttermilk and soda and add to cornmeal mixture. Fold in beaten egg whites. Pour batter into a greased 9-inch square pan and bake until golden brown, 25 to 30 minutes. Makes 6 servings; 1 serving = one 4 1/2 × 3-inch square.

PER SERVING: 142 CALORIES			
MENU EXCHANGE PATTERN			
Dairy ..... —	Fruit ..... —		
Bread 1/2	Meat ..... —		
Fat 2	Veg. .... —		
NUTRITIONAL INFORMATION			
Carbohydrate 10	g
Protein 4	g
Total fat 10	g
Saturated fat 0.9	g
Cholesterol 1	mg
Sodium 380	mg
Potassium 129	mg
Fiber 0.3	g
Calcium 82	mg
Iron 0.3	mg

Frozen Yogurt with Rum

3 cups low-fat frozen vanilla
 yogurt
6 tablespoons dark rum
1/2 cup finely chopped pecans

- Place 1/2 cup yogurt in each of 6 dessert bowls. Top with 1 tablespoon rum and 1 1/2 tablespoons chopped pecans.

PER SERVING: 181 CALORIES			
MENU EXCHANGE PATTERN			
Dairy 1/2	Fruit ..... —		
Bread 1	Meat ..... —		
Fat 1 1/2	Veg. .... —		
NUTRITIONAL INFORMATION			
Carbohydrate 19	g
Protein 4	g
Total fat 8	g
Saturated fat 1.8	g
Cholesterol 8	mg
Sodium 55	mg
Potassium 221	mg
Fiber 0.2	g
Calcium 118	mg
Iron 0.3	mg

FIN FISH

16

Spiked Cold Shrimp

Tomato, Green Onion, and Avocado Salad

Lemon-Broiled Swordfish

Green Beans

Stuffed Acorn Squash

Peach Crisp

Serves 8

PER SERVING: 809 CALORIES		
MENU EXCHANGE PATTERN		
Dairy . . . . . —	Fruit 2	
Bread 1	Meat 6½	
Fat 5	Veg. 3	
NUTRITIONAL INFORMATION		
Carbohydrate 57	g	
Protein 61	g	
Total fat 38	g	
Saturated fat 2.8	g	
Cholesterol 228	mg	
Sodium 283	mg	
Potassium 1392	mg	
Fiber 3.6	g	
Calcium 221	mg	
Iron 6.4	mg	

Spiked Cold Shrimp

1 pound shrimp
1 1/3 cups lemon juice
8 teaspoons cognac

- Boil the shrimp just until opaque and pink, about 3 to 5 minutes; do not overcook. Drop shrimp into a bowl of ice water and let stand until cold, then drain well. Shell and devein the shrimp. Combine lemon juice and cognac in a nonaluminum bowl. Add shrimp and marinate in the refrigerator for at least 30 minutes before serving.

PER SERVING: 125 CALORIES		
MENU EXCHANGE PATTERN		
Dairy . . . . . —	Fruit . . . . . —	
Bread . . . . . —	Meat 2	
Fat . . . . —	Veg. . . . . . . —	
NUTRITIONAL INFORMATION		
Carbohydrate 5	g	
Protein 20	g	
Total fat 1	g	
Saturated fat 0	g	
Cholesterol 158	mg	
Sodium 158	mg	
Potassium 300	mg	
Fiber 0	g	
Calcium 74	mg	
Iron 2	mg	

Tomato, Green Onion, and Avocado Salad

8 red-leaf lettuce leaves
4 tomatoes, each cut in 6 wedges
1 avocado, peeled, pitted, and thinly sliced

3 green onions, thinly sliced at an angle
1/2 cup Cumin Dressing (recipe follows)

- Place lettuce leaves on individual salad plates. Arrange the tomato and avocado attractively on lettuce. Sprinkle with green onion and top with dressing.

Note: To reduce fat intake, substitute a commercial low-calorie Italian dressing for the Cumin Dressing. Adjusted analysis for dressing: calories = 16; exchange = 1/2 Fat.

PER SERVING: 66 CALORIES		
MENU EXCHANGE PATTERN		
Dairy . . . . . —	Fruit . . . . . —	
Bread . . . . . —	Meat . . . . . —	
Fat 1	Veg. 1	
NUTRITIONAL INFORMATION		
Carbohydrate 7	g	
Protein 2	g	
Total fat 4	g	
Saturated fat 0.6	g	
Cholesterol 0	mg	
Sodium 7	mg	
Potassium 430	mg	
Fiber 1.2	g	
Calcium 24	mg	
Iron 1.1	mg	

Cumin Dressing

2/3 cup safflower oil
1/4 cup red wine vinegar
1/8 teaspoon ground cumin

Black pepper
Juice of 1 lemon

- Combine all ingredients in a jar and shake well. Makes 1 cup; 1 serving = 1 tablespoon.

PER SERVING: 80 CALORIES		
MENU EXCHANGE PATTERN		
Dairy . . . . . —	Fruit . . . . . —	
Bread . . . . . —	Meat . . . . . —	
Fat 2	Veg. . . . . . . —	
NUTRITIONAL INFORMATION		
Carbohydrate 0	g	
Protein 1	g	
Total fat 9	g	
Saturated fat 1	g	
Cholesterol 0	mg	
Sodium 0	mg	
Potassium 9	mg	
Fiber 0	g	
Calcium 1	mg	
Iron 0	mg	

Lemon-Broiled Swordfish

⅔ cup lemon juice
⅔ cup safflower oil
3 small cloves garlic, chopped
¼ teaspoon dried oregano

2 teaspoons grated lemon rind
Black pepper
*8 swordfish steaks, 6 ounces
   each*

- Blend all ingredients except swordfish. Add fish steaks and marinate for 30 to 40 minutes.

- Preheat broiler. Broil steaks just until firm and opaque, 4 to 5 minutes on each side, basting with the marinade. Serve immediately.

PER SERVING: 286 CALORIES		
MENU EXCHANGE PATTERN		
Dairy . . . . . —	Fruit . . . . . —	
Bread . . . . —	Meat 4½	
Fat . . . . ½	Veg. . . . . . . —	
NUTRITIONAL INFORMATION		
Carbohydrate 2	g	
Protein 32	g	
Total fat 16	g	
Saturated fat 1	g	
Cholesterol 70	mg	
Sodium 60	mg	
Potassium 25	mg	
Fiber 0	g	
Calcium 33	mg	
Iron 1.5	mg	

Green Beans

*6 cups green beans, ends
   trimmed*
Black pepper

- Bring 2 quarts water to a rapid boil in a large saucepan. Drop in beans, return to a boil, and cook uncovered until beans are crisp-tender, 10 to 15 minutes. Transfer beans to a large skillet and toss over medium heat until most of the water has evaporated. Season with pepper to taste and serve.

PER SERVING: 23 CALORIES		
MENU EXCHANGE PATTERN		
Dairy . . . . . —	Fruit . . . . . —	
Bread . . . . . . —	Meat . . . . . —	
Fat . . . . —	Veg. 1	
NUTRITIONAL INFORMATION		
Carbohydrate 5	g	
Protein 2	g	
Total fat 0	g	
Saturated fat 0	g	
Cholesterol 0	mg	
Sodium 4	mg	
Potassium 142	mg	
Fiber 0.9	g	
Calcium 47	mg	
Iron 0.6	mg	

Stuffed Acorn Squash

*4 acorn squash, halved and
   seeded*
4 teaspoons margarine, melted
Ground cinnamon
⅓ cup raisins

- Preheat oven to 350°F. Brush cut side of each squash half with 1 teaspoon margarine; sprinkle with cinnamon and divide raisins among the cavities. Cover and bake until tender, about 45 minutes.

PER SERVING: 44 CALORIES		
MENU EXCHANGE PATTERN		
Dairy . . . . . —	Fruit . . . . . —	
Bread . . . . —	Meat . . . . . —	
Fat . . . . ½	Veg. 1	
NUTRITIONAL INFORMATION		
Carbohydrate 7	g	
Protein 1	g	
Total fat 2	g	
Saturated fat 0.4	g	
Cholesterol 0	mg	
Sodium 1	mg	
Potassium 117	mg	
Fiber 0.3	g	
Calcium 13	mg	
Iron 0.3	mg	

Peach Crisp

1 cup rolled oats
½ cup walnuts
10 peaches, peeled, pitted, and
sliced

Pinch of salt
2 tablespoons arrowroot
¼ cup water
2 tablespoons barley malt

- Preheat oven to 400°F. Spread oats and nuts separately on 2 cookie sheets and toast in oven until golden, about 5 to 10 minutes. Cool slightly, then chop nuts.

- Reduce oven temperature to 375°F. Combine peaches, salt, arrowroot, and water in a large bowl and toss to distribute ingredients. Transfer to a 2-quart baking dish coated with nonstick spray, and spread evenly. Mix oats, walnuts, and barley malt and spread evenly over peach mixture. Cover dish and bake until peaches are cooked, about 20 minutes. Remove cover and brown topping under the broiler for 5 to 10 minutes. Serve warm.

Note: Barley malt is available in natural food stores and supermarkets in some parts of the country.

PER SERVING: 185 CALORIES			
MENU EXCHANGE PATTERN			
Dairy	—	Fruit	2
Bread	1	Meat	—
Fat	1	Veg.	—
NUTRITIONAL INFORMATION			
Carbohydrate	31		g
Protein	4		g
Total fat	6		g
Saturated fat	0.3		g
Cholesterol	0		mg
Sodium	53		mg
Potassium	369		mg
Fiber	1.2		g
Calcium	29		mg
Iron	1		mg

FIN FISH

17

Italian Mussel Soup

Poppyseed Bread

Swordfish with Salmoriglio Sauce

Herbed Eggplant and Tomatoes

Almond Pastry Ligurian Style

Serves 6

PER SERVING: 816 CALORIES			
MENU EXCHANGE PATTERN			
Dairy	—	Fruit	—
Bread	3	Meat	5½
Fat	5	Veg.	3
NUTRITIONAL INFORMATION			
Carbohydrate	43	g	
Protein	52	g	
Total fat	3	g	
Saturated fat	2.9	g	
Cholesterol	208	mg	
Sodium	104	mg	
Potassium	1116	mg	
Fiber	2.5	g	
Calcium	198	mg	
Iron	9.4	mg	

Italian Mussel Soup

2 teaspoons chopped garlic
½ cup safflower oil
1 tablespoon coarsely chopped fresh parsley
1½ cups cut-up fresh plum tomatoes (about 4)

⅛ teaspoon chopped red chili pepper
2 pounds fresh mussels, cleaned
½ cup dry white wine

- In a large Dutch oven, sauté garlic in the oil over medium heat until lightly colored. Add the parsley and stir once or twice, then add tomatoes and chili pepper. Simmer uncovered until tomatoes and oil separate, about 25 minutes.

- Add the mussels and wine, cover, raise heat to high, and cook until the mussels open, about 3 to 5 minutes. (To help all the mussels cook evenly, grasp the pot with both hands, holding the cover down tightly, and shake it 2 or 3 times while cooking.) If necessary, simmer 3 to 4 additional minutes uncovered to thicken sauce. Serve immediately.

Note: To clean mussels, scrub them thoroughly under cold running water with a stiff brush until you have removed all traces of dirt and slime. Discard all mussels that are not tightly closed and any that feel much lighter or heavier than the rest. With a sharp paring knife, cut off the "beards"—the hairlike tufts protruding from the shells.

PER SERVING: 178 CALORIES		
MENU EXCHANGE PATTERN		
Dairy ..... —	Fruit ..... —	
Bread ..... ½	Meat 1	
Fat 1½	Veg. 1	
NUTRITIONAL INFORMATION		
Carbohydrate 9	g	
Protein 10	g	
Total fat 10	g	
Saturated fat 0.8	g	
Cholesterol 90	mg	
Sodium 4	mg	
Potassium 414	mg	
Fiber 0.5	g	
Calcium 78	mg	
Iron 5.2	mg	

Poppyseed Bread

1 envelope active dry yeast
½ cup warm water
1 egg, beaten
1 cup whole wheat flour, sifted
2 cups all-purpose flour, sifted
½ teaspoon salt

1 tablespoon sugar
½ cup low-fat milk
3 tablespoons margarine, at room temperature
2 tablespoons poppyseed

- Stir yeast into warm water with egg in a small bowl and let stand for about 2 minutes. Mix the flours, salt, and sugar in a large bowl. Make a well in the center and pour in the yeast mixture. Stir in the milk and margarine, then knead for 10 minutes. Place in a warm area, cover with a damp towel, and let rise until doubled in volume, about 1 hour.

- Punch dough down and form into 2 long, narrow loaves. Cover with a damp cloth and let rise again for 1 hour.

- Preheat oven to 400°F. Cut diagonal slashes in the loaves and sprinkle the tops with poppyseed. Bake for 10 minutes, then reduce heat to 325°F and bake until loaves are golden and sound hollow when tapped, about 40 more minutes. Cool on racks before slicing. Each loaf makes 8 slices; 1 serving = 1 slice.

PER SERVING: 119 CALORIES		
MENU EXCHANGE PATTERN		
Dairy ..... —	Fruit ..... —	
Bread 1½	Meat ..... —	
Fat .... ½	Veg. ..... —	
NUTRITIONAL INFORMATION		
Carbohydrate 18	g	
Protein 4	g	
Total fat 4	g	
Saturated fat 0.8	g	
Cholesterol 18	mg	
Sodium 77	mg	
Potassium 116	mg	
Fiber 0.4	g	
Calcium 2	mg	
Iron 0.9	mg	

Swordfish with Salmoriglio Sauce

3 tablespoons lemon juice
1½ tablespoons fresh oregano,
*   or 1 teaspoon dried*
⅓ cup safflower oil

Black pepper
2 pounds swordfish steaks,
*   ½ inch thick*

- Preheat broiler 20 to 30 minutes before you are ready to cook.

- Combine lemon juice and oregano in a medium bowl. Add the oil drop by drop, whisking with a fork until well blended. Stir in a few grindings of pepper.

- Place the fish under the broiler as close as possible to the heat source; it must broil quickly, at a very high heat. Broil 1 to 1½ minutes on one side, then turn and cook another 1½ minutes on the other side (fish need not brown). Transfer the fish to a warm platter. Pour the sauce over the fish, moistening it thoroughly. Serve at once, spooning a bit of sauce from the platter over the fish as it is placed on individual plates.

PER SERVING: 308 CALORIES		
MENU EXCHANGE PATTERN		
Dairy .... —	Fruit ..... —	
Bread .... —	Meat 4½	
Fat 1	Veg. ..... —	
NUTRITIONAL INFORMATION		
Carbohydrate 1	g	
Protein 33	g	
Total fat 19	g	
Saturated fat 0	g	
Cholesterol 100	mg	
Sodium 0	mg	
Potassium 10	mg	
Fiber 0	g	
Calcium 33	mg	
Iron 1.5	mg	

Herbed Eggplant and Tomatoes

½ cup finely chopped onion
2 cloves garlic, minced
6 zucchini, thinly sliced
1 tablespoon safflower oil
1 eggplant, peeled and diced
1 green bell pepper, cored,
*   seeded, and chopped*
3 tomatoes, peeled and coarsely
*   chopped*

2 tablespoons chopped fresh
*   basil*
1 tablespoon fresh oregano
Black pepper
2 tablespoons chopped fresh
*   parsley*

PER SERVING: 71 CALORIES		
MENU EXCHANGE PATTERN		
Dairy ..... —	Fruit ..... —	
Bread .... —	Meat ..... —	
Fat .... ½	Veg. 2	
NUTRITIONAL INFORMATION		
Carbohydrate 11	g	
Protein 3	g	
Total fat 3	g	
Saturated fat 0.2	g	
Cholesterol 0	mg	
Sodium 7	mg	
Potassium 490	mg	
Fiber 1.5	g	
Calcium 42	mg	
Iron 1.2	mg	

- In a large nonstick skillet, sauté onion, garlic, and zucchini in safflower oil over high heat for about 2 minutes. Add all remaining ingredients except parsley. Reduce heat, cover, and simmer for 15 minutes. Uncover and continue to simmer until sauce thickens, about 20 to 30 minutes. Add parsley just before serving.

Almond Pastry Ligurian Style

¾ cup blanched almonds
6 tablespoons margarine
⅔ cup sugar
3 egg substitutes

½ cup sifted all-purpose flour
3 tablespoons brandy
Confectioners sugar

- Preheat oven to 350°F. Toast almonds in a skillet over low heat until richly browned, stirring constantly. Chop very finely. Melt margarine in a saucepan. Stir in sugar and egg substitutes, then gradually stir in flour, almonds, and brandy. Pour batter into a greased and floured 8-inch square pan and bake until lightly browned, about 20 to 25 minutes. Let cake cool in pan. Cut into 16 small squares or diamonds. Arrange on a serving platter and sprinkle with confectioners sugar. Makes 16 pieces; 1 serving = 1 piece.

PER SERVING: 140 CALORIES			
MENU EXCHANGE PATTERN			
Dairy	—	Fruit	—
Bread	1	Meat	—
Fat	1½	Veg.	—
NUTRITIONAL INFORMATION			
Carbohydrate	13	g	
Protein	3	g	
Total fat	8	g	
Saturated fat	1.1	g	
Cholesterol	0	mg	
Sodium	16	mg	
Potassium	86	mg	
Fiber	0.1	g	
Calcium	22	mg	
Iron	0.6	mg	

FIN FISH

18

Grilled Sardines with Lime

Whole Wheat Breadsticks

Salad of Spinach, Red Peppers, and Hearts of Palm

Grilled Swordfish with Parsley Almonds

Deep-Dish Apple Charlottes

Serves 6

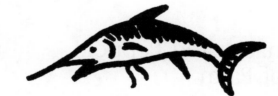

PER SERVING: 881 CALORIES		
MENU EXCHANGE PATTERN		
Dairy ..... —	Fruit 4½	
Bread 2½	Meat 5½	
Fat 5	Veg........ 1	
NUTRITIONAL INFORMATION		
Carbohydrate 90	g	
Protein 50	g	
Total fat 35	g	
Saturated fat 3.9	g	
Cholesterol 89	mg	
Sodium 809	mg	
Potassium 1812	mg	
Fiber 2.3	g	
Calcium 322	mg	
Iron 6.6	mg	

Grilled Sardines with Lime

18 fresh sardines
1 tablespoon safflower oil
Coarsely ground black pepper

Grated rind of 1 lemon
Grated rind of 1 lime
1 lime, cut in wedges

- Brush the sardines with safflower oil. Mix pepper and grated rinds and sprinkle over sardines. Grill over hot coals or broil until cooked through, about 5 minutes. Garnish with lime wedges.

PER SERVING: 57 CALORIES

MENU EXCHANGE PATTERN

Dairy	—	Fruit	—
Bread	—	Meat	1
Fat	—	Veg.	—

NUTRITIONAL INFORMATION

Carbohydrate	1	g
Protein	7	g
Total fat	3	g
Saturated fat	0	g
Cholesterol	39	mg
Sodium	232	mg
Potassium	168	mg
Fiber	0	g
Calcium	125	mg
Iron	0.8	mg

Whole Wheat Breadsticks

3 slices whole wheat bread
1 tablespoon margarine
2 tablespoons sesame seed

- Preheat oven to 300°F. Remove crust from bread and slice bread into strips. Melt margarine in a saucepan. Coat bread lightly in melted margarine and then in sesame seed. Bake until crisp, about 45 minutes. Serve warm.

PER SERVING: 68 CALORIES

MENU EXCHANGE PATTERN

Dairy	—	Fruit	—
Bread	½	Meat	—
Fat	½	Veg.	—

NUTRITIONAL INFORMATION

Carbohydrate	7	g
Protein	2	g
Total fat	4	g
Saturated fat	0.6	g
Cholesterol	0	mg
Sodium	74	mg
Potassium	37	mg
Fiber	0.3	g
Calcium	16	mg
Iron	0.5	mg

Salad of Spinach, Red Peppers, and Hearts of Palm

6 cups fresh spinach leaves
1 red bell pepper, cored, seeded, and sliced into julienne
3 hearts of palm, diced
6 tablespoons Red Pepper Vinaigrette (recipe follows)

- Tear spinach into bite-size pieces and place in a large mixing bowl. Add red pepper and hearts of palm. Toss with vinaigrette and serve.

Note: To reduce fat, substitute a commercial low-calorie Italian dressing for the vinaigrette. Adjusted analysis for dressing: calories = 16; exchange = ½ Fat.

PER SERVING: 24 CALORIES

MENU EXCHANGE PATTERN

Dairy	—	Fruit	—
Bread	—	Meat	—
Fat	—	Veg.	1

NUTRITIONAL INFORMATION

Carbohydrate	4	g
Protein	0	g
Total fat	0	g
Saturated fat	0	g
Cholesterol	0	mg
Sodium	41	mg
Potassium	356	mg
Fiber	1.7	g
Calcium	60	mg
Iron	2	mg

Red Pepper Vinaigrette

¼ cup chopped red onion
¼ cup chopped red bell pepper
¼ cup capers
⅓ cup red wine vinegar
1 cup safflower oil
1 tablespoon Dijon-style
mustard

1 teaspoon black pepper
1 teaspoon dried tarragon
1 teaspoon dry mustard
2 tablespoons chopped fresh
parsley
2 tablespoons lemon juice

• Mix all ingredients in a food processor or blender. Makes about 1¾ cups; 1 serving = 1 tablespoon.

PER SERVING: 49 CALORIES			
MENU EXCHANGE PATTERN			
Dairy	—	Fruit	—
Bread	—	Meat	—
Fat	1	Veg.	—
NUTRITIONAL INFORMATION			
Carbohydrate	0		g
Protein	0		g
Total fat	5		g
Saturated fat	0.5		g
Cholesterol	0		mg
Sodium	5		mg
Potassium	7		mg
Fiber	0		g
Calcium	1		mg
Iron	0		mg

Grilled Swordfish

6 swordfish steaks, 6 ounces
each
Coarsely ground black pepper
Parsley Almonds (recipe
follows)

• Sprinkle fish with pepper and grill over hot coals until cooked through, about 20 minutes. Top with Parsley Almonds and place under broiler until topping is melted. Serve immediately.

PER SERVING: 200 CALORIES			
MENU EXCHANGE PATTERN			
Dairy	—	Fruit	—
Bread	—	Meat	4½
Fat	—	Veg.	—
NUTRITIONAL INFORMATION			
Carbohydrate	0		g
Protein	32		g
Total fat	7		g
Saturated fat	0		g
Cholesterol	50		mg
Sodium	119		mg
Potassium	554		mg
Fiber	0		g
Calcium	32		mg
Iron	1.5		mg

Parsley Almonds

1 cup margarine, at room
temperature
½ cup toasted slivered almonds

½ cup chopped fresh parsley
1 teaspoon white pepper
Juice of ½ lemon

• Combine all ingredients in a food processor and blend just until almonds are chopped. Form mixture into a roll, wrap in plastic or foil and freeze. Cut into thin slices and top each serving of fish with 1 slice. Makes 2 cups; 1 serving = 1 tablespoon.

PER SERVING: 65 CALORIES			
MENU EXCHANGE PATTERN			
Dairy	—	Fruit	—
Bread	—	Meat	—
Fat	1½	Veg.	—
NUTRITIONAL INFORMATION			
Carbohydrate	1		g
Protein	1		g
Total fat	7		g
Saturated fat	1.2		g
Cholesterol	0		mg
Sodium	67		mg
Potassium	28		mg
Fiber	0.1		g
Calcium	9.4		mg
Iron	0.2		mg

Deep-Dish Apple Charlottes

½ teaspoon ground cinnamon
½ teaspoon ground allspice
¼ teaspoon ground nutmeg
¼ teaspoon ground cloves
⅔ cup frozen apple juice
    concentrate
⅔ cup frozen orange juice
    concentrate
⅔ cup dry white wine

¼ cup dry sherry
¼ cup water
2 large Red Delicious apples,
    peeled and very coarsely
    chopped
½ cup raisins
12 slices whole wheat bread
¼ cup margarine, melted
Ground cinnamon

- Combine first 9 ingredients in a saucepan, bring to a boil and simmer until mixture thickens a bit, about 10 minutes. Add apples and raisins and simmer for 15 minutes longer. Cool, then refrigerate overnight.

- Preheat oven to 350°F. Cut crusts from bread and cut 6 of the slices into 4 squares each. Dip squares in margarine and place 4 squares in each of 6 individual custard cups or charlotte molds with margarine side against glass; overlap squares of bread to cover the entire inside of the mold. Fill with apple mixture. Top cup with the remaining bread slices, trimmed to fit. Bake until bread is toasted, about 15 to 20 minutes. Unmold charlottes and run under the broiler briefly to crisp the tops. Sprinkle with cinnamon and serve.

PER SERVING: 418 CALORIES

MENU EXCHANGE PATTERN

Dairy	—	Fruit	4½
Bread	2	Meat	—
Fat	2	Veg.	—

NUTRITIONAL INFORMATION

Carbohydrate	76	g
Protein	6	g
Total fat	9	g
Saturated fat	1.7	g
Cholesterol	0	mg
Sodium	271	mg
Potassium	662	mg
Fiber	1.2	g
Calcium	79	mg
Iron	1.6	mg

CHICKEN

1

Watercress and Mushroom Salad

Grilled Chicken with Peppers

Scalloped Potatoes (page 200)

Pineapple Boats with Fresh Fruit

Serves 4

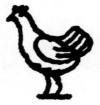

PER SERVING: 790 CALORIES			
MENU EXCHANGE PATTERN			
Dairy	½	Fruit	4
Bread	1	Meat	4
Fat	4	Veg.	3½
NUTRITIONAL INFORMATION			
Carbohydrate		83	g
Protein		44	g
Total fat		34	g
Saturated fat		7.2	g
Cholesterol		94	mg
Sodium		561	mg
Potassium		2219	mg
Fiber		5.6	g
Calcium		398	mg
Iron		5.4	mg

Watercress and Mushroom Salad

⅔ cup plain low-fat yogurt
2 tablespoons mayonnaise
⅓ cup watercress leaves
1 tablespoon chopped shallot

Black pepper
Pinch of paprika
4 cups sliced mushrooms
4 cups watercress

- Combine yogurt, mayonnaise, ⅓ cup watercress, shallot, pepper, and paprika in a blender and mix. Combine mushrooms and watercress in a bowl. Dress and serve.

PER SERVING: 103 CALORIES		
MENU EXCHANGE PATTERN		
Dairy . . . . . —	Fruit . . . . . —	
Bread . . . . —	Meat . . . . . —	
Fat 1	Veg. 2	
NUTRITIONAL INFORMATION		
Carbohydrate 8	g	
Protein 5	g	
Total fat 6	g	
Saturated fat 0.9	g	
Cholesterol 2	mg	
Sodium 96	mg	
Potassium 495	mg	
Fiber 0.8	g	
Calcium 132	mg	
Iron . . . . 1.4 mg		

Grilled Chicken with Peppers

4 green bell peppers
4 red bell peppers
¼ teaspoon finely chopped
    garlic

4 teaspoons Oriental sesame oil
¼ teaspoon dried thyme
4 chicken breasts, 6 ounces
    each, skinned

Marinade

1 teaspoon chopped garlic
¼ teaspoon crushed red pepper
¼ teaspoon ground ginger

4 teaspoons Oriental sesame oil
1 teaspoon teriyaki sauce

- Prepare marinade. Combine marinade ingredients. Spread over chicken breasts and let stand for 30 minutes.

- Blacken peppers under broiler, turning frequently until charred on all sides. Place in a plastic bag and let stand for 10 to 15 minutes. Rub skins off under running water; discard seeds and stem. Chop peppers coarsely. Sauté with garlic in sesame oil over medium-high heat until tender, about 5 minutes. Season with thyme. Grill chicken over charcoal or mesquite fire until cooked through, about 15 to 20 minutes. Serve with peppers.

PER SERVING: 353 CALORIES		
MENU EXCHANGE PATTERN		
Dairy . . . . . —	Fruit . . . . . —	
Bread . . . . —	Meat 4	
Fat 2	Veg. 1½	
NUTRITIONAL INFORMATION		
Carbohydrate 8	g	
Protein 30	g	
Total fat 22	g	
Saturated fat 4.8	g	
Cholesterol 87	mg	
Sodium 118	mg	
Potassium 654	mg	
Fiber 2.2	g	
Calcium 30	mg	
Iron . . . . 2.3 mg		

Pineapple Boats with Fresh Fruit

1 fresh pineapple, with stem
1 peach, peeled, pitted, and cut
    into chunks
⅔ cup strawberries, hulled
⅔ cup blueberries

1 papaya, peeled, seeded, and
    cut into chunks
1 cup plain low-fat yogurt
Juice of 2 limes
2 tablespoons honey

- Cut pineapple in half lengthwise, and then again into quarters. Hollow out shells and cut fruit into chunks. Mix remaining fruit with pineapple chunks. Refill pineapple quarters with fruit mixture. Mix yogurt, lime juice, and honey and serve on the side in a sauceboat.

PER SERVING: 214 CALORIES		
MENU EXCHANGE PATTERN		
Dairy . . . . . . ½	Fruit 4	
Bread . . . . —	Meat . . . . . —	
Fat . . . . —	Veg. . . . . . . —	
NUTRITIONAL INFORMATION		
Carbohydrate 50	g	
Protein 5	g	
Total fat 2	g	
Saturated fat 0.7	g	
Cholesterol 4	mg	
Sodium 46	mg	
Potassium 647	mg	
Fiber 2.2	g	
Calcium 150	mg	
Iron . . . . 1.1 mg		

CHICKEN

2

Vegi-Nachos

Chicken Pechugas

Pico de Gallo (page 90)

Mexican Rice (page 91)

Refried Beans

Frozen Yogurt with Kahlúa

Serves 4

PER SERVING: 953 CALORIES

MENU EXCHANGE PATTERN

Dairy	1	Fruit	½
Bread	4	Meat	5½
Fat	4	Veg.	3½

NUTRITIONAL INFORMATION

Carbohydrate	93	g
Protein	44	g
Total fat	41	g
Saturated fat	8.4	g
Cholesterol	73	mg
Sodium	1551	mg
Potassium	1518	mg
Fiber	3.7	g
Calcium	473	mg
Iron	6.5	mg

Vegi-Nachos

3 tablespoons margarine
2 teaspoons dry sherry
1/4 cup chopped onion
1 bell pepper, chopped
1/2 cup chopped fresh
    mushrooms

4 corn tortillas
4 ounces low-fat Monterey Jack
    cheese, grated
Jalapeño chilies, sliced

- Preheat oven to 400°F. Melt margarine in a nonstick skillet over medium heat. Add sherry, onion, bell pepper, and mushrooms. Heat, stirring occasionally, until vegetables are warmed through and coated with sauce. Cut each tortilla into 4 triangles and arrange on baking sheet coated with nonstick spray. Bake until crisp, 5 to 7 minutes. Spread with vegetable mixture. Sprinkle with cheese and top with a slice of jalapeño. Return to oven until cheese melts, then serve immediately.

Photo opposite page 242.

PER SERVING: 214 CALORIES		
MENU EXCHANGE PATTERN		
Dairy . . . . . —	Fruit . . . . . —	
Bread 1	Meat 1	
Fat 1½	Veg. 1	
NUTRITIONAL INFORMATION		
Carbohydrate 18	g	
Protein 10	g	
Total fat 12	g	
Saturated fat 1.6	g	
Cholesterol 9	mg	
Sodium 643	mg	
Potassium 163	mg	
Fiber 0.6	g	
Calcium 252	mg	
Iron 1.2	mg	

Chicken Pechugas

1 pound chicken breasts, boned
    and skinned
1/4 cup margarine
2 cloves garlic, mashed
Black pepper
3 tablespoons dry sherry

3 tablespoons low-sodium soy
    sauce
2/3 onion, sliced and grilled
1 1/2 bell peppers, cored, seeded,
    and sliced
2 tomatoes, sliced

- Place chicken between 2 pieces of wax paper or plastic wrap and pound to 1/4-inch thickness. Combine margarine, garlic, pepper, sherry, and soy sauce in a large skillet and place over medium-high heat. Add chicken breasts and cook for 2 minutes on each side. Transfer to grill or broiler to finish cooking, if desired, or continue cooking in the skillet for about 5 to 7 minutes on each side. Garnish with grilled onion, bell pepper, and tomato slices. Serve with Pico de Gallo (page 90) and Mexican Rice (page 91).

PER SERVING: 329 CALORIES		
MENU EXCHANGE PATTERN		
Dairy . . . . . —	Fruit . . . . . —	
Bread . . . . —	Meat 4	
Fat 1½	Veg. 2	
NUTRITIONAL INFORMATION		
Carbohydrate 12	g	
Protein 22	g	
Total fat 20	g	
Saturated fat 4.5	g	
Cholesterol 58	mg	
Sodium 841	mg	
Potassium 642	mg	
Fiber 1.3	g	
Calcium 43	mg	
Iron 2	mg	

Refried Beans

2 teaspoons safflower oil
²/₃ onion, chopped
1 clove garlic, minced
1 cup drained cooked kidney
   or pinto beans

2 tablespoons low-sodium
   tomato paste
2 teaspoons chili powder
¼ teaspoon ground cumin

- Heat oil in a saucepan over medium heat. Add onion and garlic and sauté until translucent, about 10 minutes. Add beans, tomato paste, chili powder, and cumin and simmer, stirring constantly, for 10 minutes. Serve hot.

PER SERVING: 99 CALORIES		
MENU EXCHANGE PATTERN		
Dairy . . . . . —	Fruit . . . . . —	
Bread 1	Meat . . . . . . ½	
Fat . . . . —	Veg. . . . . . . —	
NUTRITIONAL INFORMATION		
Carbohydrate 15		g
Protein 5		g
Total fat 3		g
Saturated fat 0.2		g
Cholesterol 0		mg
Sodium 7		mg
Potassium 284		mg
Fiber 1		g
Calcium 36		mg
Iron 1.7		mg

Frozen Yogurt with Kahlúa

2 cups low-fat frozen vanilla
   yogurt
4 tablespoons Kahlúa

- Place ½ cup frozen yogurt in each of 4 champagne glasses. Top with 1 tablespoon Kahlúa.

PER SERVING: 133 CALORIES		
MENU EXCHANGE PATTERN		
Dairy 1	Fruit . . . . . . ½	
Bread . . . . . ½	Meat . . . . . —	
Fat . . . . —	Veg. . . . . . . —	
NUTRITIONAL INFORMATION		
Carbohydrate 17		g
Protein 3		g
Total fat 2		g
Saturated fat 1		g
Cholesterol 8		mg
Sodium 54		mg
Potassium 155		mg
Fiber 0		g
Calcium 110		mg
Iron 0.1		mg

CHICKEN

3

Marinated Vegetable Salad

Cuban Chicken

Risotto Primavera

Tossed Salad with Classic Herb Dressing

Texas Sunrise

Serves 4

PER SERVING: 905 CALORIES		
MENU EXCHANGE PATTERN		
Dairy . . . . . —	Fruit 5½	
Bread 2	Meat 3	
Fat 6½	Veg. 3	
NUTRITIONAL INFORMATION		
Carbohydrate 94	g	
Protein 32	g	
Total fat 42	g	
Saturated fat 5.3	g	
Cholesterol 58	mg	
Sodium 1232	mg	
Potassium 1879	mg	
Fiber 4	g	
Calcium 186	mg	
Iron 7	mg	

Marinated Vegetable Salad

¾ pound whole mushrooms, stems trimmed
¾ cup sliced bell pepper
¾ cup sliced red or green onion
1 tablespoon chopped fresh basil
2 teaspoons chopped fresh parsley
1 clove garlic, mashed
¼ cup white wine vinegar
¼ cup low-sodium soy sauce
3 tablespoons safflower oil
¼ teaspoon black pepper

- Combine mushrooms, pepper, and onion in a large bowl. Combine all remaining ingredients and pour over vegetables. Marinate at least 2 hours before serving.

Note: To reduce fat, eliminate vinegar, soy sauce, and safflower oil and substitute ½ cup of a commercial low-calorie Italian dressing. Adjusted analysis: calories = 41; exchange = 2 Vegetable.

PER SERVING: 144 CALORIES		
MENU EXCHANGE PATTERN		
Dairy ..... —	Fruit ..... —	
Bread .... —	Meat ..... —	
Fat 2	Veg. 2	
NUTRITIONAL INFORMATION		
Carbohydrate 10	g	
Protein 5	g	
Total fat 10	g	
Saturated fat 0.9	g	
Cholesterol 0	mg	
Sodium 1046	mg	
Potassium 524	mg	
Fiber 1.1	g	
Calcium 21	mg	
Iron 1.6	mg	

Cuban Chicken

1 pound chicken parts, skinned
2 tablespoons safflower oil
1 onion, chopped
2 cloves garlic, mashed
2 fresh tomatoes, chopped
¼ cup dry white wine
¼ teaspoon ground cumin
1 tablespoon chopped fresh oregano
½ teaspoon ground cinnamon
¼ teaspoon black pepper
2 tablespoons sliced almonds
2 tablespoons raisins
4 ripe olives, rinsed and sliced
Parsley sprigs (garnish)

- Preheat oven to 500°F. Arrange chicken pieces on flat baking or broiling pan and roast until brown, about 15 minutes. While chicken is browning, heat oil in a nonstick skillet and sauté onion and garlic over medium heat until soft, about 10 minutes. Stir in tomatoes and cook briefly. Add wine and seasonings and cook over medium heat for 15 minutes.

- When chicken is brown, remove from oven and reduce temperature to 325°F. Add a small amount of water to pan to loosen browned bits. Spoon tomato sauce over chicken and return to oven. Bake, basting often, until chicken is very tender, about 30 minutes; add water or chicken stock if liquid evaporates. Sprinkle almonds, raisins, and olives over chicken and moisten with sauce. Garnish with parsley and serve.

PER SERVING: 314 CALORIES		
MENU EXCHANGE PATTERN		
Dairy ..... —	Fruit 2	
Bread .... —	Meat 3	
Fat 1½	Veg. .... —	
NUTRITIONAL INFORMATION		
Carbohydrate 14	g	
Protein 22	g	
Total fat 18	g	
Saturated fat 3.3	g	
Cholesterol 58	mg	
Sodium 158	mg	
Potassium 585	mg	
Fiber 1	g	
Calcium 51	mg	
Iron 1.8	mg	

Risotto Primavera

3 tablespoons chopped green
   onion
4 teaspoons safflower oil
²/₃ cup white rice
¹/₄ cup dry white wine
1¹/₄ cups water
1¹/₂ teaspoons fresh thyme
2 teaspoons chopped fresh
   marjoram

2 tablespoons chopped fresh
   parsley
¹/₃ cup shredded carrot
²/₃ cup green vegetable:
   broccoli, zucchini, green
   beans, asparagus, or green
   peas, chopped if necessary

- Heat oil in a large nonstick skillet over medium heat. Add onion and sauté until soft, about 10 minutes. Stir in rice and sauté briefly. Add wine and cook, stirring often, until absorbed, about 10 minutes. Add water, thyme, and marjoram, bring to a boil and stir through once. Reduce heat, cover and cook until rice is tender and liquid is absorbed, about 15 to 20 minutes. Steam vegetables to crisp-tender and then stir into rice and serve. (Risotto can be covered and kept warm over hot water; stir occasionally.)

PER SERVING: 192 CALORIES

MENU EXCHANGE PATTERN

Dairy	—	Fruit	—
Bread	2	Meat	—
Fat	1	Veg.	—

NUTRITIONAL INFORMATION

Carbohydrate	31	g
Protein	4	g
Total fat	5	g
Saturated fat	0.4	g
Cholesterol	0	mg
Sodium	18	mg
Potassium	280	mg
Fiber	1	g
Calcium	63	mg
Iron	1.7	mg

Tossed Salad

¹/₂ head romaine or red-leaf
   lettuce (about 2 cups)
¹/₂ head Boston or Bibb lettuce
   (about 2 cups)
1¹/₂ large tomatoes, quartered

¹/₃ cup sliced mushrooms
¹/₃ cup chopped green onion
¹/₄ cup Classic Herb Dressing
   (recipe follows)

- Toss all ingredients lightly in salad bowl. Top with dressing.

Note: To reduce fat, substitute a commercial low-calorie Italian dressing for the Classic Herb Dressing. Adjusted analysis for dressing: calories = 16; exchange = ¹/₂ Fat.

PER SERVING: 29 CALORIES

MENU EXCHANGE PATTERN

Dairy	—	Fruit	—
Bread	—	Meat	—
Fat	—	Veg.	1

NUTRITIONAL INFORMATION

Carbohydrate	6	g
Protein	2	g
Total fat	0	g
Saturated fat	0	g
Cholesterol	0	mg
Sodium	8	mg
Potassium	354	mg
Fiber	0.9	g
Calcium	42	mg
Iron	1.4	mg

Classic Herb Dressing

1 cup safflower or sunflower
  oil
1/4 cup lemon juice or red wine
  vinegar
1/4 cup water
1/4 cup fresh parsley, sprigs and
  tender stems
1 tablespoon fresh marjoram,
  or 1 teaspoon dried

1 tablespoon fresh thyme, or
  1 teaspoon dried
1 tablespoon fresh basil, or
  1 teaspoon dried
1/2 teaspoon celery seed
1 clove garlic, halved
1/8 teaspoon Tabasco sauce

PER SERVING: 81 CALORIES		
MENU EXCHANGE PATTERN		
Dairy ..... —	Fruit ..... —	
Bread ..... —	Meat ..... —	
Fat 2	Veg. ...... —	
NUTRITIONAL INFORMATION		
Carbohydrate 0	g	
Protein 0	g	
Total fat 9	g	
Saturated fat 0.8	g	
Cholesterol 0	mg	
Sodium 1	mg	
Potassium 7	mg	
Fiber 0	g	
Calcium 1	mg	
Iron .... 0.3 mg		

- Combine all ingredients in blender and mix at low speed until nearly smooth, then at high speed for about 30 seconds. Use on salad greens or to marinate cooked or raw vegetables. Makes about 1¾ cups; 1 serving = 1 tablespoon.

Note: ½ cup white wine vinegar can be substituted for lemon juice (or red wine vinegar) and water.

Texas Sunrise

1 envelope unflavored gelatin
1/2 cup cold water
3/4 cup water
1/4 cup lemon juice

1/2 cup sugar
1/2 cup dry white wine
1/4 cup undiluted frozen orange
  juice concentrate

PER SERVING: 146 CALORIES		
MENU EXCHANGE PATTERN		
Dairy ..... —	Fruit 3½	
Bread ..... —	Meat ..... —	
Fat .... —	Veg. ...... —	
NUTRITIONAL INFORMATION		
Carbohydrate 32	g	
Protein 0	g	
Total fat 0	g	
Saturated fat 0	g	
Cholesterol 0	mg	
Sodium 1	mg	
Potassium 136	mg	
Fiber 0	g	
Calcium 8	mg	
Iron .... 0.2 mg		

- Sprinkle gelatin over ½ cup cold water and let soften for 5 minutes. Combine softened gelatin, ¾ cup water, lemon juice, sugar, and wine in a nonaluminum saucepan and bring to a boil, making sure sugar is dissolved.

- Remove from heat and stir in orange juice concentrate. Let cool, pour into serving dishes and chill until set, about 1 hour.

CHICKEN

4

Spanish Fish Soup

Deviled Rosemary Chicken

New Potatoes Florentine

Cauliflower with Vegetable Sauce

Fruit Feast

Serves 6

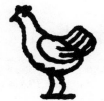

PER SERVING: 708 CALORIES		
MENU EXCHANGE PATTERN		
Dairy . . . . . —	Fruit 1½	
Bread 1½	Meat 6	
Fat 2½	Veg. 3½	
NUTRITIONAL INFORMATION		
Carbohydrate 59	g	
Protein 62	g	
Total fat 24	g	
Saturated fat 3.7	g	
Cholesterol 125	mg	
Sodium 454	mg	
Potassium 2174	mg	
Fiber 3.6	g	
Calcium 246	mg	
Iron 6.7	mg	

Spanish Fish Soup

1/4 cup margarine
3/4 cup chopped onion
2 cloves garlic, minced
1/2 cup shredded carrot
1/2 cup green bell pepper sliced
   into thin 1-inch-long strips
1 cup chopped tomato
4 cups fish stock or Homemade
   Chicken Stock (page 36)
1 bay leaf
1/4 teaspoon cayenne pepper
1 tablespoon chopped fresh
   basil, or 1 scant teaspoon
   dried

2 teaspoons chopped fresh
   rosemary, or 1 scant
   teaspoon dried
2 teaspoons coriander seed,
   bruised
2 tablespoons lemon juice
1/2 cup dry white wine
1 pound red snapper, redfish,
   flounder, catfish, or trout,
   cut into 1-inch pieces
2 tablespoons chopped fresh
   parsley

PER SERVING: 234 CALORIES		
MENU EXCHANGE PATTERN		
Dairy ..... —	Fruit ..... —	
Bread .... —	Meat 2	
Fat 2	Veg. 1	
NUTRITIONAL INFORMATION		
Carbohydrate 6	g	
Protein 15	g	
Total fat 15	g	
Saturated fat 1.7	g	
Cholesterol 28	mg	
Sodium 181	mg	
Potassium 452	mg	
Fiber 0.5	g	
Calcium 56	mg	
Iron 1.3	mg	

- Melt margarine in a large Dutch oven or deep roaster over medium heat and sauté onion, garlic, carrot, and pepper until soft, about 10 minutes. Add tomato, stock, seasonings, and lemon juice, bring to a boil, cover, and simmer for 30 to 40 minutes. Add wine and fish, return to simmer, cover, and cook just until fish flakes easily, about 10 minutes. Add parsley and serve immediately. Makes about 7 cups; 1 serving = 1 generous cup.

Deviled Rosemary Chicken

1 1/2 pounds chicken parts
1/3 cup Dijon-style mustard
1/4 cup red wine vinegar
2 tablespoons lemon juice
2 teaspoons Worcestershire
   sauce
3 cloves garlic, 1 crushed
1/8 teaspoon Tabasco sauce

2 tablespoons chopped fresh
   rosemary, or 2 teaspoons
   dried
1 cup soft breadcrumbs
2 tablespoons chopped fresh
   parsley
Chopped fresh parsley (garnish)
Rosemary sprigs (garnish)

- Preheat oven to 450°F. Remove skin and all visible fat from chicken. Arrange pieces on a flat pan and brown in oven for 15 minutes. Meanwhile, combine mustard, vinegar, lemon juice, Worcestershire, 2 whole garlic cloves, Tabasco and 1 tablespoon rosemary in a blender and mix well.

- When chicken is lightly browned, pour 1 cup hot water into pan to loosen browned juices. Remove chicken and transfer to heavy baking pan. Pour liquid in browning pan into measuring cup and allow fat to rise. Skim fat from broth. Add ¼ cup broth to blender mixture and combine. Reduce oven to 275°F.

- Baste chicken with blended mixture. Return to oven and bake until cooked through, basting frequently, about 40 more minutes.

- While chicken is cooking, combine breadcrumbs, remaining 1 tablespoon rosemary, parsley, and crushed garlic. Gradually add ¼ cup chicken broth and rub with fingers or pastry blender to moisten evenly. Place on cookie sheet in oven and let mixture brown lightly. When chicken is done, sprinkle with crumbs and drizzle with any juices. Garnish with chopped parsley and rosemary sprigs.

PER SERVING: 260 CALORIES

MENU EXCHANGE PATTERN

Dairy	—	Fruit	—
Bread	½	Meat	4
Fat	—	Veg.	—

NUTRITIONAL INFORMATION

Carbohydrate	9	g
Protein	38	g
Total fat	6	g
Saturated fat	1.5	g
Cholesterol	96	mg
Sodium	199	mg
Potassium	385	mg
Fiber	0.3	g
Calcium	50	mg
Iron	2.1	mg

New Potatoes Florentine

*3 pounds new potatoes,
   scrubbed*
1 tablespoon chopped shallot
1 tablespoon margarine
*1½ tablespoons all-purpose
   flour*
1 cup skim milk

¼ teaspoon ground nutmeg
*1 tablespoon chopped fresh herb
   (see note)*
*4 packed cups chopped fresh
   spinach*
Pinch of white pepper

- Boil potatoes in water to cover until tender, about 20 minutes. Meanwhile, sauté shallot in margarine over medium heat until soft. Add flour, stirring constantly until shallot is evenly coated. Add milk and simmer, stirring constantly, until flour taste is gone, about 10 minutes. Blend in seasonings. Add spinach, a little at a time, until well mixed and wilted. Cover and let stand 5 minutes off heat. Serve over new potatoes.

Note: Any of the following could be used in this recipe: lemon thyme, marjoram, Spanish oregano, dill, tarragon, or rosemary.

PER SERVING: 105 CALORIES

MENU EXCHANGE PATTERN

Dairy	—	Fruit	—
Bread	1	Meat	—
Fat	½	Veg.	½

NUTRITIONAL INFORMATION

Carbohydrate	18	g
Protein	4	g
Total fat	2	g
Saturated fat	0.4	g
Cholesterol	0	mg
Sodium	49	mg
Potassium	553	mg
Fiber	0.6	g
Calcium	91	mg
Iron	1.6	mg

Cauliflower with Vegetable Sauce

⅓ cup green or white onion,
    thinly sliced
1 large clove garlic, mashed
½ cup chopped celery
¼ cup chopped or sliced green
    bell pepper
½ cup sliced fresh mushrooms
1 cup eggplant cut into ½-inch
    cubes

1½ cups chopped fresh tomato
2 teaspoons chopped fresh
    rosemary
1 tablespoon chopped fresh
    oregano
2 tablespoons chopped fresh
    parsley
¼ teaspoon black pepper
3 cups cauliflower, cooked

- Coat a large nonstick skillet with cooking spray. Sauté onion, garlic, celery, and bell pepper over medium heat until soft, about 10 to 15 minutes; do not brown. Stir in mushrooms, eggplant, tomato, and seasonings. Cover, reduce heat, and simmer gently until vegetables are tender, about 10 minutes. Serve over cooked cauliflower.

PER SERVING: 51 CALORIES

MENU EXCHANGE PATTERN

Dairy	—	Fruit	—
Bread	—	Meat	—
Fat	—	Veg.	2

NUTRITIONAL INFORMATION

Carbohydrate	10	g
Protein	3	g
Total fat	0	g
Saturated fat	0	g
Cholesterol	0	mg
Sodium	24	mg
Potassium	514	mg
Fiber	1.6	g
Calcium	40	mg
Iron	1.3	mg

Fruit Feast

1 envelope unflavored gelatin
3 bananas, peeled
2 cups fresh strawberries, hulled
3 large peaches or nectarines,
    peeled and pitted
⅛ teaspoon mace

2 teaspoons lemon juice
2 tablespoons finely chopped
    fresh spearmint, lemon balm,
    lemon verbena,
    pineapplemint, or rose
    geranium leaves

- Combine all ingredients except herb in blender and mix until smooth. Stir in chopped herb. Pour into a serving bowl and chill.

PER SERVING: 58 CALORIES

MENU EXCHANGE PATTERN

Dairy	—	Fruit	1½
Bread	—	Meat	—
Fat	—	Veg.	—

NUTRITIONAL INFORMATION

Carbohydrate	15	g
Protein	1	g
Total fat	0	g
Saturated fat	0	g
Cholesterol	0	mg
Sodium	0	mg
Potassium	270	mg
Fiber	0.6	g
Calcium	9	mg
Iron	0.3	mg

CHICKEN

5

Wilhelmina Salad

Baked Chicken in White Wine

Lyonnaise Potatoes

Creamed Spinach

Strawberries with Yogurt and Grand Marnier

Serves 6

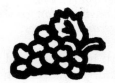

PER SERVING: 799 CALORIES		
MENU EXCHANGE PATTERN		
Dairy ...... ½	Fruit 1	
Bread 1½	Meat 6	
Fat 3½	Veg. 4	
NUTRITIONAL INFORMATION		
Carbohydrate 62	g	
Protein 60	g	
Total fat 29	g	
Saturated fat 7.5	g	
Cholesterol 136	mg	
Sodium 571	mg	
Potassium 1917	mg	
Fiber 2.6	g	
Calcium 479	mg	
Iron 6.4	mg	

Wilhelmina Salad

1 head romaine lettuce, torn
    into pieces
2 tomatoes, cut in wedges
2 ounces Roquefort cheese,
    finely crumbled
1/2 avocado, peeled, pitted, and
    thinly sliced
1/2 bunch watercress, chopped
6 tablespoons commercial low-
    calorie Italian dressing
Black pepper

- Combine lettuce, tomatoes, cheese, avocado, and watercress in a large salad bowl. Toss salad lightly with dressing and season with pepper to taste.

Note: Analysis includes salad dressing.

Photo opposite page 243.

PER SERVING: 102 CALORIES			
MENU EXCHANGE PATTERN			
Dairy	—	Fruit	—
Bread	—	Meat	—
Fat	1½	Veg.	1½
NUTRITIONAL INFORMATION			
Carbohydrate	....	7	g
Protein	....	4	g
Total fat	....	7	g
Saturated fat	......	2.4	g
Cholesterol	....	9	mg
Sodium	....	299	mg
Potassium	....	412	mg
Fiber	....	1	g
Calcium	....	114	mg
Iron	....	1.3	mg

Baked Chicken in White Wine

1/2 cup all-purpose flour
1 teaspoon paprika
1/2 teaspoon black pepper
1/2 teaspoon garlic powder
3 whole chicken breasts (about
    10 ounces each), split and
    skinned
1 1/2 cups dry white wine
2 tablespoons margarine
2 tablespoons drained capers

- Preheat oven to 450°F. Combine flour with seasonings; dredge chicken in flour mixture. Arrange chicken breasts in baking dish and pour wine over. Dot with margarine and sprinkle with capers. Cover with foil. Bake 20 minutes, then reduce heat to 325°F and continue baking until chicken is cooked through, about 1 hour.

PER SERVING: 364 CALORIES			
MENU EXCHANGE PATTERN			
Dairy	—	Fruit	—
Bread	½	Meat	6
Fat	—	Veg.	—
NUTRITIONAL INFORMATION			
Carbohydrate	....	10	g
Protein	....	45	g
Total fat	....	10	g
Saturated fat	......	3	g
Cholesterol	....	120	mg
Sodium	....	111	mg
Potassium	....	415	mg
Fiber	....	0	g
Calcium	....	30	mg
Iron	....	2	mg

Lyonnaise Potatoes

4 Idaho potatoes, peeled and
    cut into 1/4-inch slices
2 onions, chopped
1/4 cup margarine
2 tablespoons dry sherry
Paprika

- Boil potato slices in water to cover until tender, about 15 minutes. Drain potatoes and cool in cold water; drain again.

- While potatoes are cooling, sauté onion in margarine in a nonstick skillet until translucent. Stir in sherry.

- Preheat oven to 350°F. Layer half the potato slices in the bottom of a 2-quart casserole. Cover with onion and top with remaining potatoes. Sprinkle with paprika. Bake until heated thoroughly, about 20–25 minutes.

PER SERVING: 154 CALORIES			
MENU EXCHANGE PATTERN			
Dairy	—	Fruit	—
Bread	1	Meat	—
Fat	½	Veg.	1½
NUTRITIONAL INFORMATION			
Carbohydrate	....	19	g
Protein	....	2	g
Total fat	....	8	g
Saturated fat	......	1	g
Cholesterol	....	0	mg
Sodium	....	7	mg
Potassium	....	431	mg
Fiber	....	1	g
Calcium	....	21	mg
Iron	....	0.7	mg

Creamed Spinach

1 tablespoon margarine
3 cups chopped cooked spinach
¾ cup evaporated skim milk

Black pepper
2 tablespoons grated Parmesan
  cheese

- Melt margarine in saucepan over medium-high heat. Add spinach and heat, stirring constantly, to remove any residual moisture. Add milk, pepper, and cheese and stir constantly over medium heat until mixture thickens. Serve immediately.

PER SERVING: 70 CALORIES		
MENU EXCHANGE PATTERN		
Dairy . . . . . —	Fruit . . . . . —	
Bread . . . . —	Meat . . . . . —	
Fat . . . . ½	Veg. 2	
NUTRITIONAL INFORMATION		
Carbohydrate 7	g	
Protein 6	g	
Total fat 3	g	
Saturated fat 0.7	g	
Cholesterol 7	mg	
Sodium 113	mg	
Potassium 399	mg	
Fiber 0.5	g	
Calcium 199	mg	
Iron 2.1	mg	

Strawberries with Yogurt and Grand Marnier

3 cups fresh strawberries
2 tablespoons Grand Marnier
2 cups low-fat vanilla yogurt

- Hull and chill strawberries. Add Grand Marnier to yogurt and mix well. Pour over strawberries and serve cold in dessert glasses.

Note: Fresh cherries may be substituted for strawberries.

PER SERVING: 109 CALORIES		
MENU EXCHANGE PATTERN		
Dairy . . . . . . ½	Fruit 1	
Bread . . . . —	Meat . . . . . —	
Fat . . . . —	Veg. . . . . . . —	
NUTRITIONAL INFORMATION		
Carbohydrate 19	g	
Protein 3	g	
Total fat 1	g	
Saturated fat 0.5	g	
Cholesterol 3	mg	
Sodium 41	mg	
Potassium 257	mg	
Fiber 0	g	
Calcium 115	mg	
Iron 0	mg	

CHICKEN

6

Crabmeat Salad

Grilled Chicken Martin

Potato Pancakes

Corn Relish

Grilled Tomatillos

Strawberries Romanoff

Serves 4

PER SERVING: 1010 CALORIES			
MENU EXCHANGE PATTERN			
Dairy	1	Fruit	½
Bread	3½	Meat	5½
Fat	5	Veg.	3½
NUTRITIONAL INFORMATION			
Carbohydrate	83	g	
Protein	62	g	
Total fat	41	g	
Saturated fat	7.7	g	
Cholesterol	173	mg	
Sodium	971	mg	
Potassium	2213	mg	
Fiber	2.9	g	
Calcium	443	mg	
Iron	5.5	mg	

Crabmeat Salad

8 leaves spinach
8 leaves radicchio
8 leaves Boston lettuce
3/4 pound crabmeat
4 mushrooms
4 cherry tomatoes

2 hearts of palm, sliced
1/2 red bell pepper, cored,
    seeded, and sliced into
    julienne (garnish)
Sherry Horseradish Dressing
    (page 170)

PER SERVING: 92 CALORIES		
MENU EXCHANGE PATTERN		
Dairy . . . . . —	Fruit . . . . . —	
Bread . . . . —	Meat 1½	
Fat . . . . —	Veg. 1	
NUTRITIONAL INFORMATION		
Carbohydrate 4	g	
Protein 15	g	
Total fat 2	g	
Saturated fat 0	g	
Cholesterol 76	mg	
Sodium 429	mg	
Potassium 371	mg	
Fiber 0.7	g	
Calcium 56	mg	
Iron 1.7	mg	

- Arrange lettuce leaves on individual salad plates. Place crab-meat in center and surround with mushrooms, cherry tomatoes, and hearts of palm. Garnish with red pepper. Top with dressing.

Note: Analysis does not include dressing.

Grilled Chicken Martin

4 boned chicken breasts,
    6 ounces each

Corn Marinade

Kernels from 5 cooked ears of
    corn (about 2½ cups)
1/3 cup finely chopped onion
2⅔ cups dry white wine
1½ teaspoons chopped fresh
    coriander (cilantro)

1/3 cup honey
1/3 cup brandy
1 teaspoon minced garlic
2¼ teaspoons onion powder
Black pepper

PER SERVING: 328 CALORIES		
MENU EXCHANGE PATTERN		
Dairy . . . . . —	Fruit . . . . . . ½	
Bread . . . . —	Meat 4	
Fat . . . . —	Veg. . . . . . . —	
NUTRITIONAL INFORMATION		
Carbohydrate 5	g	
Protein 29	g	
Total fat 13	g	
Saturated fat 3.6	g	
Cholesterol 87	mg	
Sodium 85	mg	
Potassium 427	mg	
Fiber 0.3	g	
Calcium 16	mg	
Iron 1.2	mg	

- Prepare marinade. Combine all ingredients in a saucepan and simmer for 20 minutes. Cool.

- Marinate chicken breasts in corn marinade for at least 4 hours. Drain. Grill chicken over charcoal fire just until firm and opaque, turning several times.

Note: Frozen corn kernels can be substituted for the fresh in the marinade. Do not use canned because of the added salt.

Potato Pancakes

2 egg substitutes
1 onion, chopped
3 tablespoons all-purpose flour
Black pepper

½ teaspoon salt
3 cups peeled and grated Idaho
  potatoes
2 tablespoons safflower oil

- Mix egg substitute, onion, flour, and seasonings. Add potatoes and shape into pancakes, using ¼ cup of mixture for each. Flatten with a spoon.

- Preheat oven to 350°F. Heat oil in a nonstick skillet over medium high heat. Lightly brown pancakes on both sides and transfer to a baking sheet that has been lightly coated with nonstick spray. Bake pancakes for about 15 minutes, turn over, and bake another 10 minutes to finish cooking, then serve immediately.

PER SERVING: 202 CALORIES

MENU EXCHANGE PATTERN

Dairy	—	Fruit	—
Bread	2	Meat	—
Fat	1½	Veg.	—

NUTRITIONAL INFORMATION

Carbohydrate	27 g
Protein	6 g
Total fat	8 g
Saturated fat	0.8 g
Cholesterol	0 mg
Sodium	316 mg
Potassium	608 mg
Fiber	0.8 g
Calcium	35 mg
Iron	1.4 mg

Corn Relish

¼ cup cider vinegar
2 tablespoons sugar
¼ teaspoon celery seed
⅛ teaspoon mustard seed
⅛ teaspoon Tabasco sauce
¾ cup cooked fresh corn

2 tablespoons minced green
  bell pepper
2 tablespoons minced red bell
  pepper
2 tablespoons minced onion

- Combine vinegar, sugar, celery seed, mustard seed, and Tabasco in nonaluminum saucepan, bring to boil, and simmer 3 to 5 minutes. Add vegetables, bring to boil, and remove from heat. Cool, then chill. Let stand 24 hours before serving.

PER SERVING: 55 CALORIES

MENU EXCHANGE PATTERN

Dairy	—	Fruit	—
Bread	½	Meat	—
Fat	—	Veg.	1

NUTRITIONAL INFORMATION

Carbohydrate	14 g
Protein	1 g
Total fat	0 g
Saturated fat	0 g
Cholesterol	0 mg
Sodium	1 mg
Potassium	85 mg
Fiber	0.3 g
Calcium	4 mg
Iron	0.4 mg

Grilled Tomatillos

8 tomatillos
2 teaspoons margarine, melted

- Grill tomatillos over charcoal fire for about 10 minutes, rotating frequently. Cut in half and drizzle with margarine. Serve immediately.

  Note: Tomatillos are green tomatoes from Mexico. When fresh, they have a paper-thin husk, which should be removed before cooking. They are also sold in cans, available in Spanish or Mexican groceries or supermarkets in the southwest.

PER SERVING: 36 CALORIES	
MENU EXCHANGE PATTERN	
Dairy ..... —	Fruit ..... —
Bread .... —	Meat ..... —
Fat .... ½	Veg. 1
NUTRITIONAL INFORMATION	
Carbohydrate 4	g
Protein 1	g
Total fat 2	g
Saturated fat 0.4	g
Cholesterol 0	mg
Sodium 2	mg
Potassium 222	mg
Fiber 0.5	g
Calcium 12	mg
Iron .... 0.4 mg	

Strawberries Romanoff

24 very ripe strawberries
(2 cups), hulled
2 teaspoons sugar
4 cups plain low-fat yogurt

1 teaspoon vanilla extract
½ cup Triple Sec or Grand Marnier

- Set aside 4 perfect strawberries for garnish; with a fork, crush remaining berries with sugar in a mixing bowl. Add yogurt and vanilla and fold together gently. Fold in liqueur and spoon into wine glasses. Garnish each serving with a strawberry. Serve immediately.

PER SERVING: 201 CALORIES	
MENU EXCHANGE PATTERN	
Dairy 1	Fruit .....½
Bread .... —	Meat ..... —
Fat .... ½	Veg. ...... —
NUTRITIONAL INFORMATION	
Carbohydrate 18	g
Protein 9	g
Total fat 3	g
Saturated fat 1.7	g
Cholesterol 10	mg
Sodium 120	mg
Potassium 480	mg
Fiber 0.3	g
Calcium 314	mg
Iron .... 0.3 mg	

CHICKEN

7

Scallop and Shrimp Ceviche

Chicken Enchiladas with Green
and Red Sauces

Pico de Gallo (page 90)

Refried Beans (page 270)

Tequila Sherbet

Serves 6

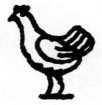

PER SERVING: 840 CALORIES			
MENU EXCHANGE PATTERN			
Dairy	—	Fruit	1
Bread	5	Meat	5½
Fat	1½	Veg.	2½
NUTRITIONAL INFORMATION			
Carbohydrate	105	g	
Protein	51	g	
Total fat	22	g	
Saturated fat	4.3	g	
Cholesterol	130	mg	
Sodium	681	mg	
Potassium	1774	mg	
Fiber	2.6	g	
Calcium	310	mg	
Iron	6.4	mg	

Scallop and Shrimp Ceviche

$1/3$ cup chopped onion
$1/2$ pound scallops
$1/4$ pound shrimp, shelled and
   deveined
$2^1/_2$ jalapeño or serrano chilies,
   chopped
$2/3$ cup lemon juice

4 sprigs fresh coriander
   (cilantro)
1 clove garlic, crushed
6 lettuce leaves
Lemon or lime wedges
   (garnish)

Ceviche Sauce

1 cup low-sodium tomato
   sauce
$1/4$ teaspoon ground coriander
Dash of Tabasco sauce
1 teaspoon low-sodium soy
   sauce

2 tablespoons lemon juice
2 tablespoons water
$1/2$ teaspoon Worcestershire
   sauce
Pinch of black pepper

- Soak chopped onion in 1 cup water for 20 minutes; drain. Combine onion with scallops, shrimp, chilies, lemon juice, cilantro, and garlic. Marinate in refrigerator for at least 5 hours, stirring occasionally. (Ceviche can be made a day ahead of serving.)

- Combine all ingredients for sauce and adjust seasoning to taste. For each serving, place ½ cup of seafood mixture on a lettuce leaf. Garnish with a lemon or lime wedge and serve sauce alongside.

PER SERVING: 77 CALORIES		
MENU EXCHANGE PATTERN		
Dairy . . . . . —	Fruit . . . . . —	
Bread . . . . —	Meat 1	
Fat . . . . —	Veg. 1	
NUTRITIONAL INFORMATION		
Carbohydrate 9	g	
Protein 10	g	
Total fat 0	g	
Saturated fat 0	g	
Cholesterol 41	mg	
Sodium 404	mg	
Potassium 462	mg	
Fiber 0.2	g	
Calcium 33	mg	
Iron . . . . 1.4 mg		

Chicken Enchiladas with Green and Red Sauces

4 cups water
1 chicken (about $2^1/_4$ pounds),
   boned and skinned
2 cloves garlic, mashed
1 jalapeño chili
2 green tomatillos, boiled until
   tender (about 10 minutes)

$1/4$ teaspoon minced garlic
1 tablespoon plain low-fat
   yogurt
2 tablespoons safflower oil
6 corn tortillas
3 cups Red Sauce (recipe
   follows)

- Boil chicken in water until cooked through, about 15 minutes. Finely chop chicken and set aside.

- Preheat oven to 350°F. Combine garlic, jalapeño, tomatillos, and yogurt in a blender and mix well. Heat 1 tablespoon oil in a saucepan over medium heat, add contents of blender and sauté until tender, about 5 minutes. Heat the remaining tablespoon of oil briefly in a small skillet large enough to hold one tortilla. Dip the tortillas in the sauce and then in the heated oil. Top each tortilla with chopped chicken, roll up, and arrange in a baking dish. Cover with the remaining sauce. Bake until heated through, about 15 minutes. Serve immediately, with Red Sauce on side.

PER SERVING: 355 CALORIES		
MENU EXCHANGE PATTERN		
Dairy ..... —	Fruit ..... —	
Bread 1	Meat 4	
Fat 1½	Veg. ...... —	
NUTRITIONAL INFORMATION		
Carbohydrate 17	g	
Protein 31	g	
Total fat 18	g	
Saturated fat 4.0	g	
Cholesterol 87	mg	
Sodium 123	mg	
Potassium 469	mg	
Fiber 0.6	g	
Calcium 92	mg	
Iron 2.2	mg	

Red Sauce

5 tomatoes
1 tablespoon safflower oil
2 Arbol chilies
2 Serrano chilies

1 tablespoon chopped fresh
  coriander (cilantro) leaves
½ teaspoon minced garlic

- Cover tomatoes with water and boil until tender, about 15 minutes. Drain well. Heat oil in a small skillet and fry the árbol chilies about 5 to 10 minutes. Combine all ingredients in a blender and blend to desired consistency. Makes about 6 cups; 1 serving = ½ cup.

PER SERVING: 27 CALORIES		
MENU EXCHANGE PATTERN		
Dairy ..... —	Fruit ..... —	
Bread ..... —	Meat ..... —	
Fat .... —	Veg. 1	
NUTRITIONAL INFORMATION		
Carbohydrate 4	g	
Protein 1	g	
Total fat 1	g	
Saturated fat 0	g	
Cholesterol 0	mg	
Sodium 91	mg	
Potassium 190	mg	
Fiber 0.4	g	
Calcium 11	mg	
Iron 0.3	mg	

Tequila Sherbet

1 envelope unflavored gelatin
1 cup water
1½ cups sugar
⅓ cup tequila

⅓ cup lime juice
1 tablespoon grated lemon rind
1 cup evaporated skim milk

- Sprinkle gelatin over ¼ cup water and let stand until gelatin is softened, about 5 minutes. Combine remaining ¾ cup water and sugar in a saucepan and bring to a boil; boil for 5 minutes. Remove from heat, add softened gelatin, and stir until dissolved. Add tequila, lime juice, and rind. Transfer to ice cube tray and freeze until ice crystals begin to form.

- Freeze evaporated skim milk until crystals begin to form. Whip until thick and slowly beat in lime mixture. Return to freezer until thoroughly frozen, beating with electric mixer every 30 minutes to prevent formation of coarse ice crystals.

- Sherbet is best if made 2 to 3 days in advance. Remove from refrigerator 10 minutes before serving.

PER SERVING: 259 CALORIES		
MENU EXCHANGE PATTERN		
Dairy ..... —	Fruit 1	
Bread 3	Meat ..... —	
Fat .... —	Veg. ..... —	
NUTRITIONAL INFORMATION		
Carbohydrate 55	g	
Protein 3	g	
Total fat 0	g	
Saturated fat 0	g	
Cholesterol 2	mg	
Sodium 49	mg	
Potassium 161	mg	
Fiber 0	g	
Calcium 125	mg	
Iron 0.2	mg	

MEAT

1

Sangría

Tortilla Soup

Carne Guisada

Mixed Mexican Vegetables

Corn Tortillas

Orange-Mango Mousse

Serves 4

PER SERVING: 974 CALORIES			
MENU EXCHANGE PATTERN			
Dairy	½	Fruit	2½
Bread	6	Meat	4
Fat	1½	Veg.	3½
NUTRITIONAL INFORMATION			
Carbohydrate	115	g	
Protein	45	g	
Total fat	26	g	
Saturated fat	4.7	g	
Cholesterol	84	mg	
Sodium	639	mg	
Potassium	2105	mg	
Fiber	3.7	g	
Calcium	415	mg	
Iron	8.5	mg	

Sangría

1/3 cup orange juice
1²/3 cups red wine
1/4 cup brandy
1 small orange, sliced

- Combine all ingredients and chill thoroughly. Serve in wine glasses.

PER SERVING: 137 CALORIES			
MENU EXCHANGE PATTERN			
Dairy	—	Fruit	. . . . . —
Bread	2	Meat	. . . . . —
Fat	—	Veg.	. . . . . . —

NUTRITIONAL INFORMATION		
Carbohydrate	9	g
Protein	0	g
Total fat	0	g
Saturated fat	0	g
Cholesterol	0	mg
Sodium	3	mg
Potassium	169	mg
Fiber	0	g
Calcium	20	mg
Iron	0.4	mg

Tortilla Soup

4 teaspoons safflower oil
1 onion, thinly sliced at an
   angle
2 cloves garlic, finely chopped
4 teaspoons chopped fresh
   coriander (cilantro) leaves
1 teaspoon dried oregano
1/3 teaspoon ground cloves
1/2 teaspoon black pepper
1/2 teaspoon ground cumin
1/4 teaspoon ground coriander

1/2 green bell pepper, sliced into
   1/4-inch strips
1 cup sliced mushrooms
2 cups diced tomato
1/3 cup low-sodium tomato
   puree
6 cups Caldo de Pollo
   (page 153)
2 corn tortillas
2 ounces low-fat Monterey Jack
   cheese, shredded

- Heat oil in heavy large saucepan over medium heat. Add onion and garlic and sauté until tender but not browned, about 10 minutes. Add cilantro, seasonings, and green pepper and saute for 2 to 3 minutes. Add mushrooms and tomato and sauté 10 to 12 minutes. Add tomato puree and Caldo de Pollo and simmer for 10 to 20 minutes.

- Preheat oven to 400°F. Slice tortillas into ½-inch strips and arrange them on a baking sheet coated with nonstick spray and bake for 4 to 5 minutes. Divide toasted strips among individual soup bowls. Ladle in soup and top each serving with shredded cheese. Serve immediately.

PER SERVING: 172 CALORIES			
MENU EXCHANGE PATTERN			
Dairy	—	Fruit	. . . . . —
Bread	1	Meat	. . . . . . ½
Fat	1	Veg.	 1

NUTRITIONAL INFORMATION		
Carbohydrate	18	g
Protein	7	g
Total fat	9	g
Saturated fat	0.4	g
Cholesterol	0	mg
Sodium	462	mg
Potassium	463	mg
Fiber	1.1	g
Calcium	148	mg
Iron	1.6	mg

Carne Guisada

1 pound lean flank steak
    (trimmed fat), cut into
    1 × ¼-inch pieces
⅓ cup dry sherry
4 teaspoons safflower oil
½ teaspoon minced garlic
¼ teaspoon whole cumin seed
¼ teaspoon black pepper
2 teaspoons low-sodium tomato
    paste

2 teaspoons low-sodium beef
    broth concentrate
¼ tomato
¼ onion
½ bell pepper, cored, seeded,
    and sliced
Juice of ½ lemon

- Cook steak with sherry in oil over low heat until brown and tender, about 5 to 10 minutes, turning once. Drain any excess fat. Combine the garlic, cumin, pepper, tomato paste, beef broth concentrate, tomato, and onion in a blender and blend for 2 minutes. Add to the meat and cook over low heat for 15 minutes, arranging bell pepper slices over meat about halfway through cooking. Sprinkle with lemon juice and serve.

PER SERVING: 245 CALORIES

MENU EXCHANGE PATTERN

Dairy	—	Fruit	—
Bread	½	Meat	3½
Fat	—	Veg.	½

NUTRITIONAL INFORMATION

Carbohydrate	5	g
Protein	25	g
Total fat	11	g
Saturated fat	3.5	g
Cholesterol	80	mg
Sodium	124	mg
Potassium	517	mg
Fiber	0.3	g
Calcium	25	mg
Iron	4.0	mg

Mixed Mexican Vegetables

2 teaspoons safflower oil
⅔ cup chopped onion
⅔ cup green beans, ends
    trimmed
⅔ green bell pepper, cored,
    seeded, and chopped
1⅓ cups sliced zucchini

1⅓ cups fresh corn kernels
⅔ cup chopped fresh or low-
    sodium canned tomatoes
⅓ cup water
½ teaspoon dried oregano
½ teaspoon dried basil
Black pepper

- Heat oil in a large saucepan over medium heat. Add onion and sauté until translucent, about 10 minutes. Add beans, green pepper, and zucchini and cook for 5 minutes. Add corn, tomatoes, water, and seasonings and simmer until vegetables are cooked through but not mushy, about 10 minutes. Serve immediately.

PER SERVING: 107 CALORIES

MENU EXCHANGE PATTERN

Dairy	—	Fruit	—
Bread	½	Meat	—
Fat	½	Veg.	2

NUTRITIONAL INFORMATION

Carbohydrate	20	g
Protein	4	g
Total fat	3	g
Saturated fat	0.2	g
Cholesterol	0	mg
Sodium	8	mg
Potassium	440	mg
Fiber	1.6	g
Calcium	44	mg
Iron	1.2	mg

Corn Tortillas

4 corn tortillas

- Wrap tortillas in aluminum foil and heat in 350°F oven for about 10 minutes. Serve warm with Carne Guisada.

PER SERVING: 63 CALORIES			
MENU EXCHANGE PATTERN			
Dairy	—	Fruit	—
Bread	1	Meat	—
Fat	—	Veg.	—
NUTRITIONAL INFORMATION			
Carbohydrate	14		g
Protein	2		g
Total fat	1		g
Saturated fat	0		g
Cholesterol	0		mg
Sodium	33		mg
Potassium	5		mg
Fiber	0.3		g
Calcium	60		mg
Iron	0.9		mg

Orange-Mango Mousse

²/₃ cup cold water
1 envelope unflavored gelatin
¹/₃ cup sugar
1 can (6 ounces) frozen orange juice concentrate
1 very ripe mango, peeled, pitted, and diced

1 cup plain low-fat yogurt
¹/₂ teaspoon vanilla extract
6 ice cubes
6 thin orange slices
Mint leaves (garnish)

- Pour water into a small saucepan, sprinkle gelatin over the top and let stand until softened, about 5 minutes. Place saucepan over low heat until gelatin is completely dissolved. Transfer to a blender. With machine running, gradually add sugar and mix for about 1 minute. Add orange juice concentrate, mango, yogurt, and vanilla and blend well, then add ice cubes one at a time while blending. Pour into individual serving glasses and freeze. Just before serving, thaw slightly, top with an orange slice and garnish with mint.

PER SERVING: 218 CALORIES			
MENU EXCHANGE PATTERN			
Dairy	½	Fruit	2½
Bread	1	Meat	—
Fat	—	Veg.	—
NUTRITIONAL INFORMATION			
Carbohydrate	47		g
Protein	6		g
Total fat	1		g
Saturated fat	0.6		g
Cholesterol	4		mg
Sodium	42		mg
Potassium	516		mg
Fiber	0.6		g
Calcium	133		mg
Iron	0.3		mg

MEAT

2

Smoked Salmon Appetizers

Rudi's Tossed Salad

Steak Forestière

Fettuccine Alfredo

Lemon Sherbet (page 107)

Serves 6

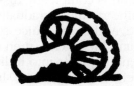

PER SERVING: 745 CALORIES		
MENU EXCHANGE PATTERN		
Dairy ..... —	Fruit ..... —	
Bread 5	Meat 5½	
Fat 1	Veg. 2	

NUTRITIONAL INFORMATION		
Carbohydrate 84	g
Protein 51	g
Total fat 23	g
Saturated fat 8.1	g
Cholesterol 112	mg
Sodium 683	mg
Potassium 1432	mg
Fiber 2	g
Calcium 295	mg
Iron 7.7	mg

Smoked Salmon Appetizers

3 ounces Neufchatel cheese
6 dry rye crackers or Wasa
  bread
6 ounces smoked salmon,
  thinly sliced

- Spread a small amount of cheese on each cracker. Top with a thin slice of salmon.

PER SERVING: 153 CALORIES		
MENU EXCHANGE PATTERN		
Dairy . . . . . —	Fruit . . . . . —	
Bread 1	Meat 1½	
Fat . . . . —	Veg. . . . . . . —	
NUTRITIONAL INFORMATION		
Carbohydrate 14	g	
Protein 11	g	
Total fat 6	g	
Saturated fat 2.2	g	
Cholesterol 20	mg	
Sodium 341	mg	
Potassium 215	mg	
Fiber 0.5	g	
Calcium 103	mg	
Iron . . . . 1.1 mg		

Rudi's Tossed Salad

3 cups iceberg lettuce torn into
  bite-size pieces
3 cups romaine lettuce torn
  into bite-size pieces
1 cucumber, sliced

3 tomatoes, cut into wedges
6 radishes, sliced
9 tablespoons Italian Dressing
  (recipe follows)

- Combine lettuces, cucumber, tomatoes, and radishes and toss lightly. Add dressing and toss again. Serve on individual salad plates.

PER SERVING: 33 CALORIES		
MENU EXCHANGE PATTERN		
Dairy . . . . . —	Fruit . . . . . —	
Bread . . . . —	Meat . . . . . —	
Fat . . . . —	Veg. 1	
NUTRITIONAL INFORMATION		
Carbohydrate 7	g	
Protein 2	g	
Total fat 0	g	
Saturated fat 0	g	
Cholesterol 0	mg	
Sodium 10	mg	
Potassium 402	mg	
Fiber 1	g	
Calcium 44	mg	
Iron . . . . 1.2 mg		

Italian Dressing

1 cup safflower oil
1 cup red wine vinegar
1 cup water
½ teaspoon dried oregano

6 drops Worcestershire sauce
1 clove garlic, minced
½ teaspoon black pepper
Juice of 1 lemon

- Combine all ingredients. Let stand for at least 1 hour before serving. Makes 3 cups; 1 serving = 1½ tablespoons.

PER SERVING: 68 CALORIES		
MENU EXCHANGE PATTERN		
Dairy . . . . —	Fruit . . . . . —	
Bread . . . . —	Meat . . . . . —	
Fat 1½	Veg. . . . . . . —	
NUTRITIONAL INFORMATION		
Carbohydrate 1	g	
Protein 0	g	
Total fat 7	g	
Saturated fat 0.6	g	
Cholesterol 0	mg	
Sodium 0	mg	
Potassium 18	mg	
Fiber 0	g	
Calcium 2	mg	
Iron . . . . 0.1 mg		

Steak Forestière

1½ pounds beef flank steak
1 tablespoon margarine
1½ cups sliced mushrooms
1½ cups diced tomato

¼ teaspoon garlic powder or
  1 clove garlic, minced
6 tablespoons chopped fresh
  chives

- Grill steak to desired doneness. Melt margarine in a skillet over medium heat. Add mushrooms, tomato, garlic, and chives and sauté until tender and most of liquid has evaporated, about 15 to 20 minutes. Spoon over steak and serve.

PER SERVING: 197 CALORIES		
MENU EXCHANGE PATTERN		
Dairy . . . . . —	Fruit . . . . . —	
Bread . . . . —	Meat 3	
Fat . . . . —	Veg. 1	
NUTRITIONAL INFORMATION		
Carbohydrate 3	g	
Protein 26	g	
Total fat 9	g	
Saturated fat 3.5	g	
Cholesterol 80	mg	
Sodium 90	mg	
Potassium 590	mg	
Fiber 0.5	g	
Calcium 25	mg	
Iron 4.1	mg	

Fettuccine Alfredo

8 ounces fettuccine
1 cup low-fat cottage cheese
1 clove garlic, halved
3 tablespoons grated Romano
  cheese

- Bring 2 quarts water to boil in a large pot. Gradually add fettuccine and cook until *al dente*, about 5 minutes. Drain. While fettuccine is cooking, combine cottage cheese, garlic, and Romano in a blender or food processor and blend until smooth. Toss cooked fettuccine with cheese mixture and serve immediately.

PER SERVING: 185 CALORIES		
MENU EXCHANGE PATTERN		
Dairy . . . . . —	Fruit . . . . . —	
Bread 2	Meat 1	
Fat . . . . —	Veg. . . . . . . —	
NUTRITIONAL INFORMATION		
Carbohydrate 30	g	
Protein 11	g	
Total fat 2	g	
Saturated fat 0.9	g	
Cholesterol 5	mg	
Sodium 200	mg	
Potassium 115	mg	
Fiber 0	g	
Calcium 71	mg	
Iron 1.1	mg	

MEAT

3

Chilled Watercress Soup with Tart Apples

Peppered Fillet of Beef with Grilled Red Onions and Ancho Pepper Preserve

Amaretto Freeze

Serves 6

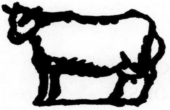

PER SERVING: 727 CALORIES		
MENU EXCHANGE PATTERN		
Dairy . . . . . . ½	Fruit 2	
Bread 2	Meat 3	
Fat 3½	Veg. 4	
NUTRITIONAL INFORMATION		
Carbohydrate 64	g	
Protein 27	g	
Total fat 33	g	
Saturated fat 15.2	g	
Cholesterol 80	mg	
Sodium 370	mg	
Potassium 1429	mg	
Fiber 2.6	g	
Calcium 243	mg	
Iron 5.1	mg	

Chilled Watercress Soup with Tart Apples

2 stalks celery, chopped
2 leeks, chopped
½ onion, chopped
1 tablespoon safflower oil
1 quart Homemade Chicken
   Stock (page 36)
2 Idaho potatoes, peeled and
   quartered
2 teaspoons fresh thyme

2 tablespoons chopped fresh
   parsley
2 tablespoons chopped fresh
   basil
4 bunches watercress
2 cups plain low-fat yogurt
White pepper
2 tart green apples, cored and
   diced

- Sauté celery, leeks, and onion in oil in a large nonstick saucepan over medium heat until translucent, about 5 minutes. Add stock, potatoes, thyme, parsley, and basil. Bring to a boil and simmer until potatoes are tender, about 10 to 15 minutes. Strain soup; puree potatoes in food processor and return puree to soup. Let cool.

- Blanch watercress for 1 to 2 seconds in boiling water; immediately plunge into ice water to cool. Chop watercress; transfer to food processor and puree until smooth. Transfer cold soup to processor. With machine running, add yogurt and pepper and blend until smooth. Add apple cubes to soup. Chill soup well. Serve in chilled bowls.

PER SERVING: 149 CALORIES		
MENU EXCHANGE PATTERN		
Dairy . . . . . —	Fruit . . . . . —	
Bread 1	Meat . . . . . —	
Fat . . . . ½	Veg. 2	
NUTRITIONAL INFORMATION		
Carbohydrate 22	g	
Protein 3	g	
Total fat 3	g	
Saturated fat 0.2	g	
Cholesterol 5	mg	
Sodium 134	mg	
Potassium 579	mg	
Fiber 1.5	g	
Calcium 79	mg	
Iron 1.3	mg	

Peppered Fillet of Beef with Grilled Red Onions

1½ pounds beef sirloin, lean
   part only
2 tablespoons black
   peppercorns, crushed
6 red onions, peeled and left
   whole
Ancho Pepper Preserve (recipe
   follows)

- Rub beef with crushed peppercorns. Grill or broil to desired doneness. Grill red onions over a hot fire or roast under broiler slowly until soft, about 20 to 25 minutes. Serve beef with Ancho Pepper Preserve and onions.

PER SERVING: 393 CALORIES		
MENU EXCHANGE PATTERN		
Dairy . . . . . —	Fruit . . . . . —	
Bread 1	Meat 3	
Fat 2½	Veg. 2	
NUTRITIONAL INFORMATION		
Carbohydrate 15	g	
Protein 20	g	
Total fat 28	g	
Saturated fat 13.5	g	
Cholesterol 67	mg	
Sodium 91	mg	
Potassium 670	mg	
Fiber 1	g	
Calcium 56	mg	
Iron 3.5	mg	

Ancho Pepper Preserve

4 ounces dried ancho chilies
1 tablespoon red wine vinegar
2 tablespoons honey
1 teaspoon minced shallot

1/2 teaspoon minced garlic
2 tablespoons red currant jelly
1/4 teaspoon salt

PER SERVING: 41 CALORIES			
MENU EXCHANGE PATTERN			
Dairy	—	Fruit	1
Bread	—	Meat	—
Fat	—	Veg.	—

NUTRITIONAL INFORMATION		
Carbohydrate	11	g
Protein	0	g
Total fat	0	g
Saturated fat	0	g
Cholesterol	0	mg
Sodium	91	mg
Potassium	30	mg
Fiber	0.1	g
Calcium	3	mg
Iron	0.2	mg

- Soak chilies in warm water to cover until soft, about 30 minutes. Drain. Puree chilies in blender with vinegar, honey, shallot, and garlic. Add currant jelly and salt and puree until very smooth and thick. Taste and adjust honey or vinegar to balance the tart/sweetness. Makes about ¾ cup; 1 serving = 2 tablespoons.

Amaretto Freeze

3 cups low-fat frozen vanilla
    yogurt
1/2 cup amaretto
Ground nutmeg

PER SERVING: 144 CALORIES			
MENU EXCHANGE PATTERN			
Dairy	½	Fruit	1
Bread	—	Meat	—
Fat	½	Veg.	—

NUTRITIONAL INFORMATION		
Carbohydrate	16	g
Protein	3	g
Total fat	2	g
Saturated fat	1.5	g
Cholesterol	8	mg
Sodium	54	mg
Potassium	150	mg
Fiber	0	g
Calcium	105	mg
Iron	0.1	mg

- In a blender mix 1½ cups frozen yogurt with ¼ cup amaretto. Transfer to 3 chilled wine glasses. Repeat with remaining yogurt and amaretto. Sprinkle lightly with nutmeg and serve.

MEAT

4

Beef and Mushroom Soup

Veal Scallopini with Lemon Sauce

"Buttered" Fettuccine

Broccoli and Carrots with Rosemary

Apple Strudel

Serves 6

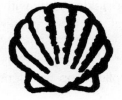

PER SERVING: 784 CALORIES		
MENU EXCHANGE PATTERN		
Dairy . . . . . —	Fruit 1	
Bread 3½	Meat 3½	
Fat 5	Veg. 3½	
NUTRITIONAL INFORMATION		
Carbohydrate 73	g	
Protein 38	g	
Total fat 37	g	
Saturated fat 9.4	g	
Cholesterol 100	mg	
Sodium 279	mg	
Potassium 1186	mg	
Fiber 2.7	g	
Calcium 148	mg	
Iron 7	mg	

Beef and Mushroom Soup

1 tablespoon margarine
2 tablespoons finely chopped
    celery
1 cup mushrooms cut into
    1/4-inch slices
1 cup shiitake mushrooms cut
    into 1/4-inch slices

1 red onion, finely chopped
1 teaspoon dried thyme
1 teaspoon cracked black
    pepper
1 bay leaf
1 1/2 quarts commercial low-
    sodium beef stock

- Melt margarine in a large nonstick skillet over medium heat. Add celery, mushrooms, and onion and sauté until golden brown, about 10 minutes. Add thyme, pepper, bay leaf, and stock and simmer 30 minutes. Serve hot.

PER SERVING: 95 CALORIES		
MENU EXCHANGE PATTERN		
Dairy . . . . . —	Fruit . . . . . —	
Bread . . . . . —	Meat . . . . . —	
Fat 1	Veg. 2	
NUTRITIONAL INFORMATION		
Carbohydrate 8	g	
Protein 4	g	
Total fat 6	g	
Saturated fat 0.4	g	
Cholesterol 0	mg	
Sodium 110	mg	
Potassium 151	mg	
Fiber 0.4	g	
Calcium 11	mg	
Iron . . . . 0.4 mg		

Veal Scallopini with Lemon Sauce

18 veal scallops, about 1 1/2
    ounces each
Black pepper
1/3 cup lemon juice

1/4 cup margarine
1 cup dry white wine
1/4 cup chopped fresh parsley

- Place veal pieces between 2 pieces of plastic wrap and pound to 1/4-inch thickness. Sprinkle with pepper and 2 tablespoons of the lemon juice.

- Melt the margarine in a large skillet over medium heat, being careful not to overheat. Add veal and sauté about 30 seconds on each side. Transfer veal to a warm platter. Add remaining lemon juice, wine, and chopped parsley to skillet and cook until sauce consistency, about 2 minutes.

- Fan 3 veal pieces on each dinner plate. Top with lemon sauce and serve.

PER SERVING: 318 CALORIES		
MENU EXCHANGE PATTERN		
Dairy . . . . . —	Fruit . . . . . —	
Bread 1/2	Meat 3 1/2	
Fat 2	Veg. . . . . . . —	
NUTRITIONAL INFORMATION		
Carbohydrate 3	g	
Protein 23	g	
Total fat 20	g	
Saturated fat 7.5	g	
Cholesterol 100	mg	
Sodium 81	mg	
Potassium 434	mg	
Fiber 0	g	
Calcium 24	mg	
Iron . . . . 3.6 mg		

"Buttered" Fettuccine

1/2 pound fettuccine
2 quarts boiling water
2 tablespoons margarine

- Gradually add fettuccine to boiling water and cook until *al dente*. Drain in a colander, stir in margarine and serve.

PER SERVING: 173 CALORIES		
MENU EXCHANGE PATTERN		
Dairy . . . . . —	Fruit . . . . . —	
Bread 2	Meat . . . . . —	
Fat 1	Veg. . . . . . . —	
NUTRITIONAL INFORMATION		
Carbohydrate 28	g	
Protein 5	g	
Total fat 4	g	
Saturated fat 0.7	g	
Cholesterol 0	mg	
Sodium 1	mg	
Potassium 76	mg	
Fiber 0	g	
Calcium 11	mg	
Iron . . . . 1.1 mg		

Broccoli and Carrots with Rosemary

1½ cups broccoli florets
1½ cups carrots, peeled and cut
   diagonally into ¼-inch slices

1 teaspoon chopped fresh
   rosemary
Juice of 1 lemon
Black pepper

- Bring broccoli and carrots to a boil in separate saucepans in ⅓ to ½ cup water. Cover and simmer until crisp-tender. Drain, toss together, and add rosemary, lemon juice, and pepper to taste.

PER SERVING: 35 CALORIES		
MENU EXCHANGE PATTERN		
Dairy ..... —	Fruit ..... —	
Bread .... —	Meat ..... —	
Fat .... —	Veg. 1½	
NUTRITIONAL INFORMATION		
Carbohydrate 7		g
Protein 3		g
Total fat 0		g
Saturated fat 0		g
Cholesterol 0		mg
Sodium 22		mg
Potassium 331		mg
Fiber 1.3		g
Calcium 77		mg
Iron 1		mg

Apple Strudel

8 Delicious apples, peeled,
   cored and sliced
cloves
¼ cup chopped walnuts
1½ tablespoons plain low-fat
   yogurt

3 tablespoons sugar
1 tablespoon ground cinnamon
8 sheets of phyllo dough
2 tablespoons margarine, melted
1 egg substitute

- Steam apple slices over boiling water containing 2 to 4 whole cloves for 5 to 8 minutes. Drain apples, spread on a cookie sheet, and cool in the refrigerator for about 5 to 10 minutes.

- Combine cooled apple slices with walnuts, yogurt, sugar, and cinnamon. Refrigerate for 30 minutes.

- Preheat oven to 350°F. Brush the surface of a nonporous work surface (such as Formica) with margarine using a pastry brush. Place 4 sheets of phyllo on the surface to form a rectangle, overlapping pieces by about 4 inches in the center. Lightly brush phyllo again with margarine.

- Spread half of the apple mixture over the dough, leaving 1 inch uncovered on each side. Fold over like a loaf of French bread and tuck seams under bottom.

- Repeat assembly procedure with remaining 4 sheets of phyllo dough and apple mixture. Transfer both strudel loaves to a cookie sheet sprayed with nonstick cooking spray. Bake until golden brown, about 25 to 30 minutes. Serve warm or at room temperature. Makes 10 servings; 1 serving = one 1-inch slice.

PER SERVING: 163 CALORIES		
MENU EXCHANGE PATTERN		
Dairy ..... —	Fruit 1	
Bread 1	Meat ..... —	
Fat 1	Veg. ...... —	
NUTRITIONAL INFORMATION		
Carbohydrate 27		g
Protein 3		g
Total fat 6		g
Saturated fat 0.8		g
Cholesterol 0		mg
Sodium 65		mg
Potassium 194		mg
Fiber 1		g
Calcium 25		mg
Iron 0.9		mg

MEAT

5

Scallops and Prawns Bercy

Veal Medallions with Crabmeat

Chilled Asparagus

Fettuccine with Parmesan

Chocolate Yogurt Pie

Serves 6

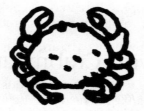

PER SERVING: 816 CALORIES			
MENU EXCHANGE PATTERN			
Dairy	½	Fruit	—
Bread	4	Meat	5½
Fat	3	Veg.	1½
NUTRITIONAL INFORMATION			
Carbohydrate	72	g	
Protein	56	g	
Total fat	31	g	
Saturated fat	10.2	g	
Cholesterol	229	mg	
Sodium	692	mg	
Potassium	1427	mg	
Fiber	1.5	g	
Calcium	246	mg	
Iron	7.7	mg	

Scallops and Prawns Bercy

½ pound scallops
½ pound prawns or large
  shrimp
1 teaspoon Worcestershire
  sauce
2 teaspoons lemon juice
Black pepper
2 tablespoons margarine

2 tablespoons chopped shallot
1 tablespoon chopped fresh
  herbs (parsley, thyme,
  tarragon, and/or oregano)
1 tablespoon brandy
1 tablespoon dry white wine
2 tablespoons skim milk

White Wine Sauce

1 tablespoon margarine
1 tablespoon all-purpose flour

¼ cup dry white wine
¼ cup skim milk

- Marinate scallops and prawns in Worcestershire, lemon juice, and pepper for 1 hour.

- Melt margarine for sauce in a small saucepan over low heat. Add flour and cook, stirring constantly, until bubbly. Slowly whisk in wine and milk and cook until mixture boils and thickens, stirring constantly. Keep warm.

- Melt 1 tablespoon margarine in a large nonstick skillet over medium heat. Add scallops and prawns and sauté until opaque, about 5 minutes. Remove from heat. Heat remaining margarine in a medium saucepan until golden brown. Stir in shallot and herbs. Add brandy and ignite, shaking pan gently until flames subside. Add wine, milk, and wine sauce and season with pepper to taste. Stir in scallops and prawns.

PER SERVING: 124 CALORIES		
MENU EXCHANGE PATTERN		
Dairy ..... —	Fruit ..... —	
Bread ..... ½	Meat 1½	
Fat .... —	Veg. ...... —	
NUTRITIONAL INFORMATION		
Carbohydrate 4	g	
Protein 13	g	
Total fat 4	g	
Saturated fat 0.8	g	
Cholesterol 68	mg	
Sodium 156	mg	
Potassium 279	mg	
Fiber 0	g	
Calcium 51	mg	
Iron 1.4	mg	

Veal Medallions with Crabmeat

4 tablespoons margarine
3 tablespoons water
3 tablespoons dry white wine
2 tablespoons brandy
1 pound king crabmeat
1½ pounds veal medallions
Black pepper
2 tablespoons all-purpose flour

2 tablespoons chopped shallot
2 tablespoons chopped fresh
  herbs (parsley, rosemary, and
  thyme)
1 tablespoon lemon juice
2 teaspoons Worcestershire
  sauce

- Melt 1 tablespoon margarine in a large saucepan over medium heat. Add water, wine, brandy, and crabmeat and cook until crab is opaque, about 5 minutes. Set aside and keep warm. Season veal with pepper and dust with flour. In a large nonstick skillet, sauté veal in 2 tablespoons margarine over medium-high heat 5 minutes per side. Set veal aside

PER SERVING: 270 CALORIES		
MENU EXCHANGE PATTERN		
Dairy ..... —	Fruit ..... —	
Bread ..... ½	Meat 4	
Fat .... —	Veg. ...... ½	
NUTRITIONAL INFORMATION		
Carbohydrate 4	g	
Protein 32	g	
Total fat 12	g	
Saturated fat 4.9	g	
Cholesterol 156	mg	
Sodium 498	mg	
Potassium 423	mg	
Fiber 0.1	g	
Calcium 50	mg	
Iron 3.6	mg	

and keep warm. Melt remaining 1 tablespoon margarine in a small saucepan over medium heat. Add shallot, herbs, lemon juice, Worcestershire, and pepper to taste and sauté until shallot is translucent, about 5 minutes.

- Transfer veal medallions to dinner plates. Toss crabmeat with shallot and herb mixture and divide into 6 equal portions. Top medallions with crab mixture.

Chilled Asparagus

1 1/2 pounds asparagus

- Trim tough ends of asparagus. Bring several inches of water to boil in a steamer. Place asparagus on a rack over water and steam until crisp-tender, about 10 minutes. Drop asparagus into ice water to cool quickly; drain well. Refrigerate until serving time.

PER SERVING: 35 CALORIES		
MENU EXCHANGE PATTERN		
Dairy ..... —	Fruit ..... —	
Bread ..... —	Meat ..... —	
Fat .... —	Veg. 1	
NUTRITIONAL INFORMATION		
Carbohydrate 7	g	
Protein 3	g	
Total fat 0.3	g	
Saturated fat 0	g	
Cholesterol 0	mg	
Sodium 3	mg	
Potassium 374	mg	
Fiber 0.9	g	
Calcium 30	mg	
Iron 1.3	mg	

Fettuccine with Parmesan

1/3 pound fresh fettuccine (without eggs)
2 tablespoons margarine
1/2 teaspoon ground nutmeg
1/2 teaspoon white pepper

1/4 cup peeled, seeded, and finely chopped tomato
2 tablespoons grated Parmesan cheese

- Cook the fettuccine until *al dente,* about 5 minutes, then rinse with cold water. Drain well. Melt the margarine in a large skillet over medium-high heat. Add the noodles and stir to coat with margarine. Add the nutmeg, pepper, and tomato and cook for 1 minute. Sprinkle with the cheese, mix lightly and serve.

PER SERVING: 131 CALORIES		
MENU EXCHANGE PATTERN		
Dairy ..... —	Fruit ..... —	
Bread 1 1/2	Meat ..... —	
Fat 1	Veg. ...... —	
NUTRITIONAL INFORMATION		
Carbohydrate 18	g	
Protein 4	g	
Total fat 5	g	
Saturated fat 1	g	
Cholesterol 1	mg	
Sodium 32	mg	
Potassium 121	mg	
Fiber 0.1	g	
Calcium 33	mg	
Iron 0.8	mg	

Chocolate Yogurt Pie

15 graham crackers
1/4 cup sugar
3 tablespoons margarine, melted

1 pint low-fat frozen chocolate yogurt
1/4 cup carob chips

- Preheat oven to 375°F. Crush graham crackers between sheets of wax paper. Combine cracker crumbs, sugar, and margarine and press firmly into 8-inch pie plate. Bake until golden brown, about 8 minutes. Let cool thoroughly. Spread frozen yogurt in crust and sprinkle with carob chips. Freeze pie until ready to serve.

PER SERVING: 256 CALORIES		
MENU EXCHANGE PATTERN		
Dairy 1/2	Fruit ..... —	
Bread 1 1/2	Meat ..... —	
Fat 2	Veg. ...... —	
NUTRITIONAL INFORMATION		
Carbohydrate 39	g	
Protein 4	g	
Total fat 10	g	
Saturated fat 3	g	
Cholesterol 3	mg	
Sodium 219	mg	
Potassium 230	mg	
Fiber 0.4	g	
Calcium 82	mg	
Iron 0.6	mg	

MEAT

6

Romaine and Watercress with
Sweet and Sour Dressing

Veal Medallions à la Grecque

Spaetzle

Sautéed Fresh Spinach

Strawberries Flambé

Serves 8

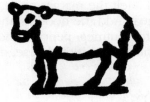

PER SERVING: 813 CALORIES		
MENU EXCHANGE PATTERN		
Dairy . . . . . . ½	Fruit 2	
Bread 3½	Meat 3½	
Fat 4½	Veg. 2½	
NUTRITIONAL INFORMATION		
Carbohydrate 83	. g	
Protein 39	g	
Total fat 33	g	
Saturated fat 10.2	g	
Cholesterol 109	mg	
Sodium 533	mg	
Potassium 1754	mg	
Fiber 2.9	g	
Calcium 315	mg	
Iron 10.8	mg	

Romaine and Watercress with Sweet and Sour Dressing

2 large heads romaine lettuce
  (about 6 cups)
3 bunches watercress
1/2 cup Sweet and Sour Dressing
  (recipe follows)

- Trim lettuce and watercress and toss gently in a large bowl. Divide among individual plates and drizzle with dressing.

  Note: To reduce fat intake, substitute a commercial low-calorie Italian dressing for the Sweet and Sour Dressing. Adjusted analysis for dressing: calories = 16; exchange = 1/2 Fat.

PER SERVING: 9 CALORIES		
MENU EXCHANGE PATTERN		
Dairy . . . . . —	Fruit . . . . . —	
Bread . . . . . —	Meat . . . . . —	
Fat . . . . —	Veg. 1/2	
NUTRITIONAL INFORMATION		
Carbohydrate 2		g
Protein 1		g
Total fat 0		g
Saturated fat 0		g
Cholesterol 0		mg
Sodium 8		mg
Potassium 133		mg
Fiber 0.3		g
Calcium 41		mg
Iron 0.7		mg

Sweet and Sour Dressing

1/2 clove garlic, chopped
2 teaspoons Dijon-style mustard
1/4 teaspoon black pepper
1/4 cup cider vinegar

1 tablespoon chopped fresh chives
2 tablespoons honey
1/2 cup safflower oil

- Combine garlic, mustard, pepper, vinegar, chives, and honey in a bowl. Gradually add the oil and whisk until smooth. Makes about 1 cup; 1 serving = 1 tablespoon.

PER SERVING: 46 CALORIES		
MENU EXCHANGE PATTERN		
Dairy . . . . —	Fruit . . . . —	
Bread . . . . —	Meat . . . . . —	
Fat 1	Veg. . . . . . . —	
NUTRITIONAL INFORMATION		
Carbohydrate 2		g
Protein 0		g
Total fat 5		g
Saturated fat 0.4		g
Cholesterol 0		mg
Sodium 5		mg
Potassium 4		mg
Fiber 0		g
Calcium 1		mg
Iron 0		mg

Veal Medallions à la Grecque

16 veal medallions, 2 1/2 ounces
  each
Black pepper
1/3 cup all-purpose flour
2 tablespoons safflower oil
2 tablespoons margarine
2 tablespoons chopped shallot

1 clove garlic, minced
8 large mushrooms, quartered
8 artichoke hearts, quartered
1 1/2 cups diced tomato
2 tablespoons lemon juice
2 tablespoons white wine
Chopped fresh parsley (garnish)

- Place veal between 2 pieces of plastic wrap and pound until thin. Season with pepper and dust with flour. Heat oil and margarine in a large nonstick skillet over medium-high heat and sauté veal for about 30 seconds on each side. Remove from skillet and keep warm.

- Add the shallot, garlic, mushrooms, artichokes, and tomato to the skillet and sauté until all vegetables are soft. Stir in the lemon juice and wine. Spoon sauce onto meat, sprinkle with parsley and serve.

Photo opposite

PER SERVING: 301 CALORIES		
MENU EXCHANGE PATTERN		
Dairy . . . . . —	Fruit . . . . . —	
Bread . . . . —	Meat 3 1/2	
Fat 2	Veg. 1	
NUTRITIONAL INFORMATION		
Carbohydrate 7		g
Protein 24		g
Total fat 19		g
Saturated fat 7		g
Cholesterol 100		mg
Sodium 82		mg
Potassium 518		mg
Fiber 0.4		g
Calcium 22		mg
Iron 3.8		mg

*Veal Medallions
à la Grecque*

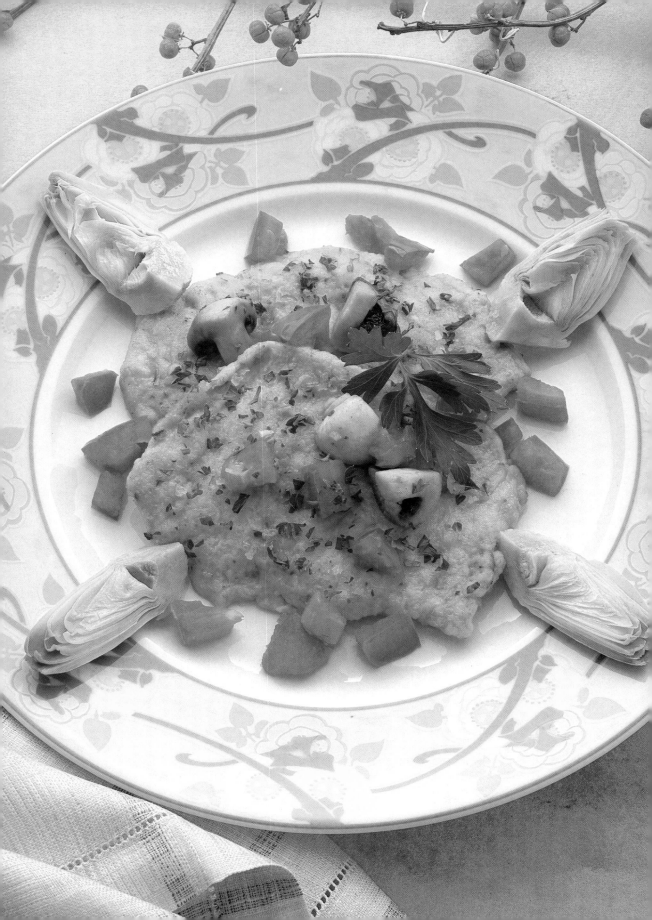

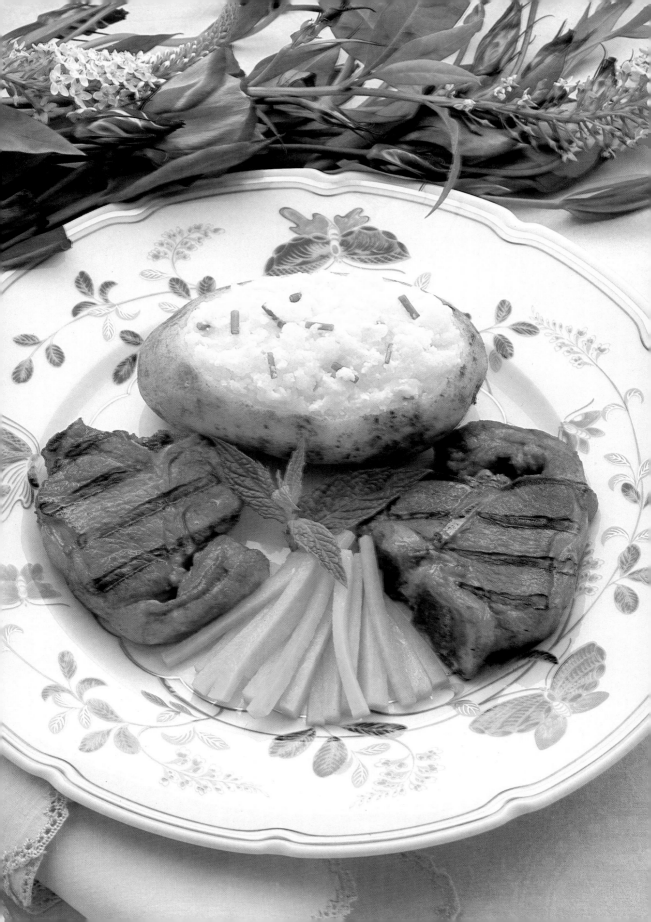

Spaetzle

2²/₃ cups all-purpose flour
1 cup water
3 egg substitutes
1 teaspoon salt
¹/₄ teaspoon white pepper
¹/₄ teaspoon nutmeg
4 teaspoons margarine, melted

- Sift the flour into a large bowl and make a well in the center. Combine the water with the egg substitute, salt, pepper, and nutmeg. Gradually stir into the flour; mix to a thick batter. Press the dough through a colander directly into boiling salted water and cook until spaetzle float, about 5 to 10 minutes. Remove spaetzle with a slotted spoon and drain. Drizzle with melted margarine and serve.

PER SERVING: 165 CALORIES

MENU EXCHANGE PATTERN

Dairy	—	Fruit	—
Bread	2	Meat	—
Fat	½	Veg.	—

NUTRITIONAL INFORMATION

Carbohydrate	28	g
Protein	7	g
Total fat	3	g
Saturated fat	0.6	g
Cholesterol	0	mg
Sodium	299	mg
Potassium	206	mg
Fiber	0.9	g
Calcium	28	mg
Iron	1.7	mg

Sautéed Fresh Spinach

4 bunches spinach, stemmed
1 medium onion, chopped
1 clove garlic, chopped
4 teaspoons margarine
Black pepper

- Bring 2 quarts of water to boil in a large pot. Drop in the spinach, cook for 1 minute, drain and plunge into cold water. Drain well. In a nonstick skillet, sauté the onion and garlic in margarine over medium heat until translucent, about 5 minutes. Add the drained spinach and sauté until heated through. Season with pepper and serve.

PER SERVING: 51 CALORIES

MENU EXCHANGE PATTERN

Dairy	—	Fruit	—
Bread	—	Meat	—
Fat	½	Veg.	1

NUTRITIONAL INFORMATION

Carbohydrate	6	g
Protein	4	g
Total fat	2	g
Saturated fat	0.4	g
Cholesterol	0	mg
Sodium	80	mg
Potassium	543	mg
Fiber	0.8	g
Calcium	106	mg
Iron	3.5	mg

Strawberries Flambé

5 cups sliced strawberries
²/₃ cup firmly packed brown sugar
¹/₂ cup strawberry liqueur
¹/₄ cup rum
4 cups frozen low-fat vanilla yogurt

- Heat the strawberries and sugar in a skillet. Add liqueur and rum and ignite, shaking pan gently until flames subside. Pour over frozen yogurt and serve immediately.

Grilled Lamb Chops with Stuffed Baked Potatoes; recipe page 329

PER SERVING: 240 CALORIES

MENU EXCHANGE PATTERN

Dairy	½	Fruit	2
Bread	1½	Meat	—
Fat	½	Veg.	—

NUTRITIONAL INFORMATION

Carbohydrate	39	g
Protein	3	g
Total fat	3	g
Saturated fat	1.8	g
Cholesterol	9	mg
Sodium	59	mg
Potassium	350	mg
Fiber	0.5	g
Calcium	117	mg
Iron	1.1	mg

MEAT

7

Crab with Belgian Endive

Veal Chops with Mushroom Sauce

Spinach Noodles with Tomatoes

Pears Poached in Burgundy

Serves 6

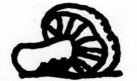

PER SERVING: 1029 CALORIES
MENU EXCHANGE PATTERN
Dairy . . . . . — Fruit 1
Bread . . . . 5½ Meat 6
Fat . . . . 5 Veg. 1½
NUTRITIONAL INFORMATION
Carbohydrate . . . . 96 g
Protein . . . . 51 g
Total fat . . . . 46 g
Saturated fat . . . . 12.2 g
Cholesterol . . . . 200 mg
Sodium . . . . 610 mg
Potassium . . . . 1920 mg
Fiber . . . . 3.1 g
Calcium . . . . 170 mg
Iron . . . . 8.0 mg

Crab with Belgian Endive

6 large leaves Bibb lettuce
3 Belgian endive
1 pound fresh crabmeat
1 cup commercial low-calorie
   Italian dressing

3 tablespoons chopped fresh dill
6 black olives
6 sprigs dill

PER SERVING: 119 CALORIES			
MENU EXCHANGE PATTERN			
Dairy	—	Fruit	—
Bread	—	Meat	2
Fat	—	Veg.	½
NUTRITIONAL INFORMATION			
Carbohydrate	3	g	
Protein	13	g	
Total fat	6	g	
Saturated fat	0.6	g	
Cholesterol	78	mg	
Sodium	457	mg	
Potassium	150	mg	
Fiber	0.2	g	
Calcium	92	mg	
Iron	5.7	mg	

- Place the Bibb lettuce on individual plates. Halve each endive lengthwise and place one half in the center of each plate. Top endive with crab. Combine the dressing with chopped dill and spoon over the crab. Set a black olive and a sprig of dill on each plate.

Note: Analysis includes dressing.

Veal Chops with Mushroom Sauce

6 veal chops, 1½ inches thick
   (about 6 ounces each), well
   trimmed
Black pepper

1 cup all-purpose flour
2 egg substitutes
¼ cup margarine
2 to 3 sprigs fresh rosemary

Mushroom Sauce

1 tablespoon margarine
1 tablespoon all-purpose flour
¾ cup low-fat milk, warmed
White pepper

½ cup dry white wine
2 cups sliced mushrooms
2 tablespoons margarine

- Preheat oven to 375°F. Season the chops with pepper, coat lightly with flour, and then egg substitute. Melt 2 tablespoons margarine ·in an ovenproof 10-inch skillet over medium-high heat; add rosemary. Arrange the chops in the skillet and brown on both sides, about 5 to 10 minutes per side. Place skillet in the oven for 12 minutes.

- For sauce, melt 1 tablespoon margarine in a small saucepan over low heat. Add flour and stir constantly for 2 minutes. Whisk in milk and heat until thickened, stirring constantly. Season with white pepper and stir in wine. In a large skillet, sauté mushrooms in 2 tablespoons margarine over high heat until juices are rendered, about 5 minutes. Stir into sauce. Keep warm.

- Transfer chops to plates and top with mushroom sauce. Serve at once.

PER SERVING: 538 CALORIES			
MENU EXCHANGE PATTERN			
Dairy	—	Fruit	—
Bread	1½	Meat	4
Fat	4½	Veg.	—
NUTRITIONAL INFORMATION			
Carbohydrate	19	g	
Protein	34	g	
Total fat	35	g	
Saturated fat	10.8	g	
Cholesterol	122	mg	
Sodium	146	mg	
Potassium	738	mg	
Fiber	0.7	g	
Calcium	83	mg	
Iron	5.4	mg	

Spinach Noodles with Tomatoes

1 tablespoon safflower oil
2 cloves garlic, minced
¹⁄₄ cup coarsely chopped fresh
*   basil*
2 large tomatoes, peeled,
*   seeded, and cut in 1-inch*
*   cubes*

Black pepper
¹⁄₂ teaspoon sugar
8 ounces spinach noodles
*   (without eggs)*
1 tablespoon margarine

PER SERVING: 191 CALORIES			
MENU EXCHANGE PATTERN			
Dairy	—	Fruit	—
Bread	2	Meat	—
Fat	1	Veg.	1
NUTRITIONAL INFORMATION			
Carbohydrate		32	g
Protein		6	g
Total fat		4	g
Saturated fat		0.7	g
Cholesterol		0	mg
Sodium		5	mg
Potassium		0	mg
Fiber		0.4	g
Calcium		25	mg
Iron		0	mg

- Heat the safflower oil in a 9-inch skillet over medium-high heat. Add the garlic and cook for 1 minute. Add basil, tomatoes, pepper, and sugar and heat through.

- Bring 2 quarts water to a boil. Add noodles and cook until *al dente*. Drain and add margarine, tossing to coat. Divide noodles among plates and top with tomato mixture.

Pears Poached in Burgundy

6 large Bartlett or Bosc pears
2 cups red wine
¹⁄₂ cup sugar

1 stick cinnamon
2 whole cloves

PER SERVING: 178 CALORIES			
MENU EXCHANGE PATTERN			
Dairy	—	Fruit	1
Bread	2	Meat	—
Fat	—	Veg.	—
NUTRITIONAL INFORMATION			
Carbohydrate		42	g
Protein		1	g
Total fat		1	g
Saturated fat		0	g
Cholesterol		0	mg
Sodium		2	mg
Potassium		226	mg
Fiber		2.3	g
Calcium		20	mg
Iron		0.5	mg

- Peel pears, halve lengthwise, and scoop out the cores. Bring wine to a boil in a large nonaluminum saucepan with sugar, cloves, and cinnamon. Add pear halves and simmer until fruit is tender but not mushy, about 15 minutes. Transfer pears to a serving dish; discard cinnamon and cloves. Boil liquid slowly until reduced to a thick syrup, then pour over the pears. Serve hot or cold.

MEAT

8

Crab Claws with Cocktail Sauce

Tomato Niçoise

Grilled Veal Chops

Peas and Carrots

Yogurt with Raspberries

Serves 6

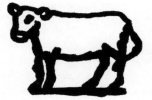

PER SERVING: 577 CALORIES			
MENU EXCHANGE PATTERN			
Dairy	½	Fruit	1
Bread	½	Meat	2½
Fat	4½	Veg.	5
NUTRITIONAL INFORMATION			
Carbohydrate	45	g	
Protein	41	g	
Total fat	28	g	
Saturated fat	8.5	g	
Cholesterol	142	mg	
Sodium	663	mg	
Potassium	1739	mg	
Fiber	6.4	g	
Calcium	349	mg	
Iron	6.3	mg	

Crab Claws with Cocktail Sauce

½ cup catsup
½ cup chili sauce
1 teaspoon prepared
  horseradish
2 drops Tabasco sauce or to
  taste

2 drops Worcestershire sauce
1 tablespoon lemon juice
30 crab claws, cooked and
  chilled

- Combine all ingredients except crab and refrigerate until well chilled. Serve sauce with crab claws.

PER SERVING: 79 CALORIES		
MENU EXCHANGE PATTERN		
Dairy . . . . . —	Fruit . . . . . —	
Bread . . . . —	Meat 1	
Fat . . . . —	Veg. 1	
NUTRITIONAL IFORMATION		
Carbohydrate 6		g
Protein 10		g
Total fat 1		g
Saturated fat 0		g
Cholesterol 56		mg
Sodium 522		mg
Potassium 141		mg
Fiber 0.4		g
Calcium 31		mg
Iron . . . . 0.7 mg		

Tomato Niçoise

6 leaves lettuce
3 tomatoes, sliced
1 avocado, peeled, pitted, and
  thinly sliced

12 artichoke hearts, cooked
6 tablespoons Tarragon
  Dressing (recipe follows)

- On 6 individual salad plates, arrange lettuce leaves, tomato slices, avocado slices, and 2 artichoke hearts. Drizzle dressing over and serve.

Note: To reduce fat, eliminate avocado from salad. Adjusted analysis: calories = 72; exchange = 3 Vegetable. To further reduce fat, substitute a commercial low-calorie dressing. Adjusted analysis for dressing: calories = 16; exchange = ½ Fat.

PER SERVING: 117 CALORIES		
MENU EXCHANGE PATTERN		
Dairy . . . . . —	Fruit . . . . . —	
Bread . . . . —	Meat . . . . . —	
Fat 1	Veg. 3	
NUTRITION INFORMATION		
Carbohydrate 17		g
Protein 4		g
Total fat 6		g
Saturated fat 0.8		g
Cholesterol 0		mg
Sodium 36		mg
Potassium 723		mg
Fiber 3.6		g
Calcium 66		mg
Iron . . . . 1.8 mg		

Tarragon Dressing

6 tablespoons safflower oil
6 tablespoons white wine
  vinegar

½ teaspoon dried tarragon
½ teaspoon black pepper
½ teaspoon dry mustard

- Combine all ingredients and blend well. Makes ¾ cup; 1 serving = 1 tablespoon.

PER SERVING: 61 CALORIES		
MENU EXCHANGE PATTERN		
Dairy . . . . . —	Fruit . . . . . —	
Bread . . . . —	Meat . . . . . —	
Fat 1½	Veg. . . . . . —	
NUTRITIONAL INFORMATION		
Carbohydrate 0		g
Protein 0		g
Total fat 7		g
Saturated fat 0.6		g
Cholesterol 0		mg
Sodium 0		mg
Potassium 9		mg
Fiber 0		g
Calcium 1		mg
Iron . . . . 0.1 mg		

Grilled Veal Chops

6 veal chops, 4 ounces each,
*   well trimmed*
½ teaspoon dried rosemary
2 tablespoons lemon juice
Pinch of garlic powder

- Sprinkle veal chops with rosemary, lemon juice, and garlic powder. Grill over medium heat until cooked to desired doneness, about 6 to 8 minutes on each side.

PER SERVING: 180 CALORIES		
MENU EXCHANGE PATTERN		
Dairy ..... —	Fruit ..... —	
Bread .... —	Meat 2½	
Fat 1	Veg. ...... —	
NUTRITIONAL INFORMATION		
Carbohydrate 0	g	
Protein 16	g	
Total fat 12	g	
Saturated fat 5.8	g	
Cholesterol 79	mg	
Sodium 57	mg	
Potassium 262	mg	
Fiber 0	g	
Calcium 9	mg	
Iron 2.4	mg	

Peas and Carrots

2 cups peas
4 medium carrots, sliced
Pinch of nutmeg

- Cook peas and carrots separately in a small amount of boiling water until just tender. Drain. Toss lightly and sprinkle with nutmeg.

PER SERVING: 61 CALORIES		
MENU EXCHANGE PATTERN		
Dairy ..... —	Fruit ..... —	
Bread .... ½	Meat ..... —	
Fat .... —	Veg. 1	
NUTRITIONAL INFORMATION		
Carbohydrate 12	g	
Protein 3	g	
Total fat 0	g	
Saturated fat 0	g	
Cholesterol 0	mg	
Sodium 24	mg	
Potassium 316	mg	
Fiber 1.5	g	
Calcium 31	mg	
Iron 1.2	mg	

Yogurt with Raspberries

1 teaspoon vanilla extract
1 cup plain low-fat yogurt
1½ cups raspberries

- Stir vanilla into yogurt and spoon into dessert dishes. Top with raspberries and serve.

PER SERVING: 87 CALORIES		
MENU EXCHANGE PATTERN		
Dairy ...... ½	Fruit 1	
Bread .... —	Meat ..... —	
Fat .... —	Veg. ...... —	
NUTRITIONAL INFORMATION		
Carbohydrate 12	g	
Protein 6	g	
Total fat 2	g	
Saturated fat 1.3	g	
Cholesterol 69	mg	
Sodium 79	mg	
Potassium 311	mg	
Fiber 0.9	g	
Calcium 213	mg	
Iron 0.3	mg	

MEAT

9

Squash Casserole

Veal Grillades

Garlic Grits

Fresh Figs with Coffee Ice Milk

Serves 6

PER SERVING: 879 CALORIES

MENU EXCHANGE PATTERN

Dairy . . . . . . ½	Fruit 2
Bread 3	Meat 5
Fat 2½	Veg. 5

NUTRITIONAL INFORMATION

Carbohydrate 98	g
Protein 43	g
Total fat 31	g
Saturated fat 7.1	g
Cholesterol 93	mg
Sodium 1340	mg
Potassium 1723	mg
Fiber 3.8	g
Calcium 572	mg
Iron 6.2	mg

Squash Casserole

1 1/2 pounds yellow squash, sliced
1/2 green bell pepper, cored, seeded, and chopped
1 small onion, chopped
1/4 teaspoon cayenne pepper
4 egg substitutes

4 ounces low-fat American-style cheese, grated
1/8 teaspoon garlic powder
1/2 cup sliced water chestnuts, drained
1 tablespoon margarine, melted
1/2 cup fresh breadcrumbs

- Preheat oven to 350°F. Steam squash, bell pepper, and onion together until tender, about 5 to 10 minutes. Drain thoroughly. Combine all remaining ingredients except breadcrumbs and add to vegetables. Pour into an ungreased 2-quart dish. Top with crumbs. Bake until crumbs are golden, about 30 minutes. Serve hot.

PER SERVING: 150 CALORIES

MENU EXCHANGE PATTERN

Dairy	—	Fruit	—
Bread	—	Meat	1
Fat	1/2	Veg.	3

NUTRITIONAL INFORMATION

Carbohydrate	15	g
Protein	12	g
Total fat	5	g
Saturated fat	0.7	g
Cholesterol	.6	mg
Sodium	531	mg
Potassium	488	mg
Fiber	1	g
Calcium	209	mg
Iron	1.8 mg	

Veal Grillades

1 1/2 pounds veal round with bones, cut 1/2-inch thick
5 tablespoons safflower oil
1/4 cup all-purpose flour
1 cup chopped onion
2 cups chopped green onion
3/4 cup chopped celery
1 1/2 cup chopped green bell pepper
2 cloves garlic, minced

1 cup water
2 cups chopped peeled tomato
1 cup red wine
1 teaspoon black pepper
2 bay leaves
1/2 teaspoon Tabasco sauce
1/2 teaspoon dried tarragon
2/3 teaspoon dried thyme
3 tablespoons chopped fresh parsley

- Remove all fat from veal. Cut meat into serving pieces and pound to 1/4-inch thickness. In a Dutch oven, brown meat well in 1 tablespoon safflower oil over medium-high heat. Transfer to a platter. Add remaining oil and flour to Dutch oven and stir constantly over high heat for about 10 minutes to make a dark brown roux. Add onion, green onion, celery, green pepper, and garlic and sauté until limp. Add water, tomato, and wine and cook, stirring, for 5 minutes. Return meat to Dutch oven and add pepper, bay leaves, and Tabasco. Reduce heat, add tarragon and thyme, and simmer for 1 hour. Stir in parsley. Let cool, then refrigerate overnight. Skim fat and reheat before serving.

PER SERVING: 353 CALORIES

MENU EXCHANGE PATTERN

Dairy	—	Fruit	—
Bread	1/2	Meat	3
Fat	2	Veg.	2

NUTRITIONAL INFORMATION

Carbohydrate	12	g
Protein	20	g
Total fat	22	g
Saturated fat	6	g
Cholesterol	79	mg
Sodium	89	mg
Potassium	629	mg
Fiber	1	g
Calcium	42	mg
Iron	3.5 mg	

Garlic Grits

1 cup grits
2 cups water
4 ounces low-sodium skim-milk
    cheddar cheese, grated

1 tablespoon margarine
2 cloves garlic, pressed
1/8 teaspoon cayenne pepper

- Cook grits in water according to package directions. Reduce heat to low and add all remaining ingredients, mixing well until all cheese has melted. Serve immediately.

PER SERVING: 122 CALORIES
MENU EXCHANGE PATTERN

Dairy	—	Fruit	—
Bread	1	Meat	1
Fat	—	Veg.	—

NUTRITIONAL INFORMATION

Carbohydrate	15	g
Protein	6	g
Total fat	3	g
Saturated fat	0.3	g
Cholesterol	.6	mg
Sodium	655	mg
Potassium	82	mg
Fiber	0.1	g
Calcium	125	mg
Iron	0.4	mg

Fresh Figs with Coffee Ice Milk

4 cups skim milk
1 cup sugar
1/2 cup Kahlúa
1 teaspoon vanilla extract

1/2 cup brewed espresso coffee
16 fresh figs
Ground cinnamon

- Combine milk, sugar, Kahlúa, vanilla, and coffee and stir until sugar is dissolved. Churn in ice cream maker according to manufacturer's instructions.

- Split figs in half and sprinkle with cinnamon. Serve in dessert dishes with ice milk. Makes about 1½ quarts ice milk; 1 serving = about ¾ cup ice milk.

PER SERVING: 254 CALORIES
MENU EXCHANGE PATTERN

Dairy	½	Fruit	2
Bread	2	Meat	—
Fat	—	Veg.	—

NUTRITIONAL INFORMATION

Carbohydrate	56	g
Protein	5	g
Total fat	1	g
Saturated fat	0.2	g
Cholesterol	2	mg
Sodium	65	mg
Potassium	524	mg
Fiber	1.5	g
Calcium	196	mg
Iron	0.5	mg

MEAT

10

Fettuccine Salad with Tomatillo-Herb Dressing

Paillard of Veal with Lemon and Tarragon

Sauterne Granita with Kiwi Coulis

Serves 6

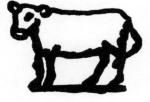

PER SERVING: 715 CALORIES			
MENU EXCHANGE PATTERN			
Dairy	—	Fruit	½
Bread	5	Meat	3
Fat	3	Veg.	2
NUTRITIONAL INFORMATION			
Carbohydrate	73	g	
Protein	31	g	
Total fat	26	g	
Saturated fat	6.6	g	
Cholesterol	99	mg	
Sodium	138	mg	
Potassium	1389	mg	
Fiber	2	g	
Calcium	86	mg	
Iron	6.4	mg	

Fettuccine Salad with Tomatillo-Herb Dressing

1 cup red wine vinegar
1 cup rice vinegar
2 cups water
$1/2$ cup fresh dill
$1^{1}/_{2}$ teaspoons white
   peppercorns
4 cloves garlic, chopped
1 cup cauliflower florets
2 carrots, sliced into julienne

1 cup zucchini sliced into
   julienne
1 cup turnips sliced into
   julienne
1 cup red bell pepper sliced
   into julienne
3 cups cooked fettuccine
   (without eggs)

Tomatillo-Herb Dressing

3 tomatillos, or 1 small red
   tomato
1 tablespoon chopped shallot
$1/4$ cup safflower oil

$1/4$ cup low-sodium tomato juice
2 tablespoons chopped fresh
   basil

- Combine vinegars, water, dill, peppercorns, and garlic in a nonaluminum saucepan, bring to a boil and simmer for 5 minutes. Let cool. Add vegetables and marinate for 2 days.

- Drop tomatillos into boiling water for 10 to 15 seconds; drain. Peel and puree in a blender. Add shallot, oil, tomato juice, and basil and blend well.

- Drain marinated vegetables, toss with fettuccine and dressing, and serve.

PER SERVING: 266 CALORIES			
MENU EXCHANGE PATTERN			
Dairy	—	Fruit	—
Bread	2	Meat	—
Fat	2	Veg.	2
NUTRITIONAL INFORMATION			
Carbohydrate		41	g
Protein		6	g
Total fat		10	g
Saturated fat		0.8	g
Cholesterol		0	mg
Sodium		55	mg
Potassium		476	mg
Fiber		1	g
Calcium		47	mg
Iron		2.4	mg

Paillard of Veal with Lemon and Tarragon

6 pieces of veal butt or veal top round, 5 ounces each
Black pepper
3½ cups thinly sliced Idaho potatoes

2 tablespoons safflower oil
1 cup lemon juice
¼ cup chopped fresh tarragon

- Place each piece of veal between 2 large squares of plastic wrap or wax paper and flatten with the flat side of a large knife or any heavy, flat object. Season with pepper and broil over mesquite just until cooked through, about 5 to 10 minutes.

- Sauté the potatoes in safflower oil over medium-high heat until tender, about 10 minutes, turning frequently. Heat lemon juice and tarragon together. Place veal in center of heated platter, surround with potatoes, and pour lemon juice and tarragon over the meat. Serve immediately.

PER SERVING: 313 CALORIES		
MENU EXCHANGE PATTERN		
Dairy ..... —	Fruit ..... —	
Bread 1½	Meat 3	
Fat 1	Veg. .... —	
NUTRITIONAL INFORMATION		
Carbohydrate 18		g
Protein 24		g
Total fat 16		g
Saturated fat 6		g
Cholesterol 99		mg
Sodium 79		mg
Potassium 758		mg
Fiber 0.4		g
Calcium 21		mg
Iron 3.8		mg

Sauterne Granita with Kiwi Coulis

4 very ripe kiwifruit
2 cups sauterne or other sweet dessert wine
¾ cup water
6 large strawberries, hulled and sliced (garnish)

- Puree kiwifruit in a blender and pass through a fine sieve to make coulis. Mix wine and water and freeze in an ice cream maker or freezer, stirring frequently until frozen into crystals to make granita.

- Divide coulis among individual plates and set 2 scoops of granita on top. Garnish with sliced strawberries.

PER SERVING: 136 CALORIES		
MENU EXCHANGE PATTERN		
Dairy ..... —	Fruit ......½	
Bread 1½	Meat ..... —	
Fat .... —	Veg. .... —	
NUTRITIONAL INFORMATION		
Carbohydrate 13		g
Protein 0		g
Total fat 0		g
Saturated fat 0		g
Cholesterol 0		mg
Sodium 3		mg
Potassium 155		mg
Fiber 0.4		g
Calcium 18		mg
Iron 0.2		mg

MEAT

11

Oysters Baccarat

Rack of Lamb Lafayette

Tarragon Potatoes

Peas and Onions

Fruit in Cassis

Serves 6

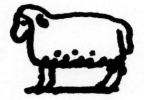

PER SERVING: 882 CALORIES		
MENU EXCHANGE PATTERN		
Dairy . . . . . —	Fruit 1	
Bread 5	Meat 4½	
Fat 4½	Veg. 2	
NUTRITIONAL INFORMATION		
Carbohydrate 80	g	
Protein 41	g	
Total fat 37	g	
Saturated fat 22.4	g	
Cholesterol 142	mg	
Sodium 585	mg	
Potassium 1799	mg	
Fiber 3.3	g	
Calcium 222	mg	
Iron 7.4	mg	

Oysters Baccarat

1 tablespoon margarine
1 tablespoon all-purpose flour
½ cup skim milk
1 cup sliced mushrooms
1 small shallot, chopped
1 teaspoon margarine

½ cup dry white wine
1 teaspoon lemon juice
Black pepper
12 whole oysters
2 ounces low-fat Monterey
   Jack-style cheese, grated

- Melt 1 tablespoon margarine in a small saucepan over low heat. Add flour and cook, stirring constantly, until bubbly. Stir in milk and cook until thickened. Let cool.

- In a medium skillet, sauté mushrooms and shallot in 1 teaspoon margarine over medium-high heat until moisture has evaporated, about 5 minutes. Add wine and lemon juice, cover, and cook over medium-low heat for 5 minutes.

- Stir in milk and flour mixture and simmer for 10 minutes. Add pepper to taste and cool. Chop the mixture. Shuck oysters, reserving half the shells. Bring 1 quart water to a boil, then add oysters and simmer over low heat until oysters change from translucent to opaque, about 5 minutes. Drain.

- Preheat oven to 350°F. Return oysters to half shells, cover with mushroom mixture and top with cheese. Bake until golden brown and cheese has melted, about 5 minutes. Serve immediately.

PER SERVING: 102 CALORIES

MENU EXCHANGE PATTERN

Dairy	—	Fruit	—
Bread	½	Meat	1
Fat	—	Veg.	—

NUTRITIONAL INFORMATION

Carbohydrate	6	g
Protein	7	g
Total fat	4	g
Saturated fat	0.4	g
Cholesterol	22	mg
Sodium	242	mg
Potassium	190	mg
Fiber	0.1	g
Calcium	127	mg
Iron	2.3	mg

Rack of Lamb Lafayette

3 racks of lamb, trimmed of all
   visible fat (2¼ pounds lean
   meat)
4 cloves garlic, chopped
1 tablespoon chopped fresh
   mint
1 teaspoon dried thyme
1 teaspoon dried rosemary

2 bay leaves, crushed
Black pepper
¼ cup safflower oil
¼ cup Dijon-style mustard
1 tablespoon dry white wine
1 cup fresh breadcrumbs
Mint sprigs (garnish)

- Have the butcher cut off the spine bone of the racks of lamb. Cut out meat halfway down between rib bones.

- Rub racks of lamb with garlic, mint, thyme, rosemary, bay leaves, and pepper. Place in a large bowl, add safflower oil, cover, and marinate in the refrigerator for at least 2 days.

- Preheat oven to 425°F. Cut each rack in half and wrap rib bones with margarine-coated wax paper so they do not burn. Place meat in a roasting pan and roast for 30 minutes.

Meanwhile, mix the mustard with the wine. Discard the greased paper. Brush mustard mixture over the meat and coat with breadcrumbs.

- Stand racks up in pan propped against each other. Reduce oven temperature to 350°F and return meat to oven for 10 minutes to brown crumbs.

- Stand meat on platter, garnish with mint and serve.

PER SERVING: 418 CALORIES			
MENU EXCHANGE PATTERN			
Dairy	—	Fruit	—
Bread	1	Meat	3½
Fat	3½	Veg.	—

NUTRITIONAL INFORMATION		
Carbohydrate	13	g
Protein	26	g
Total fat	28	g
Saturated fat	21	g
Cholesterol	120	mg
Sodium	333	mg
Potassium	434	mg
Fiber	0.2	g
Calcium	42	mg
Iron	2.5	mg

Tarragon Potatoes

6 large Idaho potatoes
1 tablespoons margarine,
  melted
1½ teaspoons finely chopped
  fresh tarragon

PER SERVING: 162 CALORIES			
MENU EXCHANGE PATTERN			
Dairy	—	Fruit	—
Bread	2	Meat	—
Fat	½	Veg.	—

NUTRITIONAL INFORMATION		
Carbohydrate	33	g
Protein	4	g
Total fat	2	g
Saturated fat	0.4	g
Cholesterol	0	mg
Sodium	6	mg
Potassium	782	mg
Fiber	1.2	g
Calcium	14	mg
Iron	1.1	mg

- Cut the potatoes in half crosswise, then halve lengthwise. Using a paring knife, cut potatoes into small barrel-shaped pieces. Cook in boiling water until easily pierced with a knife, about 5 minutes. Drain, refresh under cold water and drain well. Melt the margarine in a large skillet over high heat. Add the potatoes and sauté for 1 minute. Add tarragon, cook 1 more minute, and serve.

Peas and Onions

2 cups uncooked peas
1 quart boiling water
1 cup sliced green onion (white
  part only)

1 tablespoon margarine, melted
White pepper

PER SERVING: 64 CALORIES			
MENU EXCHANGE PATTERN			
Dairy	—	Fruit	—
Bread	—	Meat	—
Fat	½	Veg.	2

NUTRITIONAL INFORMATION		
Carbohydrate	8	g
Protein	3	g
Total fat	2	g
Saturated fat	0.3	g
Cholesterol	0	mg
Sodium	2	mg
Potassium	192	mg
Fiber	1.2	g
Calcium	22	mg
Iron	1.1	mg

- Cook peas in 1 quart boiling water until tender, about 5 minutes. In a small saucepan, sauté green onion in margarine over medium-low heat until translucent, about 5 minutes. Drain peas and add to onion. Mix well over low heat and serve immediately.

Floating Island with
Orange Sauce;
recipe page 353

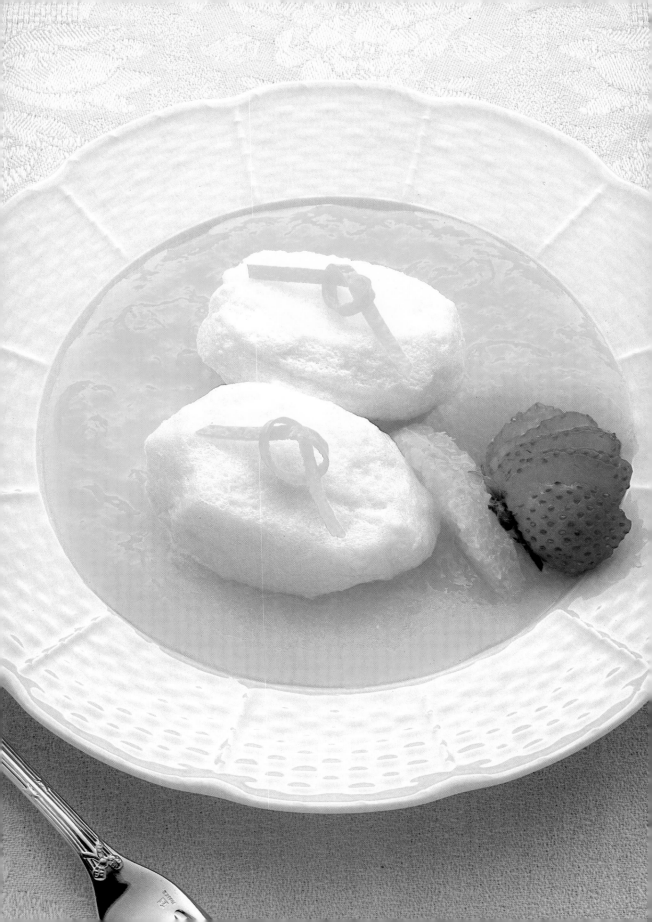

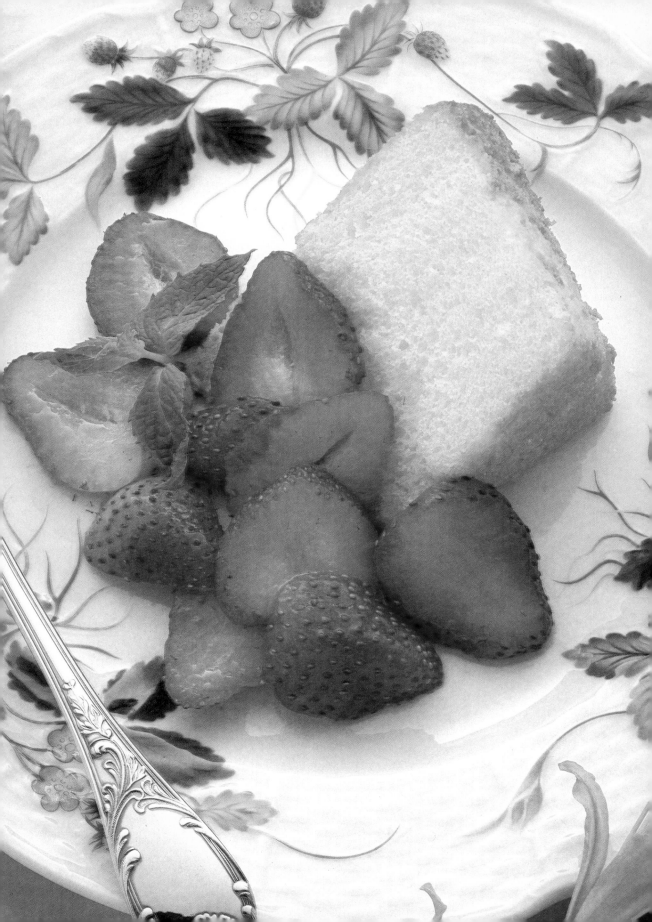

Fruit in Cassis

3 cups hulled and sliced
   strawberries
2 cups seedless green grapes or
   halved and seeded purple
   grapes

¼ cup sugar
½ cup crème de cassis
½ cup (about) white wine

- Mix the strawberries, grapes, and sugar in a large bowl. Stir in the cassis and add enough white wine to just cover the fruit. Refrigerate until ready to serve.

Note: For variation, omit the strawberries and grapes. Use a combination of 4 cups diced honeydew melon or cantaloupe, peach slices, apricot halves, and raspberries. Another variation is to use port in place of the crème de cassis and white wine. Add 2 cinnamon sticks and 4 whole cloves. Refrigerate for several hours.

PER SERVING: 137 CALORIES		
MENU EXCHANGE PATTERN		
Dairy . . . . . —	Fruit 1	
Bread . . . . . ½	Meat . . . . . —	
Fat . . . . —	Veg. . . . . . . —	
NUTRITIONAL INFORMATION		
Carbohydrate 19	g
Protein 1	g
Total fat 0	g
Saturated fat 0	g
Cholesterol 0	mg
Sodium 2	mg
Potassium 201	mg
Fiber 0.6	g
Calcium 17	mg
Iron 0.4	mg

*Angel Food Cake with
Marinated Strawberries;
recipe page 356*

MEAT

12

Marinated Oyster Salad with Corn and Bell Pepper Pickle

Lentil Soup with Fennel and Spinach

Brochette of Lamb

Wild Rice

Berries in Red Wine Jelly

Serves 8

PER SERVING: 880 CALORIES		
MENU EXCHANGE PATTERN		
Dairy . . . . . —	Fruit 1	
Bread 4½	Meat 4	
Fat 5	Veg. 4	
NUTRITIONAL INFORMATION		
Carbohydrate 59	g	
Protein 46	g	
Total fat 39	g	
Saturated fat 12.6	g	
Cholesterol 135	mg	
Sodium 965	mg	
Potassium 1356	mg	
Fiber 2.9	g	
Calcium 184	mg	
Iron 8.9	mg	

Marinated Oyster Salad with Corn and Bell Pepper Pickle

1 pint red wine vinegar
1 pint rice vinegar
1 quart water
1/4 bunch dill
1 tablespoon white peppercorns
8 cloves garlic, mashed
1 red bell pepper, cored, seeded, and quartered
1 green bell pepper, cored, seeded, and quartered

1 yellow bell pepper, cored, seeded, and quartered
1 cup cooked fresh or frozen corn kernels
16 oysters, shucked and drained
3 tablespoons safflower oil

Sherry Sauce

1 cup dry sherry
1 tablespoon grated fresh ginger

1 1/2 tablespoons sugar
1/3 cup low-sodium soy sauce
Black pepper

- Combine vinegars, water, dill, peppercorns, and garlic in a large nonaluminum saucepan, bring to a boil, and simmer for 5 minutes. Let cool. Add bell peppers and corn and marinate overnight in refrigerator. Drain peppers and corn, reserving marinade. Use liquid to marinate oysters for 30 minutes.

- Cut peppers into julienne strips. In a nonstick skillet, sauté peppers and corn in safflower oil over high heat until crisp-tender, about 5 minutes.

- Prepare sauce. Heat sherry with ginger for 2 minutes. Add sugar and soy sauce and bring to a boil. Add pepper to taste and boil over medium-high heat until reduced by 2/3. Keep warm.

- Add oysters to pan with vegetables and sauté for 2 minutes. Arrange oysters on bed of peppers and corn and top with sauce. Serve immediately.

PER SERVING: 164 CALORIES			
MENU EXCHANGE PATTERN			
Dairy	—	Fruit	—
Bread	1	Meat	1
Fat	1/2	Veg.	1

NUTRITIONAL INFORMATION		
Carbohydrate	13	g
Protein	7	g
Total fat	6	g
Saturated fat	0.5	g
Cholesterol	28	mg
Sodium	724	mg
Potassium	232	mg
Fiber	0.6	g
Calcium	60	mg
Iron	3.8	mg

Lentil Soup with Fennel and Spinach

1/3 cup coarsely chopped carrot
1/3 cup coarsely chopped celery
4 teaspoons safflower oil
1/3 cup chopped onion
2 teaspoons minced garlic
2 quarts Homemade Chicken
*   Stock (page 36)*

1 cup lentils
1 bay leaf
2 teaspoons fennel seed, tied in
*   a cheesecloth bag*
2/3 cup coarsely chopped
*   blanched spinach*
White pepper

- In a large nonstick skillet, sauté carrot and celery in oil over medium-high heat until soft, about 5 minutes. Add onion and garlic and cook until soft, 5 minutes. Add stock, lentils, bay leaf, and fennel seed pouch, bring to a slow boil, and simmer until lentils are soft, about 20 minutes. Stir in spinach and white pepper to taste. Remove fennel seed pouch and serve.

PER SERVING: 119 CALORIES	
MENU EXCHANGE PATTERN	
Dairy . . . . . — Fruit . . . . . —	
Bread . . . . . 1 Meat . . . . . —	
Fat . . . . ½ Veg. 2	
NUTRITIONAL INFORMATION	
Carbohydrate 12	g
Protein 10	g
Total fat 4	g
Saturated fat 0.2	g
Cholesterol 0	mg
Sodium 132	mg
Potassium 197	mg
Fiber 0.8	g
Calcium 23	mg
Iron . . . . 1.2 mg	

Brochette of Lamb

1 1/3 cups safflower oil
2 teaspoons chopped fresh
*   rosemary*
2 teaspoons chopped fresh
*   thyme*
1 tablespoon chopped fresh
*   basil*

1 tablespoon chopped fresh
*   oregano*
2 1/2 pounds leg of lamb, cut
*   into 1-inch cubes*
16 whole shiitake mushrooms
16 green onions, cut into
*   2-inch lengths*

- Combine oil and chopped herbs in a large bowl, add lamb, and marinate overnight.

- Alternate meat cubes, mushrooms, and green onions on skewers. Broil over mesquite charcoal, turning and basting with marinade, until lamb is cooked to desired doneness, about 10 to 15 minutes.

PER SERVING: 367 CALORIES	
MENU EXCHANGE PATTERN	
Dairy . . . . . — Fruit . . . . . —	
Bread . . . . — Meat 3	
Fat . . . . 4 Veg. 1	
NUTRITIONAL INFORMATION	
Carbohydrate 4	g
Protein 23	g
Total fat 28	g
Saturated fat 12	g
Cholesterol 105	mg
Sodium 83	mg
Potassium 602	mg
Fiber 0.7	g
Calcium 28	mg
Iron . . . . 2.3 mg	

Wild Rice

1¹/₃ cups wild rice
4 cups water

- Bring water to a boil in a large saucepan and add rice. Cover and simmer until all water is absorbed, about 45 to 50 minutes. Fluff with fork and serve.

PER SERVING: 94 CALORIES		
MENU EXCHANGE PATTERN		
Dairy . . . . . —	Fruit . . . . . —	
Bread 1	Meat . . . . . —	
Fat . . . . —	Veg. . . . . . . —	
NUTRITIONAL INFORMATION		
Carbohydrate 20		g
Protein 4		g
Total fat 0		g
Saturated fat 0		g
Cholesterol 0		mg
Sodium 2		mg
Potassium 59		mg
Fiber 0.3		g
Calcium 5		mg
Iron 1.1		mg

Berries in Red Wine Jelly

4 cups red wine
1¹/₂ envelopes unflavored gelatin
¹/₂ cup cold water
3 cups blackberries
3 cups raspberries

3 cups blueberries
1 cup plain low-fat yogurt
1 tablespoon chopped fresh mint
8 mint leaves (garnish)

- Boil wine until reduced to about 2½ cups. Meanwhile, sprinkle gelatin over water and let stand until softened, about 5 minutes. Add gelatin to the wine and stir until dissolved. Pour liquid into dessert glasses, adding the berries. Refrigerate for about 30 minutes. Combine the yogurt and mint and pour over the gelatin just before serving. Garnish with mint leaves.

PER SERVING: 136 CALORIES		
MENU EXCHANGE PATTERN		
Dairy . . . . . —	Fruit 1	
Bread 1½	Meat . . . . . —	
Fat . . . . —	Veg. . . . . . . —	
NUTRITIONAL INFORMATION		
Carbohydrate 10		g
Protein 3		g
Total fat 0		g
Saturated fat 0		g
Cholesterol 2		mg
Sodium 24		mg
Potassium 266		mg
Fiber 0.6		g
Calcium 68		mg
Iron 0.5		mg

MEAT

13

Sea Scallop and Lime Soup

Grilled Lamb Chops

Stuffed Baked Potatoes

Carrots and Onions

Cantaloupe with Berries

Serves 2

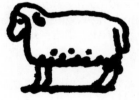

PER SERVING: 721 CALORIES			
MENU EXCHANGE PATTERN			
Dairy . . . . . . ½	Fruit 1½		
Bread 2½	Meat 3½		
Fat 5	Veg. 2		
NUTRITIONAL INFORMATION			
Carbohydrate 73		g	
Protein 35		g	
Total fat 32		g	
Saturated fat 14.7		g	
Cholesterol 89		mg	
Sodium 480		mg	
Potassium 2420		mg	
Fiber 4.5		g	
Calcium 167		mg	
Iron . . . . 5.3 mg			

Sea Scallop and Lime Soup

3 ounces sea scallops, half
   frozen
1/2 carrot, peeled
1 green onion
2 1/2 cups Homemade Chicken
   Stock (page 36)

2 slices fresh ginger
2 tablespoons dry sherry
White pepper
1/2 lime, thinly sliced

- Slice sea scallops into fine julienne. Slice carrot and onion into julienne. In a saucepan, bring stock to a boil and add ginger and sherry. Simmer over low heat for about 5 minutes, then discard ginger. Add carrot and cook for about 2 minutes. Add scallops and cook about 30 seconds. Finally add onion and cook another minute. Season to taste with white pepper, then transfer soup to bowls and garnish each with a lime slice.

PER SERVING: 74 CALORIES			
MENU EXCHANGE PATTERN			
Dairy	—	Fruit	—
Bread	—	Meat	1
Fat	—	Veg.	1
NUTRITIONAL INFORMATION			
Carbohydrate	7		g
Protein	7		g
Total fat	0		g
Saturated fat	0		g
Cholesterol	17		mg
Sodium	218		mg
Potassium	296		mg
Fiber	0.5		g
Calcium	33		mg
Iron	1.2		mg

Grilled Lamb Chops

1 tablespoon lemon juice
1 clove garlic, minced
1 teaspoon safflower oil

1/4 teaspoon dried mint leaves
4 lamb chops, 2 ounces each,
   trimmed of all visible fat

- Combine lemon juice, garlic, oil, and mint. Marinate chops in oil mixture for 30 minutes. Transfer from marinade to broiler pan or grill and cook, basting with marinade, to desired doneness.

Photo opposite page 307.

PER SERVING: 309 CALORIES			
MENU EXCHANGE PATTERN			
Dairy	—	Fruit	—
Bread	—	Meat	2 1/2
Fat	4	Veg.	—
NUTRITIONAL INFORMATION			
Carbohydrate	1		g
Protein	16		g
Total fat	26		g
Saturated fat	13.7		g
Cholesterol	70		mg
Sodium	56		mg
Potassium	266		mg
Fiber	0		g
Calcium	9		mg
Iron	1.1		mg

Stuffed Baked Potatoes

2 Idaho potatoes, baked
1/4 cup low-fat cottage cheese
1 teaspoon chopped fresh chives
White pepper

- Preheat oven to 325°F. Cut potatoes in half and carefully scoop out the pulp. Reserve 2 of the skins. Whip cottage cheese until smooth in a blender or food processor.

- Combine potato pulp, cottage cheese, chives, and pepper and blend well. Stuff into potato skins. Bake until heated through, about 20 minutes.

PER SERVING: 171 CALORIES			
MENU EXCHANGE PATTERN			
Dairy	1/2	Fruit	—
Bread	2	Meat	—
Fat	—	Veg.	—
NUTRITIONAL INFORMATION			
Carbohydrate	34		g
Protein	8		g
Total fat	1		g
Saturated fat	0.3		g
Cholesterol	2		mg
Sodium	121		mg
Potassium	812		mg
Fiber	1.2		g
Calcium	34		mg
Iron	1.2		mg

Carrots and Onions

2 teaspoons margarine
¼ onion, sliced
4 carrots, sliced into julienne

¼ cup water
2 tablespoons chopped fresh
  parsley

- Melt margarine in a nonstick skillet over medium-high heat. Add onion and carrots and sauté for 2 minutes, stirring constantly. Add water, cover and cook until vegetables are tender, about 10 minutes, stirring occasionally. Sprinkle with parsley and serve.

PER SERVING: 103 CALORIES

MENU EXCHANGE PATTERN

Dairy	—	Fruit	—
Bread	½	Meat	—
Fat	1	Veg.	1

NUTRITIONAL INFORMATION

Carbohydrate	16	g
Protein	2	g
Total fat	4	g
Saturated fat	0.7	g
Cholesterol	0	mg
Sodium	72	mg
Potassium	553	mg
Fiber	1.8	g
Calcium	68	mg
Iron	1.3	mg

Cantaloupe with Berries

½ cantaloupe, seeded
½ cup strawberries, sliced
1 kiwifruit, sliced

- Cut cantaloupe half in half again. Combine strawberries and kiwi. Place ¼ cup of sliced fruit in center of each cantaloupe wedge and serve.

PER SERVING: 64 CALORIES

MENU EXCHANGE PATTERN

Dairy	—	Fruit	1½
Bread	—	Meat	—
Fat	—	Veg.	—

NUTRITIONAL INFORMATION

Carbohydrate	15	g
Protein	2	g
Total fat	0	g
Saturated fat	0	g
Cholesterol	0	mg
Sodium	13	mg
Potassium	493	mg
Fiber	1	g
Calcium	23	mg
Iron	0.5	mg

MEAT

14

Marinated Cucumber and Mushroom Salad

Barley Soup

Broiled Pork Chops

Boiled Mustard Greens

Dilled Yellow Squash

Citrus Chiffon Cups

Serves 4

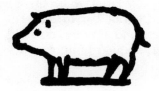

PER SERVING: 704 CALORIES		
MENU EXCHANGE PATTERN		
Dairy . . . . . —	Fruit . . . . . —	
Bread 4	Meat 2½	
Fat 3	Veg. 5½	
NUTRITIONAL INFORMATION		
Carbohydrate 88	g	
Protein 36	g	
Total fat 26	g	
Saturated fat 8	g	
Cholesterol 66	mg	
Sodium 347	mg	
Potassium 2044	mg	
Fiber 4.5	g	
Calcium 349	mg	
Iron 8.7	mg	

Marinated Cucumber and Mushroom Salad

2 cups water
3 tablespoons commercial low-
calorie Italian dressing
1 stalk fennel, minced
1 stalk celery, minced
A few coriander seeds
4 peppercorns

2 cucumbers, peeled, seeded,
and sliced diagonally
12 mushrooms, sliced ¹/₈ inch
thick
4 lettuce leaves
10 cherry tomatoes, halved

- Combine water, Italian dressing, fennel, celery, coriander, and peppercorns in a saucepan and bring to boil. Add cucumber slices and simmer 2 minutes. Remove with a slotted spoon. Add mushrooms to saucepan and simmer 2 minutes; remove. Strain liquid and pour over cucumbers and mushrooms. Chill for at least 2 hours. Arrange cucumbers and mushrooms attractively on lettuce leaves and garnish with halved cherry tomatoes.

PER SERVING: 39 CALORIES

MENU EXCHANGE PATTERN

Dairy	—	Fruit	—
Bread	—	Meat	—
Fat	—	Veg.	1½

NUTRITIONAL INFORMATION

Carbohydrate	6	g
Protein	2	g
Total fat	1	g
Saturated fat	0.1	g
Cholesterol	1	mg
Sodium	116	mg
Potassium	356	mg
Fiber	0.9	g
Calcium	31	mg
Iron	1.3	mg

Barley Soup

¹/₄ cup whole barley, washed
5 cups boiling water or
Homemade Chicken Stock
(page 36)
1 cup sliced carrot

¹/₂ cup diced celery
¹/₄ cup chopped onion
2 cups chopped peeled tomato
1 cup fresh or frozen peas
¹/₂ cup chopped fresh parsley

- Combine barley and water in a heavy large saucepan, cover and simmer until barley is tender, about 1 hour. Add remaining ingredients except parsley and simmer, covered, until vegetables are barely tender, about 10 minutes. Remove from heat, add parsley, and serve.

PER SERVING: 111 CALORIES

MENU EXCHANGE PATTERN

Dairy	—	Fruit	—
Bread	1	Meat	—
Fat	—	Veg.	2

NUTRITIONAL INFORMATION

Carbohydrate	23	g
Protein	5	g
Total fat	1	g
Saturated fat	0	g
Cholesterol	0	mg
Sodium	35	mg
Potassium	557	mg
Fiber	1.8	g
Calcium	57	mg
Iron	2.2	mg

Broiled Pork Chops

4 pork chops, 4 ounces each,
trimmed of all visible fat
2 garlic cloves, crushed
¹/₃ cup lemon juice

Black pepper
1 teaspoon dried oregano
¹/₄ teaspoon whole allspice

- Rub pork chops with mixture of garlic, lemon juice, pepper, oregano, and allspice. Broil until no longer pink in center, about 5 to 10 minutes. Serve immediately.

PER SERVING: 258 CALORIES

MENU EXCHANGE PATTERN

Dairy	—	Fruit	—
Bread	—	Meat	2½
Fat	2½	Veg.	—

NUTRITIONAL INFORMATION

Carbohydrate	1	g
Protein	17	g
Total fat	20	g
Saturated fat	7.3	g
Cholesterol	64	mg
Sodium	52	mg
Potassium	299	mg
Fiber	0	g
Calcium	5	mg
Iron	0.7	mg

Boiled Mustard Greens

1 pound mustard greens
  (about 4 cups)
1 teaspoon margarine
Black pepper

- Boil mustard greens in 1 quart water, covered, until tender, about 1 hour. Stir in margarine and pepper and serve.

PER SERVING: 44 CALORIES				
MENU EXCHANGE PATTERN				
Dairy	—		Fruit	—
Bread	—		Meat	—
Fat	½		Veg.	1
NUTRITIONAL INFORMATION				
Carbohydrate	6	g		
Protein	3	g		
Total fat	2	g		
Saturated fat	0.2	g		
Cholesterol	0	mg		
Sodium	36	mg		
Potassium	428	mg		
Fiber	1.3	g		
Calcium	208	mg		
Iron	3.4	mg		

Dilled Yellow Squash

2 cups yellow squash cut into   *1 teaspoon margarine*
  ¼-inch slices   *Pinch of white pepper*
⅓ cup chopped onion   *Pinch of dried dillweed*

- Steam sliced squash over boiling water until tender, about 4 to 5 minutes. Meanwhile, in a nonstick skillet sauté onion in margarine over medium heat until tender, about 5 minutes. Combine squash, onion, and seasonings and serve immediately.

PER SERVING: 26 CALORIES				
MENU EXCHANGE PATTERN				
Dairy	—		Fruit	—
Bread	—		Meat	—
Fat	—		Veg.	1
NUTRITIONAL INFORMATION				
Carbohydrate	4	g		
Protein	1	g		
Total fat	1	g		
Saturated fat	0.2	g		
Cholesterol	0	mg		
Sodium	2	mg		
Potassium	154	mg		
Fiber	0.5	g		
Calcium	22	mg		
Iron	0.3	mg		

Citrus Chiffon Cups

1 envelope unflavored gelatin   *½ cup orange juice*
¼ cup water   *½ teaspoon grated lemon rind*
½ cup sugar   *½ teaspoon grated orange rind*
2 egg substitutes   *4 egg whites*
½ cup lemon juice   *⅓ cup sugar*

- Soften gelatin in ¼ cup water, then mix gelatin and ½ cup sugar in a saucepan. Blend egg substitutes with fruit juices. Stir into gelatin mixture and bring just to a boil over medium heat. Remove from heat and stir in grated rind.

- Chill gelatin mixture stirring occasionally, until it mounds slightly when dropped from a spoon, about 20 minutes. Beat egg whites until soft peaks form. Gradually add ⅓ cup sugar and beat until egg whites form stiff peaks. Fold in gelatin mixture. Spoon into dessert dishes and chill until set, at least 30 minutes.

PER SERVING: 224 CALORIES				
MENU EXCHANGE PATTERN				
Dairy	—		Fruit	—
Bread	3		Meat	—
Fat	—		Veg.	—
NUTRITIONAL INFORMATION				
Carbohydrate	48	g		
Protein	7	g		
Total fat	1	g		
Saturated fat	0.2	g		
Cholesterol	0	mg		
Sodium	106	mg		
Potassium	250	mg		
Fiber	0	g		
Calcium	26	mg		
Iron	0.8	mg		

MEAT

15

Minestrone di Romagna

Saltimbocca

Spaghetti with Eggplant and Ricotta

Amaretto Coffee

Serves 4

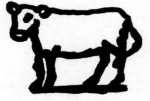

PER SERVING: 779 CALORIES

MENU EXCHANGE PATTERN

Dairy	—	Fruit	—
Bread	4	Meat	4
Fat	4	Veg.	2½

NUTRITIONAL INFORMATION

Carbohydrate	49	g
Protein	38	g
Total fat	38	g
Saturated fat	11	g
Cholesterol	121	mg
Sodium	500	mg
Potassium	1350	mg
Fiber	1.6	g
Calcium	163	mg
Iron	6.7	mg

Minestrone di Romagna

½ cup safflower oil
3 tablespoons margarine
1 cup thinly sliced onion
1 cup diced carrot
1 cup diced celery
2 cups diced peeled potatoes
2 cups diced zucchini
1 cup diced green beans
1½ cups fresh white beans (if
  available) or ¾ cup dried
  white beans, cooked

3 cups shredded cabbage,
  preferably Savoy
6 cups Homemade Chicken
  Stock (page 36) or meat
  stock
⅔ cup fresh Italian plum
  tomatoes, quartered
1 teaspoon dried basil
⅓ cup grated Parmesan cheese

- Combine the oil, margarine, and onion in a stockpot large enough for all the ingredients and cook over medium-low heat until the onion wilts and is pale gold in color but not browned. Add the carrot and cook for 2 to 3 minutes, stirring once or twice. Repeat with the celery, potatoes, zucchini, green beans, and white beans (if you are using fresh), cooking each vegetable for a few minutes and stirring. Then add the cabbage and cook for 6 minutes, giving the pot an occasional stir.

- Add the stock, tomatoes, and basil. Cover and simmer for about 3 hours (if necessary, you can stop the cooking at any time and resume it later on). Cook the soup until thick; if it is becoming too thick, add another cup of stock or water. Add the cooked dry beans (if you are not using fresh ones) 15 minutes before the soup is done. Swirl in the grated cheese just before turning off the heat. Makes about 2½ quarts; 1 serving = ¾ cup.

PER SERVING: 131 CALORIES		
MENU EXCHANGE PATTERN		
Dairy . . . . . —	Fruit . . . . . —	
Bread 1	Meat . . . . . —	
Fat 1	Veg. . . . . . . ½	
NUTRITIONAL INFORMATION		
Carbohydrate 11	g	
Protein 3	g	
Total fat 8	g	
Saturated fat 1.3	g	
Cholesterol 1	mg	
Sodium 62	mg	
Potassium 362	mg	
Fiber 0.8	g	
Calcium 60	mg	
Iron 0.1	mg	

Saltimbocca

1⅓ pounds veal scallops or
  boned, skinned chicken
  breasts
4 fresh sage leaves

4 thin slices prosciutto
2½ tablespoons margarine
6 tablespoons dry white wine

- Place veal between 2 sheets of plastic wrap and pound thin. Place a leaf of sage in the center of each piece of meat, then top with a thin slice of prosciutto. Fasten the prosciutto and sage to the meat with a toothpick (horizontally). Melt margarine in a skillet over medium heat. Add meat, prosciutto side down, and sauté almost to the point of browning, then turn and finish cooking (about 3 minutes total, a little more if using chicken). Pour in white wine during the last minute of cooking. Remove toothpick.

PER SERVING: 335 CALORIES		
MENU EXCHANGE PATTERN		
Dairy . . . . . —	Fruit . . . . . —	
Bread . . . . —	Meat 4	
Fat 2	Veg. . . . . . . —	
NUTRITIONAL INFORMATION		
Carbohydrate 1	g	
Protein 27	g	
Total fat 22	g	
Saturated fat 8.4	g	
Cholesterol 115	mg	
Sodium 274	mg	
Potassium 454	mg	
Fiber 0	g	
Calcium 18	mg	
Iron 3.8	mg	

Spaghetti with Eggplant and Ricotta

4 teaspoons safflower oil
1/3 cup very thinly sliced onion
4 cloves garlic, minced
1 1/3 cups fresh or low-sodium
   canned tomatoes, drained
   and cut into thin strips
1 small eggplant, peeled and
   cut into 1 1/2-inch cubes
1/4 teaspoon black pepper
1/3 pound spaghetti
2 tablespoons skim-milk ricotta
5 to 6 fresh basil leaves or
   2 tablespoons chopped fresh
   parsley
2 tablespoons grated Parmesan
   cheese

- Heat safflower oil in a saucepan over medium heat. Add onion and garlic and sauté for 2 minutes. Add tomatoes, eggplant, and pepper and simmer, stirring frequently, until eggplant is tender, about 15 minutes.

- Cook spaghetti until *al dente,* then drain and transfer to a warm serving bowl. Toss with eggplant sauce, ricotta, basil, and grated Parmesan cheese and serve immediately.

PER SERVING: 239 CALORIES		
MENU EXCHANGE PATTERN		
Dairy . . . . . —	Fruit . . . . . —	
Bread 2	Meat . . . . . . —	
Fat 1	Veg. 2	
NUTRITIONAL INFORMATION		
Carbohydrate 37	g	
Protein 8	g	
Total fat 7	g	
Saturated fat 1.3	g	
Cholesterol 4	mg	
Sodium 164	mg	
Potassium 401	mg	
Fiber 0.8	g	
Calcium 81	mg	
Iron 2	mg	

Amaretto Coffee

4 five-ounce cups dark-roast
   coffee
8 tablespoons amaretto

- Brew coffee by the desired method. Pour 1 ounce (2 tablespoons) amaretto into each coffee cup and fill with coffee. Serve immediately.

PER SERVING: 74 CALORIES		
MENU EXCHANGE PATTERN		
Dairy . . . . . —	Fruit . . . . . —	
Bread 1	Meat . . . . . —	
Fat . . . . —	Veg. . . . . . . —	
NUTRITIONAL INFORMATION		
Carbohydrate 0	g	
Protein 0	g	
Total fat 1	g	
Saturated fat 0	g	
Cholesterol 0	mg	
Sodium 0	mg	
Potassium 133	mg	
Fiber 0	g	
Calcium 4	mg	
Iron 0.2	mg	

MEAT

16

Sweet Potato Salad with Watercress

Grilled Pork Loin with Apple Butter

Braised Cabbage

Country Apple Tart

Serves 4

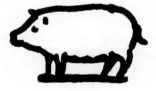

PER SERVING: 670 CALORIES			
MENU EXCHANGE PATTERN			
Dairy	—	Fruit	3½
Bread	3	Meat	2½
Fat	3½	Veg.	1
NUTRITIONAL INFORMATION			
Carbohydrate	90		g
Protein	23		g
Total fat	26		g
Saturated fat	7.9		g
Cholesterol	65		mg
Sodium	519		mg
Potassium	996		mg
Fiber	2.7		g
Calcium	97		mg
Iron	3		mg

Sweet Potato Salad with Watercress

4 small sweet potatoes with
*   skins*
4 sprigs watercress
4 teaspoons hazelnut oil
4 teaspoons lime juice

- Preheat oven to 350°F and roast sweet potatoes, turning frequently, until puffed and tender, about 1 hour. Cool potatoes to room temperature. Slice at a 45-degree angle and arrange on salad plates in pinwheel fashion. Place a sprig of watercress in the center of each pinwheel. Drizzle 1 teaspoon hazelnut oil and 1 teaspoon lime juice over potatoes and watercress.

PER SERVING: 203 CALORIES

MENU EXCHANGE PATTERN

Dairy	—	Fruit	1
Bread	2	Meat	—
Fat	1	Veg.	—

NUTRITIONAL INFORMATION

Carbohydrate	38	g
Protein	3	g
Total fat	5	g
Saturated fat	0.4	g
Cholesterol	0	mg
Sodium	14	mg
Potassium	365	mg
Fiber	1.3	g
Calcium	55	mg
Iron	1.1	mg

Grilled Pork Loin with Apple Butter

1 pound boneless pork loin,   *2 cloves garlic, minced*
*   trimmed of all visible fat*   *Black pepper*
2 teaspoons chopped fresh   *10 tablespoons apple butter*
*   rosemary*

- Preheat oven to 350°F. Rub pork loin with rosemary, garlic, and pepper. Place whole loin in oven and roast until cooked to medium or medium-well done, about 1½ hours, or until internal temperature is 185°F.

- Slice pork. Transfer slices to serving plates, arranging 4 to 5 slices into a fan on each plate. Add a small amount of water to roasting pan and scrape up juices. Pour drippings into a measuring cup and let stand until fat floats briefly, then skim. If juice is too thin, pour into small saucepan and boil until reduced to desired consistency. Drizzle juice over sliced pork. Place 2 tablespoons apple butter in center of fan of pork slices and serve.

PER SERVING: 345 CALORIES

MENU EXCHANGE PATTERN

Dairy	—	Fruit	2
Bread	—	Meat	2½
Fat	2½	Veg.	—

NUTRITIONAL INFORMATION

Carbohydrate	22	g
Protein	17	g
Total fat	20	g
Saturated fat	7.3	g
Cholesterol	65	mg
Sodium	52	mg
Potassium	409	mg
Fiber	0.5	g
Calcium	10	mg
Iron	0.9	mg

Braised Cabbage

1 medium head cabbage
   (about 2 cups shredded)
2/3 cup cider vinegar
1/2 teaspoon salt
4 teaspoons sugar

- Remove 12 outer leaves of cabbage and blanch in boiling water until flexible, about 1 minute. Drain. Chop inner leaves of cabbage. Transfer chopped cabbage to a large non-aluminum skillet. Add vinegar, salt, and sugar and cook over medium heat, stirring, until soft, about 5–10 minutes. Transfer 2 to 3 tablespoons of mixture to each blanched cabbage leaf and roll up jelly-roll fashion. Transfer cabbage rolls to a casserole and keep warm in the oven until serving time.

PER SERVING: 30 CALORIES		
MENU EXCHANGE PATTERN		
Dairy . . . . . —	Fruit . . . . . —	
Bread . . . . . —	Meat . . . . . —	
Fat . . . . —	Veg. 1	
NUTRITIONAL INFORMATION		
Carbohydrate 8	g	
Protein 0	g	
Total fat 0	g	
Saturated fat 0	g	
Cholesterol 0	mg	
Sodium 362	mg	
Potassium 122	mg	
Fiber 0.3	g	
Calcium 22	mg	
Iron 0.4	mg	

Country Apple Tart

1 1/2 cups all-purpose flour
1/2 teaspoon salt
3/4 teaspoon dry yeast
1/2 cup plus 1 1/2 teaspoons warm
   water

1/4 cup apple butter
3 tart green apples, cored and
   thinly sliced
2 tablespoons confectioners
   sugar

- Combine flour and salt in a large bowl. In a separate small bowl, combine yeast and warm water and let stand until yeast dissolves, about 5 minutes. Make a well in the flour mixture and add dissolved yeast. Mix well with a wooden spoon, then knead until dough is smooth and elastic, 5 to 10 minutes, adding a bit more flour or water as necessary.

- Return dough to the large bowl and cover with a cloth. Let rise until doubled in volume, about 1 hour. Punch down and let rise again until doubled, about 30 minutes.

- Roll dough into a 12-inch circle on a lightly floured board. Transfer to a 12-inch pizza pan. Spread with apple butter, then arrange sliced apples over top.

- Preheat oven to 450°F. Bake tart until golden brown, about 20 minutes. Remove from oven and sprinkle with confectioners sugar. Divide into 12 slices (about 2 3/4 inches wide) and serve warm. Leftovers can be reheated or served cold. Makes 12 servings; 1 serving = 1 slice.

PER SERVING: 91 CALORIES		
MENU EXCHANGE PATTERN		
Dairy . . . . . —	Fruit 1/2	
Bread 1	Meat . . . . . —	
Fat . . . . —	Veg. . . . . —	
NUTRITIONAL INFORMATION		
Carbohydrate 21	g	
Protein 2	g	
Total fat 0	g	
Saturated fat 0.2	g	
Cholesterol 0	mg	
Sodium 91	mg	
Potassium 100	mg	
Fiber 0.6	g	
Calcium 10	mg	
Iron 0.6	mg	

RABBIT AND GAME

1

Cauliflower-Asparagus Soup

Broiled Partridge

New Potatoes with Dillseed-Yogurt Sauce

Herbed Carrots

Raspberries with Zabaglione Sauce

Serves 4

PER SERVING: 973 CALORIES			
MENU EXCHANGE PATTERN			
Dairy	—	Fruit	2
Bread	4	Meat	8
Fat	2½	Veg.	2½

NUTRITIONAL INFORMATION		
Carbohydrate	89	g
Protein	70	g
Total fat	36	g
Saturated fat	5.2	g
Cholesterol	146	mg
Sodium	357	mg
Potassium	2430	mg
Fiber	6.7	g
Calcium	239	mg
Iron	6.9	mg

Cauliflower-Asparagus Soup

4 cups boiling water
2 cups cauliflower florets
2 cups chopped asparagus
1 tablespoon safflower oil
1 cup chopped onion
2 cloves garlic, minced

2 tablespoons all-purpose flour
2 cups Homemade Chicken
   Stock (page 36)
$1/4$ teaspoon ground nutmeg
$1/4$ teaspoon white pepper

- Bring the water to boil in a medium saucepan, add cauliflower florets and cook until tender, about 5 to 10 minutes. Remove cauliflower with slotted spoon and set aside. In the same water, cook asparagus until tender, about 5 minutes; drain and set aside. Reserve 1 cup of the liquid.

- Heat oil in a small skillet over medium heat and sauté onion and garlic until onion is translucent, about 5 minutes. Transfer to a blender. Add cauliflower, reserved liquid, and flour and process until smooth.

- Return pureed cauliflower to saucepan and bring to a simmer. Add stock and seasonings and simmer until slightly thickened, about 5 minutes. Add asparagus and heat through.

PER SERVING: 84 CALORIES		
MENU EXCHANGE PATTERN		
Dairy . . . . . —	Fruit . . . . . —	
Bread 1	Meat . . . . . —	
Fat . . . . ½	Veg. . . . . . . —	
NUTRITIONAL INFORMATION		
Carbohydrate 11	g	
Protein 4	g	
Total fat 4	g	
Saturated fat 0.3	g	
Cholesterol 0	mg	
Sodium 12	mg	
Potassium 328	mg	
Fiber 1.2	g	
Calcium 37	mg	
Iron . . . . 1.2 mg		

Broiled Partridge

2 partridge, $3/4$ pound each,
   dressed
$1/3$ cup safflower oil
$1/2$ teaspoon paprika

$1/2$ teaspoon dried thyme
$1/2$ cup chopped fresh parsley
$2/3$ cup cherry tomatoes

- Wash the partridge under cold running water and dry with a cheesecloth. Butterfly by cutting along the backbone of each bird with a sharp knife, then flatten so birds are spread open. Mix the oil with the paprika and thyme.

- Dip the birds into the oil mixture and grill on each side for 10 minutes. Wrap each in foil and cook for another 10 minutes, turning frequently. Arrange on a platter and garnish with parsley and cherry tomatoes.

PER SERVING: 471 CALORIES		
MENU EXCHANGE PATTERN		
Dairy . . . . . —	Fruit . . . . . —	
Bread . . . . —	Meat 7½	
Fat 1	Veg. . . . . ½	
NUTRITIONAL INFORMATION		
Carbohydrate 4	g	
Protein 54	g	
Total fat 26	g	
Saturated fat 3.7	g	
Cholesterol 144	mg	
Sodium 136	mg	
Potassium 623	mg	
Fiber 0.4	g	
Calcium 49	mg	
Iron . . . . 2.5 mg		

New Potatoes with Dillseed-Yogurt Sauce

1 1/2 pounds new potatoes
1/2 cup plain low-fat yogurt,
room temperature
1/8 teaspoon white pepper
1/2 teaspoon dillseed

- Peel potatoes and drop into a saucepan of boiling water. Cover, return to boil, and cook until tender, about 20 minutes. Combine yogurt, pepper, and dillseed. Drain potatoes and heat briefly to evaporate remaining water. Add yogurt mixture and toss potatoes to coat. Serve immediately.

PER SERVING: 147 CALORIES			
MENU EXCHANGE PATTERN			
Dairy	—	Fruit	—
Bread	2	Meat	—
Fat	—	Veg.	—
NUTRITIONAL INFORMATION			
Carbohydrate	31		g
Protein	5		g
Total fat	1		g
Saturated fat	0.3		g
Cholesterol	2		mg
Sodium	26		mg
Potassium	760		mg
Fiber	0.9		g
Calcium	64		mg
Iron	1.0		mg

Herbed Carrots

2 teaspoons margarine
1 clove garlic, minced
2 cups peeled, diagonally sliced carrots

1 cup water
2 teaspoons sugar
1/2 teaspoon dried rosemary
1/2 teaspoon white pepper

- Melt margarine in a saucepan over medium heat; add garlic and sauté until fragrant, about 2 minutes. Add carrots, water, and seasonings, cover and simmer until crisp-tender, about 10 to 20 minutes. Drain and serve.

PER SERVING: 93 CALORIES			
MENU EXCHANGE PATTERN			
Dairy	—	Fruit	—
Bread	—	Meat	—
Fat	1	Veg.	2
NUTRITIONAL INFORMATION			
Carbohydrate	14		g
Protein	1		g
Total fat	4		g
Saturated fat	0.7		g
Cholesterol	0		mg
Sodium	101		mg
Potassium	417		mg
Fiber	1.4		g
Calcium	46		mg
Iron	0.8		mg

Raspberries with Zabaglione Sauce

3 cups raspberries
2 egg substitutes
2 egg whites
1/3 cup sugar

2/3 cup dry Marsala
1/2 teaspoon vanilla extract
Grated rind of 1/2 lemon
4 sprigs mint (garnish)

- Divide raspberries among 4 champagne glasses. Combine egg substitutes, egg whites, sugar, and Marsala in the top of a double boiler and place over hot but not boiling water. Whisk constantly, scraping the sides and bottom, until the mixture begins to foam and becomes creamy, about 10 minutes. Blend in the vanilla and lemon rind and spoon over the raspberries. Garnish with mint and serve.

PER SERVING: 177 CALORIES			
MENU EXCHANGE PATTERN			
Dairy	—	Fruit	2
Bread	1	Meat	1/2
Fat	—	Veg.	—
NUTRITIONAL INFORMATION			
Carbohydrate	29		g
Protein	6		g
Total fat	2		g
Saturated fat	0.2		g
Cholesterol	0		mg
Sodium	82		mg
Potassium	302		mg
Fiber	2.8		g
Calcium	43		mg
Iron	1.4		mg

RABBIT AND GAME

2

Onion Soup Gratinée with Calvados

Breast of Pheasant with
Mushrooms and Cognac

Zucchini Casserole

Bread Pudding with Hot Whiskey Sauce

Serves 8

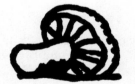

PER SERVING: 1052 CALORIES		
MENU EXCHANGE PATTERN		
Dairy 2	Fruit 1	
Bread 2½	Meat 6½	
Fat 4½	Veg. 3½	
NUTRITIONAL INFORMATION		
Carbohydrate 78	g	
Protein 61	g	
Total fat 49	g	
Saturated fat 9.2	g	
Cholesterol 138	mg	
Sodium 1212	mg	
Potassium 1285	mg	
Fiber 2.4	g	
Calcium 448	mg	
Iron . . . . 4.8 mg		

Onion Soup Gratinée with Calvados

2 large onions, thinly sliced
2 tablespoons margarine
1/4 teaspoon dried thyme
6 cups Homemade Chicken
   Stock (page 36)

Black pepper
1/4 cup Calvados or applejack
8 thin toast triangles
2/3 cup low-fat Monterey-Jack
   style cheese, grated

- In a heavy skillet, sauté onion in margarine over medium-low heat until lightly colored, about 5 minutes. Add thyme, stock, and pepper to taste and simmer over low heat for 20 minutes.

- Preheat oven to 450°F. Add Calvados to soup and pour into 6 individual ovenproof bowls. Top with toast triangles, sprinkle with grated cheese, and bake until golden brown, about 5 to 7 minutes. Serve immediately.

PER SERVING: 144 CALORIES

MENU EXCHANGE PATTERN

Dairy	—	Fruit	—
Bread	1	Meat	½
Fat	1	Veg.	—

NUTRITIONAL INFORMATION

Carbohydrate	8	g
Protein	4	g
Total fat	9	g
Saturated fat	0.6	g
Cholesterol	0	mg
Sodium	369	mg
Potassium	121	mg
Fiber	0.4	g
Calcium	89	mg
Iron	0.5	mg

Breast of Pheasant with Mushrooms and Cognac

4 pheasant breasts
3 tablespoons safflower oil
1 cup + 1 tablespoon all-
   purpose flour
3 tablespoons margarine
2 cups chopped fresh
   mushrooms

1 onion, chopped
3 tablespoons cognac
1 1/3 cups skim milk, warmed
1 cup seedless green grapes,
   sliced (garnish)

- With a sharp knife, cut along breast bone and lift away the breast meat. Remove the skin from the pheasant breasts and discard. You should have 2½ pounds breast meat. Heat the safflower oil in a heavy large skillet over low heat. Dust the pheasant with l cup flour, and sauté on both sides until brown, about 5 minutes each side. Remove the pheasant from the pan and keep warm. Discard the oil.

- In the same pan, melt 2 tablespoons margarine and sauté the mushrooms and onion over medium heat until onion is translucent, about 10 minutes. Add cognac. In a separate sauce pan, melt remaining tablespoon margarine. Add remaining 1 tablespoon flour, stirring constantly. Cook roux for about 1 to 2 minutes, then add all of the milk at once. Continue to stir constantly and bring to a boil to thicken sauce. Add mushroom mixture to sauce. Spoon over pheasant breast and serve, garnished with sliced grapes.

PER SERVING: 379 CALORIES

MENU EXCHANGE PATTERN

Dairy	—	Fruit	½
Bread	—	Meat	4
Fat	1½	Veg.	1

NUTRITIONAL INFORMATION

Carbohydrate	18	g
Protein	28	g
Total fat	20	g
Saturated fat	4.4	g
Cholesterol	73	mg
Sodium	98	mg
Potassium	506	mg
Fiber	0.7	g
Calcium	78	mg
Iron	1.7	mg

Zucchini Casserole

2 pounds zucchini, sliced
1/4 cup margarine, melted
1/2 cup plain low-fat yogurt
2 ounces low-fat American-style
  cheese

1/2 teaspoon paprika
1/2 teaspoon white pepper
1 tablespoon chopped fresh
  chives
1/2 cup fresh breadcrumbs

- Preheat oven to 350°F. Blanch zucchini in boiling water to cover for 2 minutes. Drain, then place in an oiled 1½- to 2-quart baking dish. Combine half of the melted margarine with yogurt, cheese, and paprika and simmer over low heat, stirring constantly, until cheese is melted. Remove from heat and add pepper and chives. Toss breadcrumbs with remaining margarine and sprinkle over zucchini. Bake until crumbs are golden, about 20 minutes.

PER SERVING: 122 CALORIES		
MENU EXCHANGE PATTERN		
Dairy . . . . . ½	Fruit . . . . . —	
Bread . . . . —	Meat . . . . . —	
Fat 1	Veg. 1½	
NUTRITIONAL INFORMATION		
Carbohydrate 11		g
Protein 5		g
Total fat 7		g
Saturated fat 1.3		g
Cholesterol. 3		mg
Sodium 209		mg
Potassium 300		mg
Fiber 0.7		g
Calcium 113		mg
Iron 0.7		mg

Bread Pudding

7 slices French bread, ½ inch
  thick
1/4 cup margarine
4 egg whites
2/3 cup sugar
1/4 cup dark rum

2²/₃ cups skim milk
2/3 cup plain low-fat yogurt
1 teaspoon vanilla extract
Hot Whiskey Sauce (recipe
  follows)

- Preheat oven to 375°F. Spread each slice of bread with margarine and arrange in a 2-quart baking dish, margarine side up. Beat egg whites until soft peaks form. Gradually beat in sugar and rum. Warm the milk and yogurt in a saucepan and whisk into egg whites. Add vanilla and pour over the bread. Set dish in a roasting pan filled with water to reach 1 inch from the top of the baking dish. Bake until meringue is golden brown and a knife comes out clean when inserted in center, about 1 hour. Serve with whiskey sauce.

PER SERVING: 244 CALORIES		
MENU EXCHANGE PATTERN		
Dairy 1	Fruit . . . . . —	
Bread 1½	Meat . . . . . —	
Fat 1	Veg. . . . . . —	
NUTRITIONAL INFORMATION		
Carbohydrate 34		g
Protein 8		g
Total fat 7		g
Saturated fat 1.5		g
Cholesterol 2		mg
Sodium 207		mg
Potassium 224		mg
Fiber 0		g
Calcium 147		mg
Iron 0.6		mg

Hot Whiskey Sauce

1¹/₃ cups skim milk
1/2 teaspoon cornstarch
3 tablespoons sugar

1 egg substitute
3 tablespoons bourbon

- Bring milk to a boil. Stir cornstarch into sugar; whisk with egg substitute and bourbon in a small bowl until smooth. Blend into hot milk and simmer, but do not boil, for 5 minutes.

PER SERVING: 53 CALORIES		
MENU EXCHANGE PATTERN		
Dairy . . . . . . ½	Fruit . . . . . . ½	
Bread . . . . —	Meat . . . . . —	
Fat . . . . —	Veg. . . . . . . —	
NUTRITIONAL INFORMATION		
Carbohydrate 7		g
Protein 2		g
Total fat 0		g
Saturated fat 0.1		g
Cholesterol 1		mg
Sodium 35		mg
Potassium 94		mg
Fiber 0		g
Calcium 54		mg
Iron 0.2		mg

RABBIT AND GAME

3

Red Pepper Soup with Cilantro Yogurt

Roasted Rabbit with Poblano Pepper Sauce

Corn and Pepper Relish

Pecan Torte

Serves 6

PER SERVING: 744 CALORIES			
MENU EXCHANGE PATTERN			
Dairy	—	Fruit	1½
Bread	3	Meat	5
Fat	2½	Veg.	4
NUTRITIONAL INFORMATION			
Carbohydrate	78	g	
Protein	47	g	
Total fat	31	g	
Saturated fat	6.6	g	
Cholesterol	6	mg	
Sodium	225	mg	
Potassium	2007	mg	
Fiber	4.4	g	
Calcium	351	mg	
Iron	6.1	mg	

Red Pepper Soup

2 dried ancho chilies
1 dried pasilla chili
1 dried chipotle chili
2 red bell peppers
2 tomatoes
1 red onion
2 garlic cloves
2 large sweet potatoes, peeled and chopped
2 stalks celery, coarsely chopped
1 carrot, peeled and coarsely chopped

4 cups Homemade Chicken Stock (page 36)
1 bunch fresh coriander (cilantro), chopped
2 cups plain low-fat yogurt
2 to 3 tablespoons pure maple syrup
Juice of ½ lime
¾ cup Cilantro Yogurt (recipe follows)
Cilantro leaves (garnish)

- Lightly toast the chilies in a hot nonstick skillet without oil, turning to toast all sides evenly. Roast the red peppers over an open flame or under the broiler, turning until evenly charred on all sides. Transfer peppers to a plastic bag until cool, then peel and seed under running water. Pat dry with paper towels. Roast the tomatoes, onion, and garlic in an oven until onion and garlic are soft, about 20 minutes. Combine the chilies, red peppers, tomatoes, onion, and garlic with the remaining vegetables in a stockpot and add stock and cilantro. Bring to a boil, then simmer until all of the vegetables are soft, about 30 minutes.

- Strain the soup. Transfer solids to a food processor and puree until smooth. Mix the puree back into the liquid and chill. Stir in the yogurt, maple syrup, and lime juice, adjusting the amounts to taste. Chill the soup thoroughly. Serve cold, topped with 2 tablespoons Cilantro Yogurt. (If you wish, draw a knife through the yogurt in several directions to create an interesting design.) Garnish with a few cilantro leaves. (Analysis includes Cilantro Yogurt).

PER SERVING: 164 CALORIES
MENU EXCHANGE PATTERN
Dairy ..... — Fruit ..... —
Bread ..... 2 Meat ...... ½
Fat .... — Veg. ...... —
NUTRITIONAL INFORMATION
Carbohydrate .... 32 g
Protein .... 7 g
Total fat .... 2 g
Saturated fat .... 0.8 g
Cholesterol .... 5 mg
Sodium .... 102 mg
Potassium .... 744 mg
Fiber .... 1.8 g
Calcium .... 213 mg
Iron .... 1.9 mg

Cilantro Yogurt

2 bunches fresh coriander
(cilantro); reserve some
leaves for garnish
1/2 bunch parsley
1 serrano chili

1/2 cup Homemade Chicken
Stock (page 36)
1 cup plain low-fat yogurt
Black pepper

- Combine the cilantro, parsley, chili, and chicken stock in a blender and puree. Slowly whip puree into the yogurt. Season with pepper to taste. Adjust consistency with additional stock if necessary; the mixture should be of similar consistency to the soup. Makes about 2 cups; 1 serving = 2 tablespoons.

PER SERVING: 16 CALORIES

MENU EXCHANGE PATTERN

Dairy	—	Fruit	—
Bread	—	Meat	—
Fat	—	Veg.	1/2

NUTRITIONAL INFORMATION

Carbohydrate	1	g
Protein	1	g
Total fat	0	g
Saturated fat	0.1	g
Cholesterol	1	mg
Sodium	21	mg
Potassium	74	mg
Fiber	0.1	g
Calcium	37	mg
Iron	0.4	mg

Roasted Rabbit with Poblano Pepper Sauce

2 large or 3 small poblano
chilies
2 garlic cloves
1/2 red onion
6 tomatillos
1 bunch fresh coriander
(cilantro), leaves only

1 1/2 cups Homemade Chicken
Stock (page 36)
2 teaspoons pure maple syrup
3 rabbits, 2 1/2 pounds each,
dressed (see note)
Black pepper

- Place the chilies on a grill, under the broiler, or over an open flame until browned and blistered on all sides. Place in a plastic bag and let stand 15 minutes to help loosen skins. Remove skin and seeds. Preheat oven to 350°F and roast garlic, onion, and tomatillos until soft, about 20 to 30 minutes. Combine chilies, garlic, onion, tomatillos, and cilantro in a blender, add stock and process until well blended, but still chunky.

- Transfer mixture to a saucepan and bring to a simmer; simmer 15 minutes. Stir in maple syrup and keep sauce warm. (Sauce can be prepared ahead and reheated.)

- Rub rabbits with pepper and grill over hot coals until no longer pink, about 15 to 20 minutes. Alternatively, bake in a 350°F to 400°F oven for about 20 minutes, turning at least once. Serve with sauce.

Note: Whole chickens may be substituted for the rabbits.

PER SERVING: 269 CALORIES

MENU EXCHANGE PATTERN

Dairy	—	Fruit	—
Bread	—	Meat	4
Fat	—	Veg.	2

NUTRITIONAL INFORMATION

Carbohydrate	6	g
Protein	32	g
Total fat	12	g
Saturated fat	4.6	g
Cholesterol	0	mg
Sodium	72	mg
Potassium	789	mg
Fiber	0.5	g
Calcium	63	mg
Iron	2.9	mg

Corn and Pepper Relish

Kernels from 6 ears of corn
1 tablespoon safflower oil
1 red bell pepper, cored, seeded,
and chopped
1 green bell pepper, cored,
seeded, and chopped
4 green onions, chopped

2 ancho chilies, seeded and
chopped
2 tablespoons chopped fresh
coriander (cilantro)
Juice of 1 lime
1 tablespoon pure maple syrup

PER SERVING: 122 CALORIES			
MENU EXCHANGE PATTERN			
Dairy	—	Fruit	—
Bread	1	Meat	—
Fat	½	Veg.	1
NUTRITIONAL INFORMATION			
Carbohydrate		24	g
Protein		3	g
Total fat		4	g
Saturated fat		0.2	g
Cholesterol		0	mg
Sodium		5	mg
Potassium		269	mg
Fiber		1.6	g
Calcium		23	mg
Iron		1	mg

- Sauté corn in oil in a very hot skillet until soft, about 5 to 10 minutes. Add the remaining ingredients and toss briefly over high heat until well mixed and heated through. Serve immediately.

Pecan Torte

6 egg whites
⅔ cup sugar
2 cups ground pecans

PER SERVING: 174 CALORIES			
MENU EXCHANGE PATTERN			
Dairy	—	Fruit	1½
Bread	—	Meat	½
Fat	2	Veg.	—
NUTRITIONAL INFORMATION			
Carbohydrate		14	g
Protein		3	g
Total fat		13	g
Saturated fat		0.9	g
Cholesterol		0	mg
Sodium		25	mg
Potassium		131	mg
Fiber		0.4	g
Calcium		15	mg
Iron		0.5	mg

- Preheat oven to 325°F. Beat egg whites until stiff peaks begin to form. Gradually beat in sugar. Fold in pecans and pour into an ungreased 8-inch round pan. Bake until golden brown, about 35 minutes. Let cool, then slice. Torte can be wrapped tightly and refrigerated, although it is best when served shortly after baking. Makes 12 servings; 1 serving = one 2 × 3-inch slice.

RABBIT AND GAME

4

Cape Cod Scallops with Mussels

Grilled Venison Chops and Medallions

Braised Red Cabbage with Cider Sauce

Sautéed Shiitake Mushrooms (page 142)

Floating Island with Orange Sauce

Serves 6

PER SERVING: 1090 CALORIES		
MENU EXCHANGE PATTERN		
Dairy . . . . . —	Fruit 3½	
Bread 4½	Meat 7½	
Fat 2	Veg. 4½	

NUTRITIONAL INFORMATION

Carbohydrate 87	g	
Protein 77	g	
Total fat 32	g	
Saturated fat 8.1	g	
Cholesterol 155	mg	
Sodium 371	mg	
Potassium 2015	mg	
Fiber 3.1	g	
Calcium 228	mg	
Iron . . . . 12.6 mg		

Cape Cod Scallops with Mussels

1½ cups dry white wine or
   seafood stock
½ pound mussels, cleaned (see
   page 259)
12 cloves garlic, sliced
2 tablespoons minced shallot

½ pound sea scallops
1 large tomato, diced
3 tablespoons chopped fresh
   basil, or 1 teaspoon dried
3 tablespoons margarine
Black pepper

- Bring wine to simmer in a nonstick skillet over medium heat. Add mussels, cover, and stir occasionally until shells begin to open, about 5 minutes. Remove mussels with a slotted spoon, discarding any that do not open. Add garlic and shallot to skillet, increase heat, and boil until liquid is reduced by ½. Add scallops to pan and cook about 1 minute. Add tomato and basil and return to simmer; remove from heat. Whisk in margarine 1 tablespoon at a time. Arrange mussels and scallops in bowls and top with sauce. Serve hot.

PER SERVING: 180 CALORIES		
MENU EXCHANGE PATTERN		
Dairy . . . . . —	Fruit . . . . . —	
Bread 1	Meat 1½	
Fat . . . . —	Veg. 1	
NUTRITIONAL INFORMATION		
Carbohydrate 8	g	
Protein 12	g	
Total fat 7	g	
Saturated fat 1	g	
Cholesterol 34	mg	
Sodium 115	mg	
Potassium 421	mg	
Fiber 0.3	g	
Calcium 29	mg	
Iron . . . . 2.3 mg		

Grilled Venison Chops and Medallions

6 venison chops, 3 ounces each
6 venison medallions, 3 ounces
   each

Corn Marinade (page 283)
¼ cup margarine
Pecan Sauce (recipe follows)

- Marinate chops in corn marinade for 12 hours. Grill or broil chops until center is only a light pink when cut with a knife or when medium-well done (about 4 minutes per side). In a nonstick skillet over medium-high heat, sauté medallions in margarine until center is only light pink or medium-well done (about 4 minutes per side). Top with sauce.

Note: If desired, substitute lamb for the venison but then reduce margarine to 1 tablespoon.

PER SERVING: 459 CALORIES		
MENU EXCHANGE PATTERN		
Dairy . . . . . —	Fruit . . . . . —	
Bread . . . 2½	Meat 5	
Fat . . . . —	Veg. . . . . . . —	
NUTRITIONAL INFORMATION		
Carbohydrate 25	g	
Protein 38	g	
Total fat 15	g	
Saturated fat 5.6	g	
Cholesterol 120	mg	
Sodium 121	mg	
Potassium 750	mg	
Fiber 0.7	g	
Calcium 31	mg	
Iron . . . . 8.9 mg		

Pecan Sauce

1½ pounds venison or beef
   bones
1 tablespoon juniper berries
4 cloves garlic
¼ cup coarsely chopped garlic
¼ cup coarsely chopped celery
¼ onion
1 carrot

1 bay leaf
1½ quarts Homemade Chicken
   Stock (page 36)
1 cup red wine
½ cup port
2 tablespoons Dijon-style or
   Creole mustard
¼ cup pecan halves

- Preheat oven to 400°F. In a large Dutch oven, sear bones, juniper, garlic, and vegetables in oven until brown, about 15 minutes. Add bay leaf, stock, red wine, and port and simmer, covered, over low heat for 1½ hours. Remove bones and strain liquid. Return to pan and boil until reduced to sauce consistency (about 1 to 1½ cups liquid). Whisk in mustard, spoon over venison medallions and sprinkle with pecan halves.

PER SERVING: 104 CALORIES		
MENU EXCHANGE PATTERN		
Dairy . . . . . —	Fruit 1	
Bread . . . . —	Meat . . . . . —	
Fat . . . . ½	Veg. 1½	
NUTRITIONAL INFORMATION		
Carbohydrate 6	g	
Protein 1	g	
Total fat 3	g	
Saturated fat 0.2	g	
Cholesterol 0	mg	
Sodium 26	mg	
Potassium 160	mg	
Fiber 0.4	g	
Calcium 18	mg	
Iron 0.4	mg	

Braised Red Cabbage with Cider Sauce

4 cups shredded cabbage
¼ cup red wine vinegar
2 teaspoons sugar
½ bay leaf
¼ cinnamon stick (about 1 inch)
2 tablespoons margarine
½ cup chopped onion
2 cloves garlic, chopped

2 teaspoons red currant jelly
2 tablespoons red wine
½ apple, cored and sliced into julienne
½ teaspoon coarsely crushed black pepper
½ teaspoon dried tarragon
Cider Sauce (recipe follows)

- Marinate cabbage with vinegar, sugar, bay leaf, and cinnamon stick about 2 hours. Preheat oven to 325°F. Melt margarine in Dutch oven or large ovenproof saucepan over medium heat. Add onion and garlic and sauté until translucent, about 5 minutes. Add marinated cabbage, cover, and braise in oven for 1 hour. Stir in currant jelly, wine, apple, pepper, and tarragon. Serve with sauce.

PER SERVING: 74 CALORIES		
MENU EXCHANGE PATTERN		
Dairy . . . . . —	Fruit . . . . . —	
Bread . . . . —	Meat . . . . . —	
Fat 1	Veg. 1	
NUTRITIONAL INFORMATION		
Carbohydrate 9	g	
Protein 1	g	
Total fat 4	g	
Saturated fat 0.7	g	
Cholesterol 0	mg	
Sodium 12	mg	
Potassium 166	mg	
Fiber 0.6	g	
Calcium 30	mg	
Iron 0.4	mg	

Cider Sauce

1½ tablespoons chopped shallot
1½ teaspoons margarine
⅔ cup unsweetened apple cider
¼ cup Homemade Chicken Stock (page 36)

⅔ cup evaporated skim milk
½ cup diced red bell pepper (garnish)

- In medium skillet, sauté shallot in margarine over medium heat until translucent, about 3 minutes. Add cider and simmer until reduced by ¾. Stir in stock and milk and simmer until reduced by ½. Serve over cabbage, garnishing with diced red pepper.

PER SERVING: 29 CALORIES		
MENU EXCHANGE PATTERN		
Dairy . . . . . —	Fruit . . . . . . ½	
Bread . . . . —	Meat . . . . . —	
Fat . . . . —	Veg. . . . . . —	
NUTRITIONAL INFORMATION		
Carbohydrate 4	g	
Protein 1	g	
Total fat 1	g	
Saturated fat 0.3	g	
Cholesterol 1	mg	
Sodium 44	mg	
Potassium 90	mg	
Fiber 0.1	g	
Calcium 35	mg	
Iron 0.2	mg	

Floating Island with Orange Sauce

9 oranges
3 envelopes unflavored gelatin
2 tablespoons sugar
6 egg whites
¼ cup confectioners sugar, sifted

6 strawberries, sliced vertically almost to base and slices fanned (garnish)

- Remove colored peel from ½ orange in fine julienne strips and poach in ¼ cup water until tender, about 5 minutes. Drain. Reserve 18 orange sections (3 for each serving); squeeze juice from all remaining oranges. Measure the juice.

- Pour ⅓ of the orange juice into a nonaluminum saucepan. Sprinkle in the gelatin and let stand for 10 to 15 minutes to soften. Warm over low heat to dissolve gelatin. Add remaining juice, sugar, and orange peel. Chill until set, about 1 hour.

- Shortly before serving, prepare floating islands. Whip egg whites to soft peaks. Add confectioners sugar and whip to stiff peaks. Spoon 6 mounds of meringue into a large, deep skillet of simmering water and poach 1½ minutes on each side. Remove with a slotted spoon and cover meringues with a damp towel.

- Chop orange gelatin very finely with knife. Place floating islands on dessert plates. Spoon orange mixture into a pastry bag and pipe around floating islands. Garnish with reserved orange sections and fanned strawberries.

Photo opposite page 322.

PER SERVING: 217 CALORIES		
MENU EXCHANGE PATTERN		
Dairy ..... —	Fruit 2	
Bread 1	Meat 1	
Fat .... —	Veg. ...... —	
NUTRITIONAL INFORMATION		
Carbohydrate 33	g	
Protein 23	g	
Total fat 0	g	
Saturated fat 0	g	
Cholesterol 0	mg	
Sodium 50	mg	
Potassium 421	mg	
Fiber 0.9	g	
Calcium 83	mg	
Iron 0.3	mg	

RABBIT AND GAME

5

Onion Timbale

Papaya and Lettuce Salad

Cornish Hens with Celery Apple Stuffing

Angel Food Cake with Marinated Strawberries

Serves 4

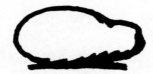

PER SERVING: 767 CALORIES			
MENU EXCHANGE PATTERN			
Dairy	—	Fruit	2
Bread	3	Meat	4
Fat	3½	Veg.	3
NUTRITIONAL INFORMATION			
Carbohydrate	82	g	
Protein	41	g	
Total fat	29	g	
Saturated fat	5.4	g	
Cholesterol	73	mg	
Sodium	605	mg	
Potassium	1543	mg	
Fiber	3.6	g	
Calcium	248	mg	
Iron	5.4	mg	

Onion Timbale

1 onion, coarsely chopped
1 1/2 cups warm skim milk
1/8 teaspoon cayenne pepper

4 egg substitutes
1/8 teaspoon garlic powder

- Preheat oven to 350°F. Cook onion in 1 cup water over medium heat until most of the water has evaporated and onion is translucent and limp, about 15 to 20 minutes (it is very important that the onion be well cooked). Puree onion in food processor. Add warm milk, cayenne, egg substitutes, and garlic powder and process until well mixed. Pour into well-oiled 2-quart mold or soufflé dish and set in a pan of warm (but not boiling) water; water should come about 2/3 up side of dish. Bake until a knife inserted in the center comes out clean, about 35 to 45 minutes. Serve immediately.

PER SERVING: 78 CALORIES			
MENU EXCHANGE PATTERN			
Dairy .... —	Fruit .... —		
Bread .... —	Meat 1		
Fat .... —	Veg. 1		
NUTRITIONAL INFORMATION			
Carbohydrate 7		g	
Protein 8		g	
Total fat 2		g	
Saturated fat 0.4		g	
Cholesterol 1		mg	
Sodium 119		mg	
Potassium 323		mg	
Fiber 0.3		g	
Calcium 112		mg	
Iron .... 1.2 mg			

Papaya and Lettuce Salad

1/2 head red-leaf lettuce (about 2 cups)
1/2 head Boston lettuce (about 2 cups)

2 ripe papayas (reserve 1/4 of seeds)
1/2 cup Tarragon Garlic Dressing (recipe follows)

- Wash and dry lettuce; tear into pieces. Peel and dice papaya. Coarsely grind papaya seeds in food processor. Combine all ingredients in a salad bowl and toss with dressing.

PER SERVING: 67 CALORIES			
MENU EXCHANGE PATTERN			
Dairy ..... —	Fruit 1		
Bread .... —	Meat ..... —		
Fat .... —	Veg. 1		
NUTRITIONAL INFORMATION			
Carbohydrate 16		g	
Protein 2		g	
Total fat 0		g	
Saturated fat 0.1		g	
Cholesterol 0		mg	
Sodium 9		mg	
Potassium 535		mg	
Fiber 1.5		g	
Calcium 55		mg	
Iron .... 1.2 mg			

Tarragon Garlic Dressing

1/2 teaspoon dried tarragon
1 to 2 cloves garlic, minced
1/2 cup tarragon vinegar
1/4 cup chopped fresh parsley

1/2 teaspoon black pepper
1 1/2 tablespoons dry sherry
1/2 cup safflower oil

- Combine all ingredients in a jar and shake to blend well. Makes about 1 1/4 cups; 1 serving = 2 tablespoons.

PER SERVING: 128 CALORIES			
MENU EXCHANGE PATTERN			
Dairy ..... —	Fruit ..... —		
Bread .... —	Meat ..... —		
Fat 2 1/2	Veg. ..... —		
NUTRITIONAL INFORMATION			
Carbohydrate 2		g	
Protein 0		g	
Total fat 13		g	
Saturated fat 1.2		g	
Cholesterol 0		mg	
Sodium 2		mg	
Potassium 36		mg	
Fiber 0.5		g	
Calcium 6		mg	
Iron .... 0.2 mg			

Cornish Hens with Celery Apple Stuffing

4 Cornish hens
Black pepper
2 bran muffins
2 celery hearts, finely chopped
1 Red Delicious apple, cored
    and chopped

1/2 onion, chopped
2 tablespoons (about) dry white
    wine
1/3 cup hoisin sauce

- Rinse hens inside and out and pat dry with paper towels. Sprinkle inside of each bird with pepper.

- Crumble muffins into a large bowl. Mix in celery, apple, onion, 1 teaspoon black pepper, and wine, using only enough wine to hold stuffing together.

- Preheat oven to 350°F. Stuff hens loosely with dressing and truss with string. Baste outside of each hen with hoisin sauce mixed with a little water. Roast uncovered until juices run clear when thigh is pierced with a fork, about 1 hour. Discard strings and serve.

PER SERVING: 302 CALORIES

MENU EXCHANGE PATTERN

Dairy	—	Fruit	—
Bread	1	Meat	3
Fat	1	Veg.	1

NUTRITIONAL INFORMATION

Carbohydrate	20	g
Protein	26	g
Total fat	13	g
Saturated fat	3.7	g
Cholesterol	72	mg
Sodium	359	mg
Potassium	528	mg
Fiber	1	g
Calcium	63	mg
Iron	2.1	mg

Angel Food Cake with Marinated Strawberries

8 egg whites
1/4 teaspoon salt
1 teaspoon cream of tartar
1 teaspoon almond extract
1 teaspoon vanilla extract

1 cup sugar
1 cup sifted cake flour
1 pint strawberries
1/4 cup Frangelico (hazelnut)
    liqueur

- Preheat oven to 325°F. Beat egg whites until foamy. Add salt and cream of tartar and beat until soft peaks form. Add almond and vanilla extracts. Gradually add sugar, beating until stiff. Sift the flour over the egg whites and fold in gently. Bake in an ungreased 10-inch tube pan until a fork inserted in center comes out clean, about 50 to 60 minutes. Invert the cake on a rack and cool completely before removing from pan.

- Slice the strawberries and mix with Frangelico. Refrigerate for several hours. Fill center of cake with marinated strawberries and serve. Makes 8 servings; 1 serving = 1 slice.

Photo opposite page 323.

PER SERVING: 193 CALORIES

MENU EXCHANGE PATTERN

Dairy	—	Fruit	1
Bread	2	Meat	—
Fat	—	Veg.	—

NUTRITIONAL INFORMATION

Carbohydrate	38	g
Protein	5	g
Total fat	1	g
Saturated fat	0.3	g
Cholesterol	0	mg
Sodium	117	mg
Potassium	121	mg
Fiber	0.2	g
Calcium	12	mg
Iron	0.6	mg

A–Exchange Patterns: 1,000 to 3,000 Calories

The following exchange patterns range from 1,000 to 3,000 calories. Diets are designed to be 15 to 20 percent protein, 50 to 55 percent carbohydrate, and 30 percent fat. When caloric intake is less than 1,500, however, the percentage of calories derived from protein may need to be higher than 15 to 20 percent. In this case, protein intake will represent a higher percentage of the day's calories to satisfy the Recommended Dietary Allowance (RDA) for protein.

1,000 CALORIES*
TOTAL DAILY INTAKE

Milk (1%) . . ½   Fruit 4   Meat (oz.) . . 4
Bread 4   Vegetable . . 5   Fat 3

	MEAL PLAN	SAMPLE MEALS
Breakfast	½ Milk 1 Bread 1 Fruit – Vegetable – Meat (ounces) – Fat	½ cup low-fat (1%) milk ¾ cup high-fiber flake cereal ½ cup orange juice
Snack	–	–
Lunch	– Milk 2 Bread 1 Fruit 2 Vegetable 1 Meat (ounces) 1 Fat	2 slices whole wheat bread 1 apple 1 cup raw carrots 1 ounce lean meat, poultry, or fish 1 teaspoon margarine or mayonnaise 1 cup iced tea
Snack	1 Fruit	1 small apple
Dinner	– Milk 1 Bread 1 Fruit 3 Vegetable 3 Meat (ounces) 2 Fat	½ cup mashed potato 1 orange 1½ cups steamed vegetables 3 ounces lean meat, poultry, or fish 2 teaspoons margarine (to season) 1 cup iced tea
Snack	–	–

Vitamin and mineral supplement advisable.

1,100 CALORIES*
TOTAL DAILY INTAKE

Milk (1%) . . ½   Fruit 4   Meat (oz.) . . 4
Bread 5   Vegetable . . 5   Fat 4

1,300 CALORIES*
TOTAL DAILY INTAKE

Milk (1%) . 1½   Fruit 4   Meat (oz.) . . 5
Bread 5   Vegetable . . 5   Fat 4

1,200 CALORIES*
TOTAL DAILY INTAKE

Milk (1%) . . 1   Fruit 4   Meat (oz.) . . 4
Bread 6   Vegetable . . 5   Fat 4

1,400 CALORIES*
TOTAL DAILY INTAKE

Milk (1%) . . 2   Fruit 4   Meat (oz.) . . 5
Bread 6   Vegetable . . 5   Fat 4

1,500 CALORIES*
TOTAL DAILY INTAKE

Milk (1%) .. 2   Fruit 4   Meat (oz.).. 5
Bread 7   Vegetable .. 5   Fat 4

	MEAL PLAN	SAMPLE MEALS
Breakfast	1 Milk 2 Bread 1 Fruit – Vegetable – Meat (ounces) 1 Fat	1 cup low-fat (1%) milk ¾ cup high-fiber flake cereal 1 slice whole wheat toast ½ cup orange juice 1 teaspoon margarine
Snack	–	–
Lunch	1 Milk 2 Bread 1 Fruit 2 Vegetable 1 Meat (ounces) 1 Fat	1 cup low-fat (1%) milk 2 slices whole wheat bread 1 apple 1 cup raw carrots 1 ounce lean meat, poultry, or fish 1 teaspoon margarine or mayonnaise
Snack	1 Fruit	1 small apple
Dinner	– Milk 3 Bread 1 Fruit 3 Vegetable 4 Meat (ounces) 2 Fat	1½ cups rice ¼ cantaloupe 1½ cups steamed vegetables 4 ounces lean meat, poultry, or fish 2 teaspoons margarine 1 cup iced tea
Snack	–	–

Vitamin and mineral supplement advisable.

1,600 CALORIES*
TOTAL DAILY INTAKE

Milk (1%) .. 2   Fruit 5   Meat (oz.).. 5
Bread 7   Vegetable .. 6   Fat 5

1,800 CALORIES*
TOTAL DAILY INTAKE

Milk (1%) .. 2   Fruit 6   Meat (oz.).. 6
Bread 8   Vegetable .. 6   Fat 6

1,700 CALORIES*
TOTAL DAILY INTAKE

Milk (1%) .. 2   Fruit 6   Meat (oz.).. 6
Bread 7   Vegetable .. 6   Fat 5

1,900 CALORIES*
TOTAL DAILY INTAKE

Milk (1%) .. 2   Fruit 5   Meat (oz.).. 7
Bread 9   Vegetable .. 6   Fat 6

2,000 CALORIES		
TOTAL DAILY INTAKE		
Milk (1%) . . 2	Fruit 5	Meat (oz.) . . 7
Bread 10	Vegetable . . 6	Fat 7

	MEAL PLAN	SAMPLE MEALS
Breakfast	1 Milk 4 Bread 2 Fruit – Vegetable – Meat (ounces) 2 Fat	1 cup low-fat (1%) milk 1½ cups high-fiber flake cereal 2 slices whole wheat toast 1 cup orange juice 2 teaspoons margarine
Snack	–	–
Lunch	1 Milk 2 Bread 1 Fruit 2 Vegetable 2 Meat (ounces) 2 Fat	1 cup low-fat (1%) milk 2 slices whole wheat bread ½ cup fresh berries 1 cup raw vegetables 2 ounces lean meat, poultry, or fish 2 teaspoons margarine or mayonnaise
Snack	1 Fruit	1 small apple
Dinner	– Milk 3 Bread 2 Fruit 4 Vegetable 5 Meat (ounces) 3 Fat	1 cup mashed potato 1 small roll 1 cup mixed fruit 1 cup steamed vegetables 1 cup lettuce salad 5 ounces lean meat, poultry, or fish 2 teaspoons margarine 1 teaspoon oil with vinegar 1 cup iced tea
Snack	1 Bread	3 cups plain air-popped popcorn

2,100 CALORIES		
TOTAL DAILY INTAKE		
Milk (1%) . . 3	Fruit 5	Meat (oz.) . . 7
Bread 10	Vegetable . . 6	Fat 7

2,300 CALORIES		
TOTAL DAILY INTAKE		
Milk (1%) . . 3	Fruit 7	Meat (oz.) . . 7
Bread 12	Vegetable . . 6	Fat 7

2,200 CALORIES		
TOTAL DAILY INTAKE		
Milk (1%) . . 2	Fruit 6	Meat (oz.) . . 7
Bread 11	Vegetable . . 6	Fat 7

2,400 CALORIES		
TOTAL DAILY INTAKE		
Milk (2%) . . 3	Fruit 7	Meat (oz.) . . 7
Bread 12	Vegetable . . 6	Fat 7

2,500 CALORIES		
TOTAL DAILY INTAKE		
Milk (2%) .. 3	Fruit 8	Meat (oz.).. 8
Bread 12	Vegetable .. 6	Fat 7

	MEAL PLAN	SAMPLE MEALS
Breakfast	1 Milk	1 cup low-fat (2%) milk
	4 Bread	1½ cups high-fiber flake cereal
	2 Fruit	2 slices whole wheat toast
	– Vegetable	½ banana
	– Meat (ounces)	½ cup orange juice
	2 Fat	2 teaspoons margarine
Snack	2 Fruit	1 cup grapefruit juice
	1 Bread	4 salt-free soda crackers
Lunch	1 Milk	1 cup low-fat (2%) milk
	2 Bread	2 slices whole wheat bread
	1 Fruit	¼ cantaloupe
	2 Vegetable	1 cup raw vegetables
	3 Meat (ounces)	3 ounces lean meat, poultry, or fish
	2 Fat	2 teaspoons margarine or mayonnaise
Snack	1 Fruit	1 small apple
Dinner	1 Milk	1 cup low-fat (2%) milk
	4 Bread	1½ cups rice
	2 Fruit	1 roll
	4 Vegetable	1 cup mixed fruit
	5 Meat (ounces)	1 cup steamed vegetables
	3 Fat	1 cup green salad
		5 ounces lean meat, poultry, or fish
		2 teaspoons margarine
		1 teaspoon oil with vinegar
Snack	1 Bread	3 cups plain air-popped popcorn

2,600 CALORIES		
TOTAL DAILY INTAKE		
Milk (2%) .. 3	Fruit 9	Meat (oz.).. 8
Bread 12	Vegetable .. 8	Fat 8

2,800 CALORIES		
TOTAL DAILY INTAKE		
Milk (2%) .. 3	Fruit 9	Meat (oz.).. 9
Bread 13	Vegetable .. 8	Fat 9

2,700 CALORIES		
TOTAL DAILY INTAKE		
Milk (2%) .. 3	Fruit 8	Meat (oz.).. 8
Bread 13	Vegetable .. 8	Fat 9

2,900 CALORIES		
TOTAL DAILY INTAKE		
Milk (2%) .. 3	Fruit 10	Meat (oz.).. 9
Bread 14	Vegetable .. 8	Fat 9

3,000 CALORIES		
TOTAL DAILY INTAKE		
Milk (2%) . . 4	Fruit 9	Meat (oz.) . . 9
Bread 14	Vegetable . . 8	Fat 9

	MEAL PLAN	SAMPLE MEALS
Breakfast	1 Milk 4 Bread 2 Fruit – Vegetable – Meat (ounces) 2 Fat	1 cup low-fat (2%) milk 1½ cups high-fiber flake cereal 2 slices whole wheat toast ½ banana ½ cup orange juice 2 teaspoons margarine
Snack	2 Fruit 1 Bread	1 cup grapefruit juice 4 salt-free soda crackers
Lunch	1 Milk 2 Bread 2 Fruit 2 Vegetable 3 Meat (ounces) 2 Fat	1 cup low-fat (2%) milk 2 slices whole wheat bread ½ cantaloupe 1 cup raw vegetables 3 ounces lean meat, poultry, or fish 2 teaspoons margarine or mayonnaise
Snack	1 Milk 1 Fruit 2 Bread 1 Meat (ounces) 1 Fat	1 cup low-fat (2%) milk 1 small apple 2 slices whole wheat bread 1 ounce lean meat, poultry, or fish 1 teaspoon margarine or mayonnaise
Dinner	1 Milk 4 Bread 2 Fruit 6 Vegetable 5 Meat (ounces) 4 Fat	1 cup low-fat (2%) milk 1½ cups rice 1 roll 1 cup mixed fruit 1 cup steamed vegetables 2 cups green salad 5 ounces lean meat, poultry, or fish 2 teaspoons margarine 2 teaspoons oil with vinegar
Snack	1 Bread	3 cups plain air-popped popcorn

B–Exchange Lists

Dairy

The following foods in the amounts indicated contain approximately 12 grams of carbo-hydrate, 8 grams of protein, a trace of fat, and 80 calories. Each is equal to 1 Dairy exchange unless otherwise indicated. Selections should be made from the "allowable" category. Foods in the "avoid" group are higher in fat and calories.

ALLOWABLE

PRODUCT	AMOUNT	EXCHANGE
Milk		
Buttermilk (skim)	1 cup	1 dairy
Buttermilk (low-fat)	1 cup	1 dairy + 1 fat
Chocolate milk (1–2%)	1 cup	1 dairy + 1 fat + 1 fruit
Evaporated skim milk	½ cup	1 dairy
Evaporated low-fat milk	½ cup	1 dairy + 1 fat
Low-fat milk (1–2%)	1 cup	1 dairy + 1 fat
Powdered skim milk	1 cup	1 dairy
Skim milk	1 cup	1 dairy
Cheese		
Creamed cottage cheese	⅓ cup	1 dairy
Low-fat, cheese (less than 15% fat)	2 ounces	1 dairy
Low-fat (1–2% fat) cottage cheese	½ cup	1 dairy
Ricotta, part-skim	½ cup	1 dairy + 1 fat
Skim milk cheese	2 ounces	1 dairy
Yogurt		
Nonfat, plain	1 cup	1 dairy
Nonfat, flavored	1 cup	1 dairy + 2 fruit
Nonfat, fruited	1 cup	1 dairy + 2 fruit
Low-fat, plain	1 cup	1½ dairy + 1 fat
Low-fat, flavored	1 cup	1½ dairy + 1 fat + 1 bread
Low-fat, fruited	1 cup	1 dairy + 1 fat + 1 bread + 2 fruit
Low-fat, frozen	⅓ cup	1 bread
Miscellaneous		
Ice milk	⅓ cup	1 bread

AVOID

PRODUCT	AMOUNT	EXCHANGE
Milk		
Buttermilk (from whole)	1 cup	1 dairy + 2 fat
Chocolate milk	1 cup	1 dairy + 2 fat + 1 fruit
Evaporated (from whole)	1 cup	1 dairy + 2 fat
Whole	1 cup	1 dairy + 2 fat
Cheeses—Aged		
Blue cheese	2 ounces	1 dairy + 2 fat
Cheddar	2 ounces	1 dairy + 2 fat
Cream	2 ounces	1 dairy + 2 fat
Mozzarrella	2 ounces	1 dairy + 2 fat
Parmesan, hard	2 ounces	1 dairy + 2 fat
Parmesan, grated	2 tablespoons	1 dairy + ½ fat
Swiss	2 ounces	1 dairy + 2 fat
Cheese—Not aged		
Ricotta	½ cup	1 dairy + 3 fat
Yogurt		
Whole, plain	1 cup	1 dairy + 1½ fat
Whole, flavored	1 cup	1 dairy + 1½ fat + 1 bread
Whole, fruited	1 cup	1 dairy + 1½ fat + 1 bread + 2 fruit
Miscellaneous		
Butter	1 teaspoon	1 fat
Half and half	2 tablespoons	1 fat
Ice cream	½ cup	1 bread + 2 fat
Light cream	2 tablespoons	1 fat
Sour cream	2 tablespoons	1 fat
Whipping (heavy) cream	1 tablespoon	1 fat

Bread

The following foods contain approximately 15 grams of carbohydrate, 2 grams of protein, and 70 calories. Each is equal to 1 bread exchange unless otherwise indicated. The bread exchange list includes cereals and starchy vegetables, as well as foods that contain an equivalent amount of carbohydrates. Alcohol is categorized as a bread rather than as a separate exchange group. Selections should be made from the "allowable category." Foods in the "avoid" group contain more saturated fat and are higher in calories.

ALLOWABLE

PRODUCT	AMOUNT	EXCHANGE
Breads		
French	1 slice	1 bread
Italian	1 slice	1 bread
Pita	½ small	1 bread
Pumpernickel	1 slice	1 bread
Raisin	1 slice	1 bread
Rye	1 slice	1 bread
Whole wheat	1 slice	1 bread
White	1 slice	1 bread
Bread products		
Bagel, small	½	1 bread
Bun, hamburger, hot dog	½ small	1 bread
Cornbread	2-inch square	1 bread + 1 fat
English muffin	½ small	1 bread
Muffin	1 small	1 bread + 1 fat
Pancake	1 5-inch diameter	1 bread
Roll, plain	1 small	1 bread
Tortilla, corn	1 6-inch diameter	1 bread
Tortilla, flour	1 6-inch diameter	1 bread
Waffle	1 5-inch square	1 bread
Cereal		
Barley, cooked	½ cup	1 bread
Bran flakes	¾ cup	1 bread
Cold cereal, flake or puff	¾ cup	1 bread
Hot cereal	½ cup	1 bread
Grits, cooked	½ cup	1 bread
Cornmeal, dry	2 tbsp.	1 bread
Flour	2½ tbsp.	1 bread
Pasta, cooked		
Macaroni	½ cup	1 bread
Noodles	½ cup	1 bread
Lasagna	½ cup	1 bread
Spaghetti	½ cup	1 bread
Crackers		
Arrowroot	3	1 bread
Bread sticks	5 7-inch length	1 bread
Graham	1 2½-inch square	1 bread
Matzo	1 6-inch square	1 bread
Oyster	20	1 bread
Pretzels, large rings	5	1 bread

ALLOWABLE (Continued)

PRODUCT	AMOUNT	EXCHANGE
Pretzels, 8-inch rods	3	1 bread
Pretzel sticks	20	1 bread
Rye wafers	3	1 bread
Saltines	6	1 bread
Soda	4	1 bread
Dried Beans, Peas, and Lentils		
Baked beans, no pork	½ cup	1 bread
Dried beans, cooked	½ cup	1 bread
Lima beans, cooked	½ cup	1 bread
Peas, cooked	½ cup	1 bread
Lentils, cooked	½ cup	1 bread
Starchy Vegetables		
Acorn squash	½ cup	1 bread
Corn	⅓ cup	1 bread
Corn on the cob	1 small	1 bread
Hominy, cooked	½ cup	1 bread
Parsnips	⅔ cup	1 bread
Peas	½ cup	1 bread
Potato, white	1 small	1 bread
Potato, mashed	½ cup	1 bread
Pumpkin	¾ cup	1 bread
Rice, cooked (white/brown)	½ cup	1 bread
Sweet potato	¼ cup	1 bread
Miscellaneous		
Bread crumbs	3 tbsp.	1 bread
Barbecue sauce	¼ cup	1 bread
Catsup	¼ cup	1 bread
Chili sauce	¼ cup	1 bread
Cornstarch	2 tbsp.	1 bread
Popcorn, air-popped	3 cups	1 bread
Desserts		
Angel food cake	1 slice	1 bread
Fruit ice	¼ cup	1 bread
Gelatin, sweetened	⅓ cup	1 bread
Frozen yogurt	⅓ cup	1 bread
Ice milk	⅓ cup	1 bread
Sherbet	¼ cup	1 bread
Alcohol		
Beer, regular	5 ounces	1 bread
Beer, light	8 ounces	1 bread
Distilled liquor (gin, rum, scotch, etc.)	1 ounce	1 bread
Dry wine	3½ ounces	1 bread
Sweet wine	2 ounces	1 bread

AVOID

PRODUCT	AMOUNT	EXCHANGE
Biscuit	1 small	1 bread + 1 fat
Butter roll	1 small	1 bread + 1 fat
Cake (with icing)	1 small slice	1½ bread + 2 fat + 2 fruit
Cereals, presweetened	1 cup	1 bread + 1½ fruit
Cereals with coconut	1 cup	1 bread + 1 fat
Cheesecake	⅙ cake	1½ bread + 3 fat
Cheesebread	1 slice	1 bread + 1 fat + 1 meat
Cookies, plain	1	½ bread + ½ fat + ½ fruit
Corn chips	1 ounce	1 bread + 2 fat
Croissants	1 small	1 bread + 1½ fat

AVOID (Continued)

PRODUCT	AMOUNT	EXCHANGE
Cupcake (with icing)	1	1 bread + 1 fat + ½ fruit
Doughnut (plain)	1	½ bread + 1½ fat + ½ fruit
Ice cream	½ cup	1 bread + 2 fat
Noodles, egg	½ cup	1 bread
Noodles, chow mein	1 cup	2 bread + 2 fat + ½ meat
Pies, fruit	1 small slice	2 bread + 3 fat + 2 fruit
Potato chips	10	1 bread + 1 fat
Potatoes, French-fried	8	1 bread + 1 fat
Sweet roll	1 small	2 bread + 3 fat

Fat

The following foods contain approximately 5 grams of fat and 45 calories. Each is equal to 1 Fat exchange unless otherwise indicated. Selections should be made from the category that contains polyunsaturated fats. Foods in the "avoid" group contain more saturated fat and are higher in calories.

ALLOWABLE

PRODUCT	AMOUNT	EXCHANGE
Avocado, 4-inch diameter	⅛	1 fat
Margarine, soft, tub, or stick	1 teaspoon	1 fat
Margarine, diet	2 teaspoons	1 fat
Nuts		
Almonds	6	1 fat
Cashews	4	1 fat
Chestnuts	5	1 fat
Filberts (Hazelnuts)	5	1 fat
Mixed	5	1 fat
Peanuts	10	1 fat
Peanut butter	1 tablespoon	1 fat
Pecans	5	1 fat
Piñon (pine)	1 tablespoon	1 fat
Pistachio	15	1 fat
Walnuts	5 halves	1 fat
Oil		
Corn oil	1 teaspoon	1 fat
Cottonseed oil	1 teaspoon	1 fat
Olive oil	1 teaspoon	1 fat
Peanut oil	1 teaspoon	1 fat
Safflower oil	1 teaspoon	1 fat
Sesame oil	1 teaspoon	1 fat
Soybean oil	1 teaspoon	1 fat
Sunflower oil	1 teaspoon	1 fat
Walnut oil	1 teaspoon	1 fat
Olives	5 small	1 fat

ALLOWABLE (Continued)

PRODUCT	AMOUNT	EXCHANGE
Salad Dressing		
Caesar	2 teaspoons	1 fat
French	2 teaspoons	1 fat
French, low-calorie	2 tablespoons	1 fat
Italian	2 teaspoons	1 fat
Italian, low-calorie	2 tablespoons	1 fat
Mayonnaise	2 teaspoons	1 fat
Mayonnaise, low-calorie	2 tablespoons	1 fat
Thousand Island	2 teaspoons	1 fat
Thousand Island, low-calorie	2 tablespoons	1 fat
Vinegar and oil	2 teaspoons	1 fat
Seeds		
Pumpkin	1 tablespoon	1 fat
Sesame	1 tablespoon	1 fat
Sunflower	1 tablespoon	1 fat

AVOID

PRODUCT	AMOUNT	EXCHANGE
Butter	1 teaspoon	1 fat
Bacon	1 slice	1 fat
Bacon fat	1 teaspoon	1 fat
Chocolate	1 ounce	2½ fat
Coconut	2 tablespoons	1 fat
Cream, light	2 tablespoons	1 fat
Cream, sour	2 tablespoons	1 fat
Cream, heavy	1 tablespoon	1 fat

AVOID *(Continued)*

PRODUCT	AMOUNT	EXCHANGE
Gravy from meat drippings	1 tablespoon	1 fat
Imitation coffee creamer, liquid	2 tablespoons	1 fat
Imitation coffee creamer, powder	1 tablespoon	1 fat
Lard	1 teaspoon	1 fat
Macadamia nuts	3	1 fat
Oil		
Coconut	1 teaspoon	1 fat
Palm oil	1 teaspoon	1 fat

AVOID *(Continued)*

PRODUCT	AMOUNT	EXCHANGE
Partially hydrogenated vegetable oils	1 teaspoon	1 fat
Salad Dressings		
Blue cheese (Roquefort)	2 teaspoons	1 fat
Creamy salad dressing	2 teaspoons	1 fat
Green goddess	2 teaspoons	1 fat
Salad dressings made with sour cream or cheese	2 teaspoons	1 fat
Tartar sauce	2 teaspoons	1 fat
White sauce	2 tablespoons	1 fat

Fruit

The following foods contain approximately 10 grams of carbohydrate and 40 calories. Each is equal to 1 Fruit exchange unless otherwise indicated. Selections should be made from the "allowable" category. Foods in the "avoid" group are higher in sugar and calories.

ALLOWABLE

PRODUCT	AMOUNT	EXCHANGE
Fruits and Juices		
Apple	1 small	1 fruit
Apple juice	⅓ cup	1 fruit
Apple sauce	½ cup	1 fruit
Apricots, fresh	2 medium	1 fruit
Apricots, dried	4 halves	1 fruit
Banana	½ small	1 fruit
Blackberries	½ cup	1 fruit
Blueberries	½ cup	1 fruit
Cantaloupe	¼ melon	1 fruit
Cherries	10 large	1 fruit
Cranberry juice cocktail, low-calorie	¾ cup	1 fruit
Cranberry juice cocktail, regular	¼ cup	1 fruit
Cranberry sauce	2 tablespoons	1 fruit
Cider	⅓ cup	1 fruit
Dates	2	1 fruit
Figs, dried	1 small	1 fruit
Figs, fresh	2 large	1 fruit
Fruit cocktail, unsweetened	½ cup	1 fruit
Grapefruit	½	1 fruit
Grapefruit juice	½ cup	1 fruit
Grapes	12	1 fruit
Grape juice	¼ cup	1 fruit
Honeydew melon	⅛ melon	1 fruit
Kiwi	1	1 fruit
Mandarin oranges	½ cup	1 fruit
Mango	½ small	1 fruit
Nectarine	1 medium	1 fruit
Orange	1 medium	1 fruit
Orange juice	½ cup	1 fruit
Papaya	¾ cup	1 fruit

ALLOWABLE *(Continued)*

PRODUCT	AMOUNT	EXCHANGE
Peach	1 medium	1 fruit
Pear	1 small	1 fruit
Persimmon	1 medium	1 fruit
Pineapple	½ cup	1 fruit
Pineapple juice	⅓ cup	1 fruit
Plums	2 medium	1 fruit
Prunes	2 medium	1 fruit
Prune juice	¼ cup	1 fruit
Raisins	2 tablespoons	1 fruit
Raspberries	½ cup	1 fruit
Strawberries	1 cup	1 fruit
Tangerine	1 medium	1 fruit
Tangerine juice	½ cup	1 fruit
Watermelon	1 cup	1 fruit
Miscellaneous		
Fruit bar	1	1½ fruit
Fruit and ice	¼ cup	1 fruit
Honey	1 tablespoon	1 fruit
Popsicle	1 bar	1 bread
Soft drink, sweetened	4 ounces	1 fruit
Sugar	1 tablespoon	1 fruit
Sherbet	¼ cup	1 bread

AVOID

PRODUCT	AMOUNT	EXCHANGE
Fruit pie filling	amount for ⅙ pie	1 fruit + 1 bread
Fruit in sugar syrup, light	½ cup	1½ fruit
Fruit in sugar syrup, heavy	½ cup	2 fruit

Meat

The following foods contain approximately 7 grams of protein, 3 grams of fat, and 55 calories per ounce. Meat exchanges are expressed in terms of ounces (cooked weight). If a particular meat has more fat than a lean meat, additional fat exchanges will be indicated. The Choice and Good grades of meat have less fat than Prime. Selections should be made from the "allowable" category. Foods in the "avoid" group are higher in fat and calories.

ALLOWABLE

PRODUCT	AMOUNT	EXCHANGE
Beef (Choice or Good)		
Baby beef	1 ounce	1 meat
Chopped beef	1 ounce	1 meat
Chuck	1 ounce	1 meat
Flank steak	1 ounce	1 meat
Ground chuck (lean, 10% fat)	1 ounce	1 meat
Ground round (lean, 10% fat)	1 ounce	1 meat
Round, bottom or top	1 ounce	1 meat
Rump, all cuts	1 ounce	1 meat
Lamb		
Leg	1 ounce	1 meat
Rib, chop or roast	1 ounce	1 meat
Fish and Shellfish		
Any fresh or frozen fish	1 ounce	1 meat
Anchovies, drained	7 small	1 meat
Clams	2 medium	1 meat
Crab	1 ounce	1 meat
Frogs' legs	1 ounce	1 meat
Lobster	1 ounce	1 meat
Oysters	1 ounce	1 meat
Salmon, canned	¼ cup	1 meat
Sardines, drained	1 ounce	1 meat
Scallops	1 ounce	1 meat
Shrimp	1 ounce	1 meat
Squid	1 ounce	1 meat
Tuna, canned in water	¼ cup	1 meat
Cheese		
Cheese, low-fat (less than 5% fat)	1 ounce	1 meat
Cottage cheese (1–2% fat)	½ cup	1 meat
Peas, dried	¼ cup	1 meat + 1 bread
Beans, dried	¼ cup	1 meat + 1 bread
Egg		
Egg substitute	1	1 meat
Egg whites	1	free
Luncheon Meat		
Beef, thin sliced	1 ounce	1 meat
Chicken, thin sliced	1 ounce	1 meat
Ham, thin sliced	1 ounce	1 meat
Turkey, thin sliced	1 ounce	1 meat
Turkey franks	1 frank	1 meat + 1 fat
Turkey ham	1 ounce	1 meat
Turkey pastrami	1 ounce	1 meat
Sirloin	1 ounce	1 meat
Loin, chops	1 ounce	1 meat

ALLOWABLE (Continued)

PRODUCT	AMOUNT	EXCHANGE
Loin, roast	1 ounce	1 meat
Shank	1 ounce	1 meat
Shoulder	1 ounce	1 meat
Pork		
Canadian bacon	1 ounce	1 meat + ½ fat
Leg, whole rump	1 ounce	1 meat
Ham, center	1 ounce	1 meat
Ham, rump	1 ounce	1 meat
Loin, rib	1 ounce	1 meat + ½ fat
Loin, chop	1 ounce	1 meat + ½ fat
Ribs, center	1 ounce	1 meat
Ribs, shank	1 ounce	1 meat
Veal		
Cutlets	1 ounce	1 meat
Leg	1 ounce	1 meat
Loin	1 ounce	1 meat
Rib	1 ounce	1 meat
Shank	1 ounce	1 meat
Shoulder	1 ounce	1 meat
Poultry (skin removed)		
Chicken	1 ounce	1 meat
Cornish hen	1 ounce	1 meat
Guinea hen	1 ounce	1 meat
Pheasant	1 ounce	1 meat
Turkey	1 ounce	1 meat

AVOID

PRODUCT	AMOUNT	EXCHANGE
Beef (Prime)		
Brisket	1 ounce	1 meat + 1 fat
Canned	1 ounce	1 meat + ½ fat
Corn	1 ounce	1 meat + ½ fat
Ground (15% fat)	1 ounce	1 meat + ½ fat
Ground (20% fat)	1 ounce	1 meat + 1 fat
Hamburger (regular)	1 ounce	1 meat + 1 fat
Roast, rib	1 ounce	1 meat + 1 fat
Round, ground	1 ounce	1 meat + ½ fat
Sausage	1 ounce	1 meat + 1 fat
Lamb		
Breast	1 ounce	1 meat + 1 fat
Ground	1 ounce	1 meat + 1 fat
Mutton	1 ounce	1 meat + 1 fat
Organ Meat (high in cholesterol)		
Heart	1 ounce	1 meat
Kidney	1 ounce	1 meat
Liver	1 ounce	1 meat
Sweetbreads, beef	1 ounce	1 meat + 1 fat

AVOID (Continued)

PRODUCT	AMOUNT	EXCHANGE
Pork		
Country-style ham	1 ounce	1 meat + 1 fat
Deviled ham	1 ounce	1 meat + 1 fat
Loin, back ribs	1 ounce	1 meat + 1 fat
Pork ground	1 ounce	1 meat + 1 fat
Sausage	1 ounce	1 meat + 1 fat
Spare ribs	1 ounce	1 meat + 1 fat
Veal		
Breast	1 ounce	1 meat + 1 fat
Poultry		
Capon	1 ounce	1 meat + ½ fat
Duck	1 ounce	1 meat + 1½ fat
Goose	1 ounce	1 meat + 1 fat
Cheese—Aged		
Blue cheese	1 ounce	1 meat + 1 fat

AVOID (Continued)

PRODUCT	AMOUNT	EXCHANGE
Cheddar	1 ounce	1 meat + 1 fat
Cream	1 ounce	1 meat + 1 fat
Mozzarella	1 ounce	1 meat + 1 fat
Parmesan, hard	1 ounce	1 meat + 1 fat
Parmesan, grated	1 tablespoon	1 meat + ½ fat
Swiss	1 ounce	1 meat + 1 fat
Egg (high in cholesterol)		
Egg (yolk)	1	1 meat
Luncheon Meat		
Bologna	1 slice	½ meat + 1 fat
Bratwurst	1 link	1½ meat + 3 fat
Frankfurters, beef and pork	1 frank	1 meat + 2 fat
Liverwurst	1 slice	½ meat + ½ fat
Salami	1 ounce	½ meat + 1 fat

Vegetable

The following foods contain approximately 5 grams of carbohydrate, 2 grams of protein, and 25 calories. Each is equal to 1 Vegetable exchange unless otherwise indicated. Starchy vegetables are found in the bread exchange list. Selections should be made from the "allowable" category. Foods in the "avoid" group are higher in fat and calories.

ALLOWABLE

PRODUCT	AMOUNT	EXCHANGE
Artichoke	large (3½ ounces)	1½ veg
Artichoke hearts	½ cup	1 veg
Asparagus	⅔ cup	1 veg
Bamboo shoots	⅔ cup	1 veg
Beans, green and wax	½ cup	1 veg
Bean sprouts	½ cup	1 veg
Beets	½ cup	1 veg
Broccoli	½ cup	1 veg
Brussels sprouts	½ cup	1 veg
Cabbage, shredded	2 cups	1 veg
Carrots	½ cup	1 veg
Cauliflower	1 cup	1 veg
Celery, diced	1 cup	1 veg
Cucumbers	1 medium	½ veg
Eggplant	½ cup	1 veg
Endive (escarole)	20 leaves	1 veg
Ginger (fresh)	1½ ounce	1 veg
Greens, all types	½ cup	1 veg
Leeks	2 medium	1 veg
Lettuce	3½ ounces	½ veg
Mushroom	½ cup	1 veg
Okra	½ cup	1 veg
Onions	½ cup	1 veg
Parsley	¼ cup	1 veg
Pepper, green or red	1 large	1 veg
Pimiento	3 medium	1 veg
Radishes	15 small	1 veg
Rutabaga	½ cup	1 veg
Sauerkraut	⅔ cup	1 veg

ALLOWABLE (Continued)

PRODUCT	AMOUNT	EXCHANGE
Shallots	1 ounce	1 veg
Spinach	½ cup	1 veg
Squash, summer	⅔ cup	1 veg
Tomatoes	½ cup	1 veg
Tomato juice	½ cup	1 veg
Tomato paste	2 tablespoons	1 veg
Tomato sauce	½ cup	½ bread
Turnips	⅔ cup	1 veg
Vegetable juice cocktail	½ cup	1 veg
Watercress	4 ounces	1 veg
Water chestnuts	5 medium	1 veg
Zucchini	⅔ cup	1 veg

AVOID

PRODUCT	AMOUNT	EXCHANGE
Fried Vegetables		
Fried eggplant	½ cup	1 veg + 1 fat
Fried okra	½ cup	1 veg + 1 fat
Fried onion rings	½ cup	1 veg + 1 fat
Vegetables, breaded and fried	½ cup	1 veg + 1 fat
Vegetables with Sauces		
Vegetables in butter sauce	½ cup	1 veg + ½ fat
Vegetables in cream sauce	½ cup	1 veg + 1½ fat
Vegetables in cheese sauce	½ cup	1 veg + 1½ fat

C–Dietary Guidelines and Tips

General Dietary Guidelines

Bakery and Dessert Items
1. Avoid high-fat doughnuts, cakes, candy, cookies, pies, sweet rolls.
2. Bake with vegetable oil and margarine rather than butter or lard.
3. Use cocoa powder in place of solid chocolate.
4. Reduce sugar content of recipes to ⅓ to ½ of original level.

Eggs
1. Limit egg yolks to two per week.

Fats and Oils
1. Substitute margarine for butter.
2. Use margarine or vegetable oil in place of shortening.
3. Use safflower oil as a vegetable oil when possible.
4. Use nonstick vegetable sprays.
5. Season vegetables with margarine or oil instead of butter.

Milk and Cheese
1. Use 1-percent-fat milk in place of whole milk.
2. Substitute low-fat cheese (less than 12 percent fat) for higher-fat cheese.

3. Avoid cream.
4. Use sherbet, fruit ices, frozen yogurt, or ice milk instead of ice cream.

Meat, Fish, and Poultry
1. Use only lean meat, fish, and poultry.
2. Avoid Prime cuts of meat; lesser grades have less fat.
3. Trim all visible fat.
4. Use more veal instead of beef.
5. Remove skin from poultry.
6. Limit meat, fish, or poultry to 7 to 8 ounces per day.

Snacks
1. Avoid high-fat crackers.
2. Use low-fat crackers such as rye toast and whole wheat rusk.
3. Avoid salted, high-fat snack items such as chips, nuts, pretzels.

Tips for Decreasing Fat

1. Use more poultry and fish instead of red meat.
2. Broil, bake, steam, poach, or "oven fry" instead of pan frying or deep-fat frying.
3. Roast meat on racks to allow drainage of fat. Discard drippings.
4. Trim all visible fat.
5. Use nonstick skillets to minimize the use of additional fat when sautéing or browning.
6. When browning meat, spoon off or drain away all excess fat released ("pan broiling"). Blot cooked meat in a double thickness of paper towels to remove excess fat.
7. Substitute nonstick vegetable sprays for grease on baking pans and in casserole dishes.
8. Remove the skin from poultry (about ⅓ of the fat is in and immediately under the skin).
9. When purchasing canned fish (tuna, sardines, salmon, etc.), select items packed in water, mustard, or other oil-free dressings.
10. Chill meat drippings and remove the hardened fat that collects at the top before making gravy. Use the same technique to remove fat from stews and soups.

11. If onions begin to stick to the pan when sautéing, add a small amount of water and continue cooking until water evaporates.
12. Decrease the use of high-fat salad dressings, gravies, and sauces.
13. Use low-fat yogurt, low-fat buttermilk, and flavored vinegars to reduce fat in salad dressings. Try a mixture of half oil and half vinegar to decrease the amount of fat.
14. When selecting dairy products, choose low-fat or nonfat items.
15. For baking, substitute low-fat plain yogurt for sour cream.
16. Whip well-chilled evaporated milk to substitute for whipped cream.
17. Avoid nuts and seeds, which are high in fat and calories. Purchase dry-roasted, unsalted nuts to help decrease fat.
18. In baking, substitute 2 large egg whites for 1 whole large egg or 3 egg whites for 2 whole eggs.
19. Use unsweetened plain cocoa powder instead of baking chocolate.

Tips for Decreasing Sodium

Success or failure in reducing sodium intake and controlling weight may have a great impact on blood pressure. Because table salt and processed foods are the two major contributors of dietary sodium, the easiest way to limit intake is by restricting the use of the salt shaker and reducing the consumption of processed food. Other major sources of sodium are foods themselves, softened water and medications.

The taste for salt is acquired; we are not born with a craving for salt. After a few months of adherence to a low-salt diet, many find that salty food becomes objectionable. The suggestions below may be helpful in learning to break the salt habit.

1. Do not add salt to food before tasting.
2. Remove salt shakers from the table.
3. Gradually reduce the amount of salt used in baking and cooking.
4. Use herbs and spices in place of salt to season food.
5. Buy processed foods labeled "low-sodium," "low-salt," or "no salt added."
6. Follow Table C.1, Low-Sodium Guide that lists foods that are considered acceptable and those that are not.
7. When eating away from home, be selective and follow the Low-Sodium Guide. Whenever possible, avoid fast-food establishments that offer a limited menu of salty food.

No food, regardless of salt content, needs to be avoided entirely with a moderate sodium restriction. The important point to remember is to decrease the frequency of use. There are often alternate items that can substitute for a food high in sodium.

Table C.1 Low-Sodium Guide

TYPE OF FOOD	ALLOWABLE	AVOID
Beverages	Coffee, decaffeinated coffee; carbonated beverages limited to 2 per day	Instant chocolate drinks, buttermilk
Breads	Unsalted crackers, bread made without salt, flour	Breads or rolls with salt toppings
Cereals	Unsalted cooked cereals, puffed rice, puffed wheat, shredded wheat, dry cereal	Other dry cereals, quick-cooking or instant cooked cereals
Desserts	Gelatin desserts, sherbet, fruit ices and frozen bars, desserts made with milk and eggs in amounts allowed	Rich pastries
Fats	Unsalted butter or margarine, vegetable oil, vegetable shortening, unsalted salad dressing or mayonnaise	Bacon, bacon fat, salt pork, commercial salad dressing or mayonnaise in excess of amount allowed, olives, salted nuts, regular peanut butter
Fruits and Juices	All fresh, canned or frozen fruits and juices (except tomato juice), salt-free tomato juice	Tomato juice
Eggs, Cheese, Fish, Meats, and Poultry	Low-fat cottage cheese, cream cheese, low-sodium cheese, eggs according to dietary restrictions, unsalted meat and poultry	Aged cheese (greater than 12% butter fat), fish, meat, or poultry that has been cured, brined, or canned with salt (sausage, ham, luncheon meat; corned beef, frankfurters, bacon)
Starches	Grits, macaroni, noodles, potatoes, rice, pasta, unsalted popcorn	Pretzels, corn chips, snack chips, salted popcorn
Vegetables	Unsalted broth or bouillon, homemade soups using allowed seasonings, low-sodium canned soups	Bouillon cubes, broth bases, canned, commercial, or dehydrated soups, pickles, sauerkraut
Sweets	Pure sugar candy, honey, jam, jelly, preserves, marmalade, white or brown sugar, syrup, chocolate	Candy with salted nuts
Condiments/spices	Herbs, garlic powder, onion powder, vinegar, low-sodium soy sauce (avoid if following a strict low-sodium diet)	Cooking wine, celery salt, garlic salt, salt, catsup, chili sauce, barbecue and meat sauces, meat tenderizers, mustard, soy sauce, Worcestershire sauce

Tips for Decreasing Sugar

1. Try using ⅔ to ¾ of the sugar called for in recipes.
2. Avoid soft drinks containing sugar. Substitute unsweetened fruit juices mixed with seltzer or club soda.
3. Avoid snacks and cereals with added sugar.
4. Decrease intake of sugar in coffee and tea by adding ground cinnamon or other spices.
5. Use fresh fruit purees with chopped fruit to add natural sweetness to baked goods or plain low-fat yogurt.
6. Make your own frozen fruit bars by freezing pure fruit juice (orange juice is particularly good).
7. Serve seasonal fresh fruit with thin slices of low-fat cheese for dessert.
8. Plain frozen bananas are naturally sweet snacks. Peel ripe bananas and cut in half crosswise. Insert a stick if desired, wrap tightly in plastic, and freeze in an airtight container. (They will not darken if kept tightly wrapped.)
9. Use unsweetened apple butter or apple spread instead of jam for sandwiches and toast.
10. When purchasing frozen fruit, select fresh frozen types without added sugar.
11. Flavor pancakes, waffles, French toast, muffins, and quick breads with spices such as cinnamon, cardamom, or nutmeg, or with extracts—vanilla, almond, orange, or maple. They will taste sweeter.
12. Avoid commercial gelatin or pudding desserts containing sugar.
13. Replace cocoa with carob powder in baked goods and decrease the sugar by 25 percent.
14. Dilute pancake syrup with water.

Tips for Increasing Fruits and Vegetables

1. Steam vegetables. Use leftover cooking water for broth.
2. Do not overcook vegetables. Nutrients are preserved and vegetables taste better if they are cooked just until crisp-tender.
3. Prepare more vegetable combination meals by increasing the use of stews, soups, and casseroles. Gradually increase the variety and quantity of vegetables and reduce the quantity of meat.
4. Use small amounts of ground, finely chopped, or grated vegetable to stretch ground meat. Increase the use of vitamin A-rich vegetables such as carrots, pumpkin, and squash in baked goods.
5. Serve vegetable appetizers and snacks.
6. Keep washed vegetables in the refrigerator for snacks.
7. Stretch meals with side dishes that emphasize vegetables and fruits.
8. Puree vegetables to thicken soups and add flavor.
9. Substitute frozen vegetables and fruits when fresh produce is unavailable.
10. Use chopped vegetables and fruits along with or instead of bread as poultry stuffing.
11. Use fresh fruit to create tempting desserts.

Tips for Increasing Whole Grains and Legumes

1. Use whole grain breads; try whole grain English muffins, pita bread, rolls, and muffins. Read labels and look for "whole wheat" flour.
2. Substitute whole wheat flour for some all-purpose flour in baking.
3. Serve whole grain side dishes as a substitute for pasta or potatoes. Try whole wheat pasta.
4. Substitute brown rice for white rice.
5. Use whole grain crackers.
6. Use a small amount of bran along with whole wheat bread crumbs as toppings for casseroles and as a filler for meat loaf. Bread crumbs can be made in a food processor and stored in an airtight container in the freezer.
7. Make whole wheat croutons by slicing whole wheat bread into cubes and toasting them in a 300°F oven until dry.
8. When selecting breakfast cereals, emphasize unsweetened whole grains such as bran flakes and shredded wheat. For hot cereals, select cooked rolled oats, bulgur wheat, millet, buckwheat, or rye flakes.

High-Fiber Foods

Dietary fiber is primarily found in fresh fruits and vegetables, dried peas and beans, and whole grains. Bran, which is particularly high in fiber, is the outer coating of the wheat kernel. Foods high in fiber are listed below by food group. Refer also to Table C.2, which lists some high-fiber foods.

BREADS AND CEREALS Whole grains; cracked or crushed wheat breads, rolls, or crackers; bran or whole grain cereals; wheat germ, which can be added to casseroles, meat loaf, meat sauces, or soups; snack items such as popcorn and granola bars. Begin with two servings of these high-fiber foods per day plus 1 tablespoon of wheat germ or bran added in cooking. Progress to 4 to 8 servings per day plus 4 to 6 tablespoons of wheat germ. One of these servings should consist of at least ¾ cup bran or whole grain cereal.

VEGETABLES AND FRUITS   All raw fruits and vegetables. Include edible skin—on apples, potatoes, cucumbers, squash, etc. Begin with three servings per day; progress to 6 to 8 servings per day.

WATER   Another important aspect of a high-fiber diet is water. Drink plenty of fluids, especially water. Your daily fluid intake should be at least eight 8-ounce glasses.

Table C.2   Suggested High-Fiber Foods

	HIGH-FIBER FOOD	SUBSTITUTED FOR
Breads	100% whole wheat bread Wheat berry bread	Regular white bread
	Whole wheat English muffins	Plain English muffins
	Whole wheat crackers	Plain crackers
	Whole wheat hamburger and hot dog rolls	Commercial rolls
	Whole wheat croutons	Regular croutons
Grains	Brown rice	White rice
	Bulgur Millet	White rice or potatoes
	Whole wheat pasta	Regular pasta
Dry Ingredients	Wheat germ Bran (unprocessed) Whole wheat flours	Add these ingredients in cooking and baking in place of all or part of regular all-purpose flour
	Cracked wheat Cornmeal Wheat berries Rolled oats and wheat	Add to casseroles or use as toppings
Cereals	Old-fashioned oatmeal Ralston whole wheat cereal	Quick-cooking oatmeal
	40% Bran Flakes Raisin Bran Shredded Wheat Grape Nuts Granolas All-Bran or 100% Bran	Other dry cereals
Raw Fruit	Orange, grapefruit, tangerine sections (with membranes) Apples, pears, peaches with skins Grapes	Sugary snacks and desserts
Dried Fruit	Prunes, raisins, apricots, apples	Use as toppings for cereals and baked goods
Raw Vegetables	Celery sticks Carrot sticks Broccoli Cucumber Zucchini Lettuce salads	Use as appetizers and snacks; add grated vegetables to ground meat
Cooked Vegetables	Celery Carrots Broccoli Green Beans Peas Cabbage Asparagus Cauliflower Corn	Use fresh vegetables whenever possible instead of canned; use frozen if fresh are unavailable. Steam vegetables until crisp-tender

High-Potassium Foods

Potassium helps increase sodium loss in urine and may contribute to a lowering of high blood pressure. Fruits and vegetables are good sources of potassium.

FRUIT		VEGETABLES	
RICH SOURCE		**RICH SOURCE**	
Apricots	Honeydew melon	Artichokes	Leeks
Avocados	Oranges	Bamboo shoots	Mushrooms
Bananas	Peaches	Beans (white, dry red,	Parsnips
Cantaloupe	Prune juice	limas, fordhook)	Potatoes
Dates	Prunes	Beet greens	Spinach
Figs	Raisins	Chard	Squash (winter)
		Chickpeas	Sweet potatoes
		Cowpeas	Tomatoes (raw)
		Escarole	Tomato juice
GOOD SOURCE		**GOOD SOURCE**	
Apricot juice	Pineapple juice	Asparagus	Kohlrabi
Fruit cocktail	Plums	Bell peppers	Lentils
Grapefruit juice	Pomegranates	Broccoli (cooked)	Lettuce
Kumquats	Raspberries	Brussels sprouts	Mustard greens
Mango	Rhubarb	Carrots	Okra
Orange juice	Strawberries	Cauliflower	Peas
Papaya	Tangerine juice	Collards (cooked)	Pumpkin
Pears	Watermelon	Corn on the cob	Tomatoes (canned)
Persimmons		Eggplant	Turnip greens
		Kale	Vegetable juice cocktail

D–Reference Tables

Table D.1 Distribution of Plasma Total Cholesterol (mg/dl)

Age (years)	WHITE MALES PERCENTILES							WHITE FEMALES PERCENTILES						
	5	10	25	50	75	90	95	5	10	25	50	75	90	95
0–4	—	—	—	—	—	—	—	—	—	—	—	—	—	—
5–9	125	131	141	153	168	183	189	131	136	151	164	176	190	197
10–14	124	131	144	160	173	188	202	125	131	142	159	171	191	205
15–19	118	123	136	152	168	183	191	118	126	140	157	176	198	207
20–24	118	126	142	159	179	197	212	121	132	147	165	186	220	237
25–29	130	137	154	176	199	223	234	130	142	158	178	198	217	231
30–34	142	152	171	190	213	237	258	133	141	158	178	199	215	228
35–39	147	157	176	195	222	248	267	139	149	165	186	209	233	249
40–44	150	160	179	204	229	251	260	146	156	172	193	220	241	259
45–49	163	171	188	210	235	258	275	148	162	182	204	231	256	268
50–54	157	168	189	211	237	263	274	163	171	188	214	240	267	281
55–59	161	172	188	214	236	260	280	167	182	201	229	251	278	294
60–64	163	170	191	215	237	262	287	172	186	207	226	251	282	300
65–69	166	174	192	213	250	275	288	167	179	212	233	259	282	291
70 +	144	160	185	214	236	253	265	173	181	196	226	249	268	280

Adapted from the Lipid Research Clinics Population Studies Data Book *as published in* Circulation 69:1065 A (1984).

Moderate Risk for Heart Disease: Total cholesterol levels between 75th and 90th percentiles.
High Risk for Heart Disease: Total cholesterol greater than the 90th percentile.

Table D.2
Cholesterol Content of Foods

FOOD	CHOLESTEROL (Milligrams)
Whole milk, 1 cup	34
Cheddar cheese, 1 ounce	30
Ice cream, 1 cup	88
Egg	274
Butter, 1 tablespoon	33
Bacon, 1 slice	19
Mayonnaise, 1 tablespoon	10
Hot dog, beef	22
Lean meat, cooked, 1 ounce	25
Liver, cooked, 1 ounce	20
Fish, light-flesh, cooked, 1 ounce	20
Fish, dark-flesh, cooked, 1 ounce	40
Lobster, 1 ounce	57
Oyster, 1 ounce	66
Shrimp, 1 ounce	43
Other shellfish, 1 ounce	15–25

Adapted from Pennington, J.T. and H.N. Church. Food Values of Portions Commonly Used, *14th ed. Harper & Row, New York (1985).*

Table D.3
Common Sources of Caffeine in Food

PRODUCT	CAFFEINE (Milligrams)
Soft drinks (12 ounces)	33–54
Coffee	
Drip (5 ounces)	146
Percolated (5 ounces)	110
Instant, regular (5 ounces)	53
Decaffeinated (5 ounces)	2
Tea	
One-minute brew (5 ounces)	9–33
Three-minute brew (5 ounces)	20–46
Five-minute brew (5 ounces)	20–50
Cocoa and Chocolate	
Cocoa beverage (6 ounces)	10
Milk chocolate (1 ounce)	6
Baking chocolate (1 ounce)	35

Adapted from Pennington, J.T. and H.N. Church. Food Values of Portions Commonly Used, *14th ed. Harper & Row, New York (1985); and from Bunker, M.L. and M. McWilliams.* Caffeine Content of Common Beverages. *J. Amer. Dietetic Assoc. 74:28(1979).*

Table D.4 Vegetable Proteins

Food	Serving Size	Protein (grams)	Food	Serving Size	Protein (grams)
Banana	1 medium	1.2	Lentils	½ cup cooked	5.9
Bean, curd	1 piece	9.4	Macaroni	1 cup cooked	6.0
Beans, kidney	½ cup cooked	9.8	Oatmeal	1 cup cooked	4.8
Beans, lima	½ cup cooked	6.0	Peas, green	½ cup cooked	4.2
Beans, navy	½ cup cooked	7.4	Potato	1 medium	2.1
Bean sprouts, mung	3½ oz.	3.8	Rice, brown	1 cup cooked	4.8
Bran flakes, 40%	1 cup	4.4	Rice, white	1 cup cooked	3.8
Bread, white	1 slice	2.0	Shredded wheat	2 biscuits	5.2
Bread, whole wheat	1 slice	2.3	Soybeans	½ cup cooked	7.4
Broccoli	⅔ cup	3.1	Spaghetti	1 cup cooked	7.3
Bulgur	1 cup cooked	8.4	Squash, acorn	½ medium	3.0
Corn	½ cup kernels, cooked	3.1	Sweet potato	1 small	2.1
			Walnuts	10 large	5.4

From Pennington, J.T. and H.N. Church. Food Values of Portions Commonly Used, *14th ed. Harper and Row, New York (1985).*

Table D.5 The Exercise Cost of Eating*

Food	Calories	Walking (min.)	Biking (min.)	Jogging (min.)	Swimming (min.)
Apple	87	17	11	9	8
Bacon, 2 slices	96	19	12	10	9
Beer, 8 ounces	115	22	14	12	10
Cake, ¹⁄₁₆ of 9-inch	250	48	31	25	22
Carrot	42	8	5	4	4
Cereal, with milk and sugar	212	41	26	21	19
Cheese, American, 1 slice	112	22	14	11	10
Cheeseburger	350	67	43	35	31
Chicken breast, fried	232	45	28	23	21
Cola, 8 ounces	105	20	13	11	9
Cookie, chocolate chip	50	10	6	5	5
Cookie, vanilla wafer	15	3	2	2	1
Doughnut	125	24	15	13	11
Egg, boiled	78	15	10	8	7
Egg, fried or scrambled	108	21	13	11	10
French dressing, 1 tablespoon	57	11	7	6	5
Ham, 2 slices, cooked	254	49	31	25	23
Ice cream, ⅔ cup	186	36	23	19	19
Ice milk, ⅔ cup	137	26	17	14	12
Mayonnaise, 1 tablespoon	100	19	12	10	9
Milk, skim, 8 ounces	88	17	11	9	8
Milk, whole, 8 ounces	160	36	20	16	14
Milk shake, 8 ounces	420	81	51	42	38
Orange	73	14	9	7	7
Pancake, with 2 tablespoons syrup	204	39	25	20	18
Peach	38	7	5	4	3
Peach shortcake	266	51	32	27	24
Pie, fruit, ⅙ of 9-inch	400	77	49	40	36
Pie, pecan, ⅙ of 9-inch	670	129	82	67	60
Pizza, ⅛ of 14-inch	185	36	23	19	17
Potato chips, 5	54	10	7	5	5
Roast beef with gravy sandwich	430	83	52	43	38
Sherbet, ⅔ cup	120	23	15	12	11
Shrimp, fried, 3½ ounces	225	43	27	23	20
Spaghetti with meat sauce	396	76	48	40	35
Tuna salad sandwich	278	54	34	28	25
T-bone steak, 4 ounces cooked	235	45	29	24	21

Energy costs estimated for a 154-pound individual.
Adapted from Pollock, M.L., J.H. Wilmore, and S.M. Fox. Exercise in Health and Disease. *W.B. Saunders Company, Philadelphia (1984).*

Glossary

adventitia   The outermost cell layer of blood vessel walls.

alcohol   A colorless liquid, produced by the fermentation of certain carbohydrates or obtained synthetically, containing 7 calories per gram.

allicin   A substance that may inhibit blood clot formation; produced when onions or garlic are cut or cooked.

amino acids   Nitrogen-containing compounds that are the building blocks of protein.

angina pectoris   Chest pain, usually associated with insufficient blood flow to the heart and often occurring with exercise.

artery   A vessel through which blood passes away from the heart to various parts of the body.

aspartame   A combination of two amino acids—aspartic acid and phenylalanine—which is a sugar substitute distributed in the United States as NutraSweet® and Equal®.

atherosclerosis   A disease in which the artery walls become narrowed as a result of the deposition of fat; the underlying cause of most heart disease.

behavior modification   A technique often used to alter a person's habits: for example, changing a person's eating and activity habits to control weight.

bran   The outer covering of cereal grains, which is high in fiber.

caffeine   A substance naturally present in coffee and tea that is a central nervous system stimulant.

calcium   The major mineral in the body; it plays an important structural role in bone and is involved in blood clot formation.

calorie   The standard unit used to measure energy.

carbohydrate   A sugar or starch containing 4 calories per gram.

cardiovascular disease   Disease of the heart and blood vessels which includes coronary artery disease, hypertension, stroke, congestive heart failure, peripheral vascular disease, congenital heart defects.

cholesterol   A waxy, fatlike substance found in all animal tissues; too much cholesterol in the blood may lead to the development of heart and blood vessel disease.

complex carbohydrates   Starches composed of sugar units linked together into chains.

coronary arteries   Blood vessels that surround the heart and supply the heart muscle with oxygen and nutrients.

coronary risk profile   A rating scale of several medical conditions and behavioral patterns that can be used to estimate an overall risk for heart disease.

diabetes   A condition in which the pancreas either does not produce enough insulin (a hormone) or produces an ineffective form of insulin; without sufficient and functioning insulin, blood sugar levels remain excessive.

eicosapentenoic acid   A fatty acid, commonly present in fish oil, that may lower blood cholesterol levels and reduce the tendency of blood to clot.

endothelium   The layer of cells lining the inner cavities of blood vessels and the chambers of the heart.

exchange system   A method of grouping foods into categories; within each exchange group, one specified amount of food can be substituted for another.

fat   A substance found in food that contains 9 calories per gram and is stored in the body as a source of energy.

fatty streaks   Deposits of fat, appearing in blood vessels, that represent an early stage of atherosclerosis.

fiber   All the components of foods (carbohydrates, cellulose, hemicellulose, pectin, lignin) that are not digested by enzymes in the intestinal tract and are not absorbed into the bloodstream.

heart attack   Heart muscle damage due to a reduced flow of oxygen and nutrients to heart tissue.

hemoglobin   A protein in the blood that carries oxygen to tissues.

high-density lipoproteins (HDLs)   Proteins in the blood that are thought to transport cholesterol from tissues to the liver for excretion; HDLs help protect against the development of atherosclerosis.

hypercholesterolemia   Elevated levels of cholesterol in the blood.

hypertension   Elevated blood pressure, which may increase the workload of the heart and the risk of heart disease.

intima   The inner layer of blood vessels.

iron   A mineral that serves as an important component of hemoglobin, the oxygen-carrying protein of the blood.

legumes   A large family of plants that have pods, such as beans and peas.

linoleic acid A fatty acid, commonly found in vegetable oils, that is effective in lowering blood cholesterol.

lipid Fat.

lipoproteins Proteins in the blood that carry fat.

low-density lipoproteins (LDLs) Proteins in the blood that normally transport 65 percent of the cholesterol and may be deposited in plaque; high LDL levels increase the risk of heart disease.

media The middle layer of blood vessels.

milligram A unit of weight; one-thousandth of a gram.

monounsaturated fat A type of fat, commonly found in olive oil, peanuts, olives, and avocados, which may help reduce blood cholesterol levels.

myocardial infarction Heart attack.

obesity Excess body fat, which increases the chance of developing two major heart disease risk factors: high blood pressure and diabetes.

oleic acid The major monounsaturated fat, present in foods and the body, that may help lower blood cholesterol levels.

osteoporosis A state of gradual demineralization of bony tissues that may be associated with a low intake of calcium over a lifetime.

pectin A water-soluble fiber, found in high amounts in the rind of citrus fruits, which may help to lower blood cholesterol levels.

plaque In the lining of an artery, a mass of smooth muscle cells containing fat, cholesterol, and calcium that may obstruct the flow of blood.

plasma The fluid portion of the blood in which the red blood cells are suspended.

platelets Sticky cells found in the blood that are involved in the clotting process.

polyunsaturated fat Usually liquid at room temperature, this type of fat is commonly found in vegetable oils such as corn, cottonseed, safflower, sesame seed, soybean, and sunflower; polyunsaturated fats tend to lower blood cholesterol.

potassium A mineral present in relatively high amounts in many fruits, fruit juices, and vegetables; loss of potassium from the body may occur when medications are taken to control high blood pressure.

protein A compound, present in all living tissue, that is made up of many relatively simple, nitrogen-containing units called amino acids; protein contains 4 calories per gram.

Recommended Dietary Allowances (RDA)   The intake of essential nutrients considered by experts to be adequate to meet the known nutritional needs of practically all healthy persons.

risk factors   Characteristics associated with an increased risk of developing coronary heart disease, such as high blood pressure, elevated blood cholesterol, cigarette smoking, etc.

saccharin   An artificial sweetener.

salt   A crystalline compound of sodium and chlorine; excessive intake may contribute to the development of high blood pressure in some individuals.

saturated fat   Usually solid at room temperature, this fat is found primarily in foods of animal origin, such as whole-milk dairy products and red meat; saturated fats raise blood cholesterol levels.

sodium   A mineral present in table salt that may contribute to elevated blood pressure when consumed in excessive amounts.

stress   Physical, mental, or emotional tension that develops as a reaction to daily life situations.

sucrose   Table sugar.

triglycerides   The major fat in food and in fatty tissues of the body; elevated levels of triglycerides are weakly associated with an increased risk of coronary artery disease.

very-low-density lipoproteins (VLDLs)   Proteins in the blood that normally transport mostly triglycerides; elevated VLDL levels may slightly increase the risk of coronary heart disease.

Conversion Table

SOLID MEASURES

For cooks measuring items by weight, here are approximate equivalents, in both Imperial and metric. So as to avoid awkward measurements, some conversions are not exact.

	U.S. CUSTOMARY	METRIC	IMPERIAL
Butter	1 cup	225 g	8 oz
	½ cup	115 g	4 oz
	¼ cup	60 g	2 oz
	1 Tbsp	15 g	½ oz
Cheese (grated)	1 cup	115 g	4 oz
Fruit (chopped fresh)	1 cup	225 g	8 oz
Herbs (chopped fresh)	¼ cup	7 g	¼ oz
Meats/Chicken (chopped, cooked)	1 cup	175 g	6 oz
Mushrooms (chopped, fresh)	1 cup	70 g	2½ oz
Nuts (chopped)	1 cup	115 g	4 oz
Raisins (and other dried chopped fruits)	1 cup	175 g	6 oz
Rice (uncooked)	1 cup	225 g	8 oz
(cooked)	3 cups	225 g	8 oz
Vegetables (chopped, raw)	1 cup	115 g	4 oz

LIQUID MEASURES

The Imperial pint is larger than the U.S. pint, therefore note the following when measuring liquid ingredients.

U.S.	IMPERIAL
1 cup = 8 fluid ounces	1 cup = 10 fluid ounces
½ cup = 4 fluid ounces	½ cup = 5 fluid ounces
1 tablespoon = ¾ fluid ounce	1 tablespoon = 1 fluid ounce

U.S. MEASURE	METRIC APPROXIMATE	IMPERIAL APPROXIMATE
1 quart (4 cups)	950 mL	1½ pints + 4 Tbsp
1 pint (2 cups)	450 mL	¾ pint
1 cup	236 mL	¼ pint + 6 Tbsp
1 Tbsp	15 mL	1 Tbsp
1 tsp	5 mL	1 tsp

DRY MEASURES

Outside the United States, the following items are measured by weight. Use the following table, but bear in mind that measurements will vary, depending on the variety of flour and moisture. Cup measurements are loosely packed; flour is measured directly from package (presifted).

	U.S. CUSTOMARY	METRIC	IMPERIAL
Flour (all-purpose)	1 cup	150 g	5 oz
Cornmeal	1 cup	175 g	6 oz
Sugar (granulated)	1 cup	190 g	6½ oz
(confectioners)	1 cup	80 g	2⅔ oz
(brown)	1 cup	160 g	5⅓ oz

OVEN TEMPERATURES

Fahrenheit	225	300	350	400	450
Celsius	110	150	180	200	230
Gas Mark	¼	2	4	6	8